What other readers are saying ab
Silence, Song & Shadow

D0117080

"Captivating and enlightening! .... touches the heart, moves the soul, and reaches
the core of our lives. I savored every page and couldn't wait to share it with others."
— Gail A. Lindsey, 1998 Chair, AIA Committee on the Environment

✧

"The healing energy of place! Silence, Song & Shadows tells of the need for our
spirits to be filled by the energy of the sacred. With clarity, simplicity, and beauty,
it raises our consciousness about why and how to bring sacred energy into the
spaces that surround us. This is a lovely book!"
— Donna Eden, author of ENERGY MEDICINE

✧

"A wondrous work about the sacred nature of place and home, a forgotten
language of design and craft that humans have used for millennia to discourse
with their gods and inner selves. This will make you ache for what we have lost,
yet guide you to finding and creating enchantment once again."
— Paul Hawken, author of NATURAL CAPITALISM

✧

"Bender reaches beneath the surface of ordinary life to find the essence of sacred
space. Simply, yet eloquently, he prepares a pathway for us to occupy the
universe as well as our intimate surroundings in a way that is meaningful and holy."
— Denise Linn, author of SACRED SPACE

✧

" . . .a wake-up call, an antidote to the banality that so often embraces our work
across the country. . . the beginnings of healthy discourse into a new way of
looking at the art of placemaking, the art of making buildings that "have souls
which nurture our own". . . of great importance to our profession."
— Susan A. Maxman, past president, American Institute of Architects

✧

"Places the central questions of our time directly on the shrine of spirit, where they
so richly belong. Here are the philosophical and spiritual foundations for a sustainable future. Everyone in the "green building" movement should read this book."
— David Rousseau, author of YOUR HOME, YOUR HEALTH

✧

"Designers need a far greater concern for exactly what Tom Bender describes.
Important concepts for all of our work."
— Louis deMoll, past president, American Institute of Architects;
past president, International Union of Architects

✧

"A lantern of hope for all concerned with the creation of a more sustainable and
balanced world."
— Sarah Susanka, author of THE NOT SO BIG HOUSE

BUILDING WITH THE BREATH OF LIFE

WORKING WITH CHI ENERGY IN OUR HOMES AND COMMUNITIES

TOM BENDER

FIRE RIVER PRESS

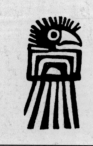

PUBLISHED BY ——

FIRE RIVER PRESS
PO Box 397
Manzanita OR 97130 USA
email: fireriverpress@nehalemtel.net

FIRE RIVER PRESS books by the same author:

ENVIRONMENTAL DESIGN PRIMER, 1973
THE HEART OF PLACE, 1993
SILENCE, SONG, AND SHADOWS, 2000
BUILDING WITH THE BREATH OF LIFE, 2000

The companion volume to this book is Tom Bender's
SILENCE, SONG, AND SHADOWS: Our Need for the Sacred in Our Surroundings.

With over 200 full-color illustrations, it explores dozens of the central concepts of energetics of place, and is designed to help you *feel* its implications. It can be applied independently of the historical and detailed material in this volume.

If you're heart-centered, and can just run with an idea once it clicks, start with that book. Fill in the details with this book as you go.

If your head likes to see things laid out more fully and get some basic comfort with new ideas first, start with this book, which is designed to help you *understand* how to work with chi energy in our surroundings. Then read SSS to give your heart and spirit touchstones from which to work.

LIBRARY OF CONGRESS CARD NUMBER 00-102944
Bender, Tom
    BUILDING WITH THE BREATH OF LIFE:
    Working with Chi Energy in Our Homes and Communities /
    by Tom Bender
    Includes index and bibliographical references
ISBN 0-9675089-1-6
    1. Body, Mind & Spirit – New Thought
    2. Feng-Shui – General
    3. Architecture – Sustainability & Ecological Design
    4. Health & Fitness – Healing
    5. Science – Chi Energy
    6. House & Home – Design and Caretaking

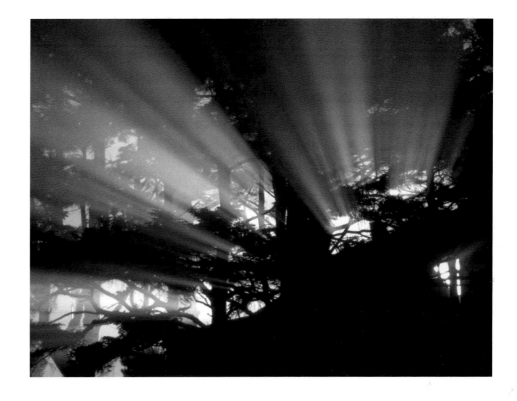

Preface

The acknowledgement of the existence of chi energy that is coming together in our culture today has profound implications beyond its specific application in acupuncture, healing and meditation. Its existence fundamentally expands and alters our basic beliefs of how the Universe works, and the basis from which we develop and focus all parts of our culture. Its transformative role in how we build and use our homes and communities is not one I sought out, but one which overwhelmed me as it slowly revealed itself piece by piece. It is a story worth examining and exploring, even if very foreign and alien to what we've grown up believing.

We are slowly learning that relationships are the core of personal health and of community – relationships with our selves, with others, and with our suroundings. As this book shows, many of the most important relationships occur on an energetic level, and their consideration in our surroundings is vital to our health.

The realms of life are vast – the standing people, the winged ones, the legged and the finned people, those who surf our inner seas; the people of earth and rock, of water, fire, air, and spirit. There are the ancestors, the beings of light and darkness from other domains, and the consciousness that inhabits the far reaches of stellar space. Each brings to us new dimensions of wisdom, ability, and beauty.

From the depths of time, we have been part of and have communicated with this vast and wonderful community. We have danced and sung together. We have shared wisdom and pain, undertaken adventures, experienced mutual awe at the wonder of Creation. Until recently, that is, when we shut ourselves off inside walls of greed and self-centeredness.

In these pages lies a story of acknowledging this wonderful room full of strangers that are really dearest friends. It is a story of learning how to again communicate and share with them. It is a story of how to rejoin Creation and accept a new and more wonderful role in its dance and its song. To these dear friends, and their role in its happening, I dedicate this book.

Our surroundings consist of far more than buildings and concrete. Aligning our individual and community intentions with that of all life brings the power of rightness and the love, support, power, and knowledge of all Creation to all we build or make.

Contents

PREFACE 5

LIST OF EXERCISES 11

✧ ENERGY, PLACE, AND THE SACRED

1. ENTERING THE UNIVERSE OF CHI 12

* LIFE FORCE ENERGY IN WORLD CULTURES   14
* CHI IN THE BODY   18
* CHI AN THE SACRED   25
* CHI AND PLACE   27
* DESIGN WITH CHI   29

2. BUILDING WITH THE BREATH OF LIFE 32

* OUR SURROUNDINGS AS MIRRORS   33
* A CHI-CENTERED UNIVERSE   34
* PRINCIPLES OF ENERGETICS OF PLACE   35

3. UNFOLDING THE PAST 44

* A NEW SENSE OF THE POSSIBLE   45
* INITIATORY TEMPLES OF EGYPT   48
* VISITS OF THE KAMI TO THE IZUMO SHRINE, JAPAN   58
* MAYA COMMUNITY PORTALS TO THE SPIRIT WORLD   59
* HINDU TEMPLES AND THE GEOMETRY OF CONSCIOUSNESS   64
* SETTING THE INTENTION OF A NATION IN HAN CHINA   66
* FENG SHUI OF CHINESE CITIES: Mirrors Of The Cosmos   68
* CHI AND THE SPIRIT WORLD IN KHMER WATER TEMPLES   69
* STEINER SCHOOLS: Learning In Spirit   76
* LEARNING FROM THE DAGARA TO HEAL OUR ANCESTORS   77
* LIVING IN THE BELLY OF A BIRD IN A KAWAKIUTL VILLAGE   80
* DIVINATION IN LOCATING RELIGIOUS STRUCTURES   84

4. RESTORING PLANETARY BALANCE 86

* AN EVOLUTIONARY PERSPECTIVE ON CHANGE   87
* CHANGING DIMENSIONS OF GROWTH   88
* THE NON-ECONOMIC BENEFITS OF SUSTAINABILITY   93
  - Curing Diseases of the Spirit   94
  - Life Without Fear   94
  - An Economy of Giving, not Taking   95
  - Living from the Heart   95

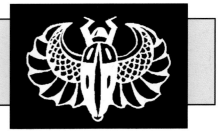

- *Sacred Surroundings   96*
- *Change from a Legal to a Sacred Society   97*
- *Life without Failure   97*
- *The Primacy of Inner Resources   100*
* CHARACTERISTICS OF AN ENDURING SOCIETY   101
* MULTICULTURAL SYNTHESIS   102

5. THE THREE "I"S 104
  * CORE ELEMENTS OF ENERGETIC DESIGN   105
  * THE THREE "I"S   105
    - *CHI: Life-Force in Our Surroundings   105*
    - *LI: Intention and Purpose   108*
    - *TUMMI: Gut Level Intuition   113*
  * RIGHT DURATION   114
  * SIGNIFICANCE   115
  * ELEMENTS OF ENERGETICS OF PLACE   116

6. ORDER AND CHANGE 120
  * CHI IN A MATERIAL WORLD   121
  * YIN and YANG: *Relationships and Transformation*   122
  * SO: *Numbers, Resonance, and Injunctive Experience*   123
  * HSING: *Outward Forms of Appearance*   134
  * CHIH CHUNG: *Relationships at a Distance*   137

✧ TOOLS

7. ENERGETIC DESIGN TOOLS 140
  * CLEAR GOALS   141
    - *Becoming Native   141*
    - *Resources and Communities   141*
    - *Free Nature   142*
    - *Affirming the World We Believe In   143*
    - *What Does Gaia Want?   144*
  * MIND TOOLS   146
    - *Looking at the World Whole   146*
    - *Following the Threads   150*
  * PLACE TOOLS   151
    - *X-Ray Vision and Empty Minds   151*
    - *Maintenance and Caring   153*
  * ENERGETIC TOOLS   153
    - *Spiritual Centering   153*

CONTENTS

- *Trance Design   154*
- *Ritual   156*
        Rituals in Building   159
        Rituals of Relationship with Place   160
- *Working with Chi   161*
- *Intention and Chi   163*
- *Earth Energy   167*

8. GETTING TO KNOW A PLACE 170
   * *SURROUNDINGS*   *171*
   - *Natural features   171*
   - *Human Elements   173*
   - *Invisible Forces   173*
   * *NEIGHBORHOOD*   *174*
   * *THE SITE AND ON-SITE BUILDINGS*   *175*
   - *Topology and Topography   175*
   - *People – Past, Present, and Future   178*
   - *Connections and Barriers   178*
   * *INSIDE BUILDINGS*   *180*
   * *POSSESSIONS*   *183*

✦ PUTTING ENERGETICS INTO PRACTICE

9. BUILDINGS WITH SOULS 186
   * *BUILDING WITH A SOUL*   *187*
   * *ENTRIES*   *192*
   * *BUILDING FROM INSIDE*   *197*

10. GARDENS OF THE SPIRIT 200
   * *HOMES FOR OUR SPIRITS*   *201*
   * *SPIRIT-OF-PLACE GARDENS*   *202*
   - *Winter Gardens   203*
   - *Wind, Water, and Star Gardens   204*
   * *GARDENS OF THE SPIRIT*   *205*
   - *Computer Zen Gardens   205*
   - *Gardens of Death   206*
   - *A Garden of Time   208*
   * *GARDENS OF CELEBRATION*   *209*
   - *Cloud Gardens   209*
   - *A Wind Garden   211*

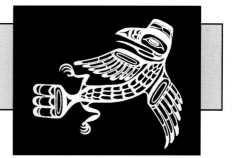

11. CITIES OF PASSION 214
    * *WHAT MAKES A CITY LOVEABLE?*   215
        - *Chi of Place* 215
        - *Community Intentions* 218
        - *Wildness* 220
        - *Roots of Community Passions* 220
    * *FINDING A PASSION*   226
    * *CHANGING COMMUNITY CHI*   228
        - *Celebrate Death* 228
        - *Heal Place-Rape* 229
        - *Make the Sacred Visible* 231
        - *Make Work Sacred* 231
        - *Transform Root Intentions* 232
        - *Honor Other Life* 232
        - *Make Space for New Creation* 232

12. SACRED PLACES 234
    * *HOLDING PLACES SACRED*   235
    * *VARIETIES OF SACRED PLACES*   236
    * *EXPRESSING SACREDNESS*   239
    * *THE SHRINE OF THE MOUNTAIN AND THE WATERS*   240

13. TAKING ACTION 252
    * *SEWAGE IS ART!*   253
    * *INSTITUTIONS HAVE HEARTS*   259
    * *THE RICHNESS OF EDGES*   260
    * *TRANSFORMING A WORKPLACE*   261
    * *THEIR OWN PLACE TO LEARN*   262
    * *THE COLOR OF LIGHT*   265
    * *HONORING THE SPIRITS OF ALL LIFE*   266
    * *TAKE CARE WHAT MIRRORS REFLECT*   267
    * *THE PEACE OF SANCTUARY*   268
    * *SILENCE AND INTENTION*   270

BIBLIOGRAPHY 272
INDEX 278

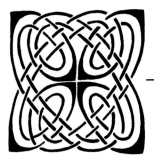

EXERCISES:

EXPERIENCING ENERGETICS OF PLACE

When I first heard about working with subtle energies, the process sounded like crazy hocus-pocus. It made my left-brained self want to scream and run the other direction. With reason – its monopolistic control of my life was being challenged. When I finally tried some things, I was totally blown away time after time when I found *it worked*! If you're like I was, take a deep breath, practice willful suspension of disbelief, step by step, and see what happens. If something feels crazy or wrong, stay away from it until your tummi feels okay. It may take a few tries at first to get solid results. Initial attempts are often easier and more successful in a group or working with an experienced person that can support, guide, monitor, give feedback, and ensure you don't make too many wrong turns. These exercises throughout the book can help get your toes wet, and connect you with other resources that can take you deeper. Once you have actually experienced chi energy, everything in this book takes on different meaning.

EXPERIENCING PERSONAL CHI	21
KINESIOLOGY	26
PLUGGING IN TO THE ENERGETIC UNIVERSE	30
EMPOWERING IMAGES	82
LETTING GO OF A GREEDY WORLD	98
CO-CREATION CONFERENCE CALLS	146
GROUP ENERGY IN RITUAL	158
CALLING AND MOVING PLACE ENERGY	162
CLEARING ENERGY IN A SPACE	164
SETTING INTENTION OF A SPACE	165
WORKING WITH INTENTION	166
DOWSING	169
SENSING CHI IN A PLACE	176
FILLING A PLACE WITH SOUL	191
FINDING THE FREEDOM TO GIVE	264

1 *ENTERING THE UNIVERSE OF CHI*

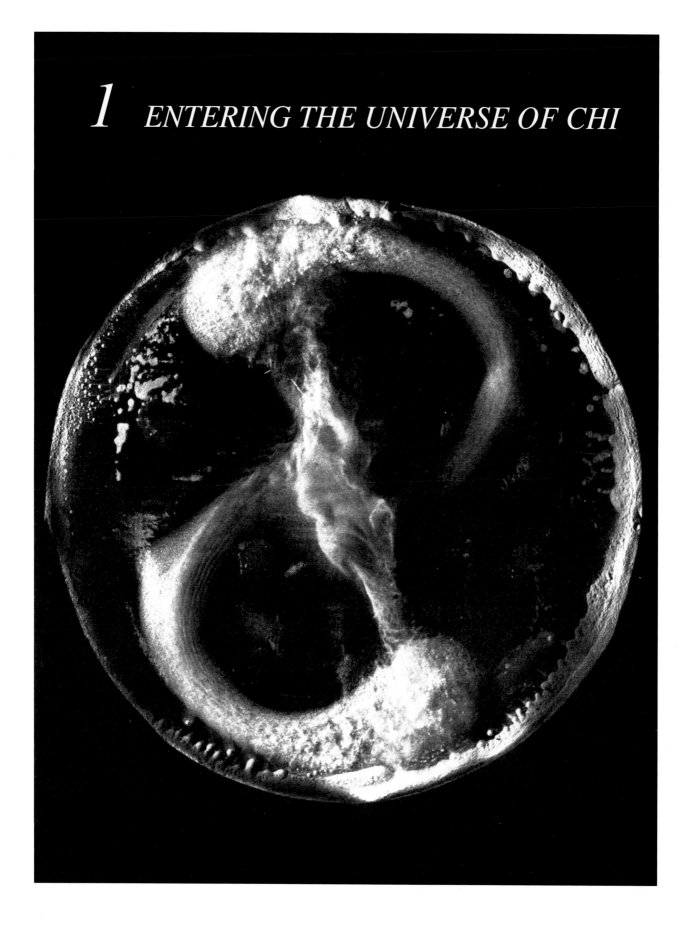

From the dawn of time, human societies on our planet have held that all of Creation is alive and intimately interconnected, that holiness resides in all things, and that our lives need to be kept in harmony with all of this vast and wonderful Creation. As Ernest Eitel, a 19th century missionary to China, said regarding the Chinese practice of feng shui:

> *They see a golden chain of spiritual life running through every form of existence and binding together, as in one living body, everything that subsists in heaven above or earth below.[1]*

He is echoed across the centuries and the miles by sacred place researcher Jim Swan:

> *Skeptical scientists comment that one cannot say the Earth is alive, for if it is, it must have a communication system, and everyone knows the Earth cannot talk. But it **can** talk. This is precisely what the research on sacred places shows. People go out to certain places and engage in interactions with nature in which information is exchanged. The Earth may not speak in English, but if we allow our minds to perceive through dreams, intuitions, animal messages, and voices that speak to us in the silence, the Earth is talking to us in words that are strong and clear.[2]*

Throughout history cultures have acknowledged the existence of a subtle life-force energy, or *chi*, underlying and connecting all material existence. Again and again, cultures have acknowledged the existence of deities within all things and all places. Again and again, people have affirmed the continuing existence of ancestors, and intentionally made connection with them. And again and again, they have honored their natural surroundings and created their built surroundings to align with the meaning and power they found in this living universe.

The universe of chi is both new and timelessly ancient. It is a vision of the energy – rather than material – basis of all Creation, of the intimate interconnectedness of all life. Verifiable through our own senses, giving deeper and more fecund power to our awareness of self and our relationship with our outer world, the contemporary rebirth of this vision is transforming all aspects of

Facing page: Hans Jenny's studies of the effects of sound vibration on the organizational structure of various materials gives a visual image of the dynamic interactions between vibration, energy, and organization as it emerges on the material level.

---

[1] Ernest Eitel, FENG-SHUI: The Rudiments of Natural Science in China, Lane, Crawford & Co., 1873. Reprinted Synergetic Press, 1993.

[2] James Swan, SACRED PLACES, Bear & Co., 1990.

our perception, experience, and living. It is a vision of the rhythmic iteration of sound, of song, of complex vibration, harmonics and overtones that give rise to and maintain all the complex interfolding structure of the universe.

Virtually every culture other than our own has experienced and incorporated an understanding of this *breath of life* into all aspects of their lives. Ours alone seems to have lost this understanding. *Chi, prana, kundalini, ki, vis medicatrix naturae, mana* . . . the names are as many as the cultures that have known it, yet the consistency and accuracy of the descriptions and practices related to this phenomenon are awesome. The personal experience of this breath of life through yoga, tai chi, qi-gong, martial arts, meditation, or spontaneous occurrence is acknowledged by increasing numbers of people in our own culture. We are experiencing it today with the same consistency and replicability as in past cultures.

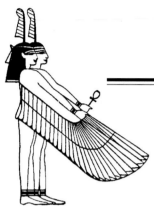

LIFE-FORCE ENERGY IN WORLD CULTURES

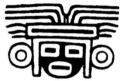

NAME	CULTURE / NATION /PERSON

AFRICA

Ntoro	Ashanti[12]
Ntu	Bantu[12]
Mulungu	Central African Yaos,[2] Ghana[12]
Mungo	Central Africa[1], Sudanese[2]
Elima	Congo[1, 2]
Njom	Ekoi[2]
Ayik	Elgonyi[2]
Wong	Gold Coast[2]
Megbe	Ituri Pygmies,[2] Hiru Pygmies[12]
N/um, Rlun	Kalahari Bushman[4, 2]
Ngai	Masai[2]
Ori	Yoruba[1]

AMERICA (N.)

Manitou	Algonquin[1, 2]
Dige	Apache[1]
Hullo	Chickasaw[1]
Maxpe	Crow[1]
Ton	Dakota[12]
Sila	Inuit[2]
Orenda, Oki	Iroquois,[1, 2] Huron[12]
Digin	Navaho[1]
Wakonda	Omaha, Sioux[1, 2]
Po-Wa-Ha	Pueblo[6]
Wakan	Sioux[1, 2]

AMERICA (S.)

Axé	Candomblé[8]
Huaca	Incan, Peruvian[2]
Itz, K'awil, Ch'ul, Ch'ulel	Maya[7]
Gana	Incan[12]

ASIA

Ch'i, Qi	China[1]
Ki, Reiki	Japan[1]
Kundalini, Prana	Hindu[4, 1]
Kundalini, Prana	Khmer[2]
Badi, Mana	Malaya[2]
Eckankar	Pali[2]
Lungta	Tibetan[14]
Tinh	Vietnam[1]

AUSTRALIA

Arunquiltha, Churinga, Kurunba	Aborigines[2, 2, 6]
Zogo	Torres Strait Tribes[2]

EUROPE

Holy Spirit	Christians[2]
Wouivre, Nwyure	Druid[6]

Elàn Vital	Early Europe[1]
Ether	Early Europe[6]
Illiaster	1500's Europe[11]
Facultas Formatrix	Galen[2], Johannes Kepler[2]
Wodan	German[2]
Dynamis	Greek[1, 5]
Entelecheia (Formative Cause)	Greek (from Aristotle)[2, 5]
Pneuma (Numia, Mumia)	Greek (from Galen)[1]
Telesma	Greek (from Hermes Trismegistus)[2]
Vis Medicatrix Naturae	Greek (from Hippocrates)[1]
Nous	Greek (from Plato)[2]
Vital Fluid	Medival Alchemists[1]
Numen	Roman[1]
Spirare	Roman[12]

MID-EAST

Napishtu	Akkadian[9]
Anima Mundi	Avicenna[2] (Arabic)
Ka, Hike, Ankh	Egyptian[1]
Ruach	Hebrews[2]

El, Manna	Israel[1]
Yesod	Jewish Kabbalah[2]
Baraka	Moroccan[1, 6], Persian[1], Sufi[2]
Shiimti	Sumerian[9]

PACIFIC

Labuni	Gelaria (N. Guinea)[2]
Tane	Hawaii[12]
Kerei	Indonesia[1]
Anut	Kusaie[2]
Andriamanitra	Malagasy (Philippines)[2]
Atua	Maoris[2]
Aka	Mauli[13]
Kasinge, Kalit	Palau[2]
Huna	Polynesian[1]
Mana	Polynesian / Hawaiian[1, 2]
Ani, Han	Ponape[2]
Tondi	Sumatra[1], Bataks[2]
Yaris	Tobi[2]
Miwi	Yaralde of the Lower Murray[10]

1. Dr. Clyde W. Ford, WHERE HEALING WATERS MEET, 1980.
2. John White & Stanley Krippner, FUTURE SCIENCE, 1977.
3. Barbara Brennan, HANDS OF LIGHT, 1987.
4. Richard Katz, quoted in KUNDALINI EXPERIENCE, Lee Sannella, 1992.
5. Vinton McCabe, LET LIKE CURE LIKE, 1997.
6. Paul Devereux, PLACES OF POWER, 1990.
7. David Freidel, Linda Schele & Joy Parker, MAYA COSMOS, 1993.
8. Robert Voeks, SACRED LEAVES OF CANDOMBLÉ, 1997.
9. Zacheria Sitchen, THE TWELFTH PLANET, 1991.
10. A.P Elkin, ABORIGINAL MEN OF HIGH DEGREE, 1946.
11. Barbara Brennan, LIGHT EMERGING, 1993.
12. William Collinge, SUBTLE ENERGIES, 1998.
13. Hank Welsselman, MEDICINEMAKER, 1998.
14. Helen Berliner, ENLIGHTENED BY DESIGN, 1999.

18th - 20th CENTURY RESEARCHERS

Anamorphosis	Ludwig von Bertalanffy[2]
Astral Light	H.P. Blavatsky[2]
Biomagnetism	George De la Warr[2]
Bioplasma	V.S. Grischenko[2]
Elan Vital	Henri Bergson[2,5]
Eloptic Energy	Thomas Galen Hieronymus[2]
Etheric Force	Radiesthists[2]
Etheric Formative Forces	Rudolf Steiner[2]
Gestaltung	Johann Wolfgang von Goethe[2]
Integrative Tendency	Arthur Koestler[2]
Kirlian Energy	Czech[1]
L-Fields (life fields)	Harold Saxon Burr[1]
Lebenskraft, Vital Force, Dynamis	Samuel Hahnemann (Homeopathy)[5]
Libido	Sigmund Freud[2]
Life Force	Luigi Galvani[2]
M-Fields (morphogenetic fields)	Rupert Sheldrake[1]
Magnetic Fluid	Anton Mesmer[1]
Magnetoelectricity	William T. Tiller[2]
Negative Entropy	Erwin Schroedinger[2]
Noetic Energy	Charles Muses[2]
Od, Odyllic, Odic Force	Karl von Reichenbach[2]
Orgone Energy	Wilhelm Reich[1]
Primary Perception	Cleve Backster[2]
Psi Faculty	J.B. Rhine[2]
Psi Plasma	Andrija Puharich[2]
Psionics	John W. Campbell[2]
Psychotronic Energy	Robert Pavlita[2]
Synchronicity	Carl Gustav Jung[2]
Synergy	Abraham Maslow[2]
Unitary Principle in Nature	L.L. Whyte[2]
Universal Energy Field	Barbara Brennan[3]
Universal Intelligence	Chiropractic[1]
Will to live	Western Medicine[1]

✧

A world based on chi and the sacred differs from one based on our customary beliefs in ways that can be extremely difficult to grasp intellectually. One piece of it can be glimpsed in the words of Malidoma Somé concerning the nature of work in a Dagara community:

> *Our vision is the starting point of a primal technological power, which is the ability to manifest, to make Spirit real in material form. . . . Spirit and work are linked among indigenous people because human work is viewed as an intensification of the work that Spirit does in nature.*

> *. . . For villagers, the product of any work must be engineered not only to serve the collective good but also to be an extension of the goodness of the collective. For instance, when women get together to make pottery, they are acknowledging that their ability to create is a part of nature's design, a part of their purpose. Before a woman participates in the work with clay, which is the earth, she will first gather the signs and images she has seen in nature, and she will bring these signs into the circle of other women. In the interest of producing something that is an extension of their wholeness, the women will begin by chanting and singing together, echoing one another.*

> *. . . They are seated in a circle, and they chant until they are in some sort of ecstatic place, and it is from that place that they begin molding the clay. It is as if the knowledge of how to make pots is not in their brains, but in their collective energy. . . . The women can sit all day in front of two dozen mounds of clay, doing nothing but chanting – until the last hours, when in a flurry of activity all kinds of pots come forth. . . . The product of work here, the pot, embodies the intimacy and wholeness experienced by the women over the course of the day. The women understand that it is necessary to reach that place of wholeness before they can bring something out of it.*

> *. . . Most work in the village is done collectively. The purpose is not so much the desire to get the job done but to raise enough energy for people to feel nourished by what they do. The nourishment does not come after the job, it comes <u>before</u> the job and <u>during</u> the job. . . . You are nourished first, and then the work flows out of your fullness.*

> *. . . As a result of our work practices, the indigenous notion of abundance is very different from that in the West. Villagers are interested not in accumulation but in a sense of <u>fullness</u>. . . . Abundance, in that sense of fullness, has a power that takes us away from worry.*[3]

In the spirit world lies the root of our existence, our purposes, our nurture, and our potentials. Restoring communion between the material and the spirit worlds is vital to the outcome and rightness of all our actions. Sourced in communion with the spirit world, our surroundings and the product of all our actions are permeated with vital energy and rightness of spirit.

---

[3] Malidoma Somé, THE HEALING WISDOM OF AFRICA, Tarcher/Putnam, 1998.

✦

Our culture is on the threshold of a quiet yet fundamental transformation. Acknowledgment of the existence and importance of chi or life force energy – the foundation of the arts, sciences, healing, and spiritual practices of virtually all cultures in history – is reaching a critical mass in our own society.

An operative definition of chi – in general and particularly in regard to placemaking – is easier to come by at this time than a precise "scientific" one, as our sciences are only beginning to study its phenomena seriously.[4] Chi in the body has generally been called "subtle energy" or "life force energy."[5] It is the energy source and medium which constitutes the auric fields underlying material existence, around which our material bodies coalesce. In the cultures that have acknowledged chi, it is considered both the energetic connection with non-material dimensions of existence and the primary energy source for the material body. Many sectors of our culture are independently coming to acknowledge varied aspects of this energy's existence.

When we acknowledge the central role of chi in our universe, some interesting transformations occur in how we see our world, how we live our lives, and the kind of culture that we develop:

In a world where no one can lie – where our innermost thoughts and feelings are known to each other – it becomes imperative to base our lives, our building, and our culture on speaking and living truth.

When we acknowledge that instant communication occurs, not only between people but among all forms of life – stars, rocks, the cells in our bodies – we need to consider the needs of other life, open to their wisdom, and honor their spirits in our surroundings.

To acknowledge that we continue to exist on an energy level after "death" is to transform our sense of our purpose on earth, of death, and as well our connection with the spirit world.

When we can call on the counsel of ancestors and other beings in the spiritual planes of life, our process of determining goals and actions, as well as the roles of our surroundings becomes very different.

When we discover that astrology can show us what kinds of surroundings are good or bad for us at different times, it becomes important for us to pay attention

---

[4] For a clear presentation of experimental and conceptual study of the nature of chi, see Richard Gerber, VIBRATIONAL MEDICINE, Bear & Co., 1996. Or see William Collinge, SUBTLE ENERGY, Warner Books, 1998. For a perspective on how our concepts of physics could be expanded to adjust to these phenomena, see William A. Tiller, SCIENCE AND HUMAN TRANSFORMATION: Subtle Energies, Intentionality and Consciousness, Pavior, 1997. Paul LaVoilette's BEYOND THE BIG BANG, Park St. Press, 1995, also provides an interesting critique of our current theories of cosmogenesis and physics, as it affects such phenomena.

[5] Barbara Brennan's HANDS OF LIGHT, Bantam Books, 1987, gives a more thorough discussion, and Rosalyn Bruyere's WHEELS OF LIGHT, Fireside Books, 1989, a slightly differing perspective.

to our connections with all of Creation, as well as the qualities of the places we make and use.

* When we discover that "magic" is practiced and can have a powerful effect for good or ill, attention to the energetics of place and community become vital.

* When we realize that the health of all Creation is essential to our well-being, the basic values underlying our culture and the making of our homes and communities must change.

* When we recognize that our minds and hearts are an integral and powerful part of our interaction with the world on both sides of our skin, and that those aspects of our existence are inseparable, we can begin to improve our surroundings by listening to the messages of our hearts.

* When we realize that sacredness is the heart of meaningful lives and an enduring society, we start to learn and practice honoring and love in our work, communities, and personal lives.

CHI IN THE BODY

Recent physical identification of the actual acupuncture meridians in our bodies, joined with new clarity on their role in moving chi energy, is leading to the development of a new discipline of energy medicine.

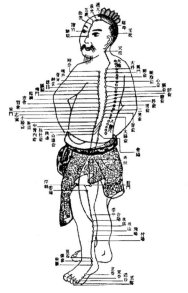

        In November, 1997, the National Institutes of Health released a strong endorsement of the use of acupuncture. In doing so, they noted "very clear-cut evidence" of its successful action and that it is less invasive, with fewer side effects, than conventional treatments. For a major governmental player in the U.S. medical establishment to make such an endorsement of a practice based on chi is remarkable – *particularly* as the panel noted "there is no evidence that confirms this theory." What is perhaps most remarkable is that in endorsing something denied by our conventional scientific concepts, they are in essence challenging the adequacy of those very concepts! The chi underlying acupuncture is the same chi in the earth which is central to the Chinese art of feng shui and the energetics of place traditions of other cultures.

        Western scientists have only recently seriously explored energy-based alternatives to traditional medical theory.[6] The sensitive instrumentation now available confirms the existence and operation of chi energy in our bodies. It has been demonstrated via MRI scans with radioactive isotopes that some form of energy is transported in our bodies along traditional acupuncture meridians, rather than through blood, lymph or any other known circulatory systems. This has been documented independently and in detail by Korean Professor Kim Bong Han[7]and by French medical researchers Jean-Claude Darras and Pierre de Vernejoul at the nuclear medicine section of Necker Hospital in Paris.[8]

---

[6] Robert O. Becker, CROSS CURRENTS: THE PERILS OF ELECTROPOLLUTION, THE PROMISE OF ELECTROMEDICINE, Tarcher, 1990; and Robert O. Becker and Gary Selden, BODY ELECTRIC: ELECTROMAGNETISM AND THE FOUNDATION OF LIFE, Morrow & Co, 1985.

[7] S. Rose-Neil, "The Work of Professor Kim Bong Ham", THE ACUPUNCTURIST, 1967; or more accessibly in Richard Gerber's VIBRATIONAL MEDICINE, Bear & Co., 1996.

[8] Research results available from World Research Foundation, 15300 Ventura Blvd., Suite 405, Sherman Oaks, CA 91403.

These researchers have demonstrated the existence of a system of extremely fine ductlike tubules in our bodies, approximately 0.5 - 1.0 microns in diameter, that follow the ancient descriptions of acupuncture meridian pathways. In subsequent studies using infrared emissions, the accuracy of the "maps" shown in ancient acupuncture texts has been confirmed.[9] Other research using ion flow[10] and light emission[11] have shown that we can assess the energy flowing through each chakra[12], meridian, and internal organ, as well as changes in that energy following acupuncture, meditation, qi gong, and other energy healing treatments.[13]

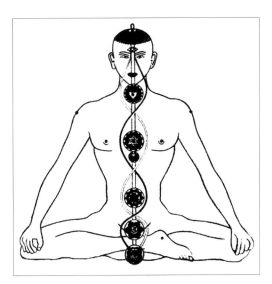

Electrical oscillations in the skin above the chakras have been found to occur in the range of 100 to 1,600 cycles per second, in contrast with 0 to 100 in the brain, 225 in the muscles, and 250 in the heart.[14] When energy is consciously projected through a chakra by advanced meditators, the strength of the electrical field emanating from that chakra multiplies.[15]

Numerous studies show that the energy state of our bodies is distinctly different during sleep, movement, meditation, and other activities. For example, brain scans of dowsers show significantly different brainwave activity than those of meditators. Dowsers show the coherent delta-wave profile of meditators, but also coherent alpha, beta, and theta waves, which are related to creative cognition, contact with the subconscious mind, and the visual component of imagery.[16]

Refinement of energy practices such as qi-gong is providing easily accessed means of personally experiencing the existence of the chakras and other energy-related dimensions of our bodies and their role in our health and well-being.

"Energy healing," "laying on of hands," qi gong, and related practices of healing that affect bodily chi have been effective enough in promoting healing in a variety of situations that they are now covered by many health insurance policies. Though rarely advertised, growing numbers of medical personnel are taking advanced training in psychic skills for diagnosis and healing. Traditional practices of energy healing have been refined and paired with manipulation of specific points

---

[9] P. Wang, X. Hu, and B. Wu, "Displaying of the Infrared Radiant Track Long Meridians on the Back of the Human Body," CHEN TZU YEN CHIU ACUPUNCTURE RESEARCH, 1993.

[10] Hiroshi Motoyama, MEASUREMENTS OF KI ENERGY, DIAGNOSIS AND TREATMENTS, Human Science Press, 1998.

[11] I. Dumitrescu and J. Kenyon, ELECTROGRAPHIC IMAGING IN MEDICINE AND BIOLOGY, Neville Spearman, 1983.

[12] (From Sanskrit) A chain of whirling vortices of subtle energy along the central axis of our bodies. See Gerber, below, for a detailed explanation.

[13] For a clear overview of these and other related studies, see Richard Gerber, VIBRATIONAL MEDICINE, Bear & Co., 1996.

[14] Based on a study by Valerie Hunt summarized in Richard Gerber, VIBRATIONAL MEDICINE, Bear & Co., 1996.

[15] H. Motoyama and R. Brown, SCIENCE AND THE EVOLUTION OF CONSCIOUSNESS: CHAKRAS, KI, AND PSI, Autumn Press, 1978.

[16] See Ed Stillman, "Dowser's Brainwave Characteristics," AMERICAN DOWSER QUARTERLY, Winter '97 and Spring '98. (See illustration on page 25.)

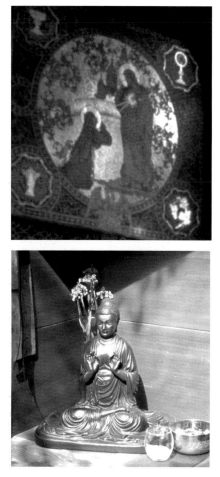

connected with our bodies' numerous specific energy systems for self-verifiable diagnosis and treatment.[17]

Nature, the British equivalent of *Scientific American*, announced in their December, 1997 issue the successful experimental demonstration of "quantum teleportation" by researchers in Austria. Quantum teleportation shows that information even on the subatomic level can be transmitted *instantly* over stellar distances (without being limited by the speed of light). With this demonstration, the informational interconnectedness of all Creation is no longer in question.[18] Related work is underway by IBM.

Reports by participants in the CIA's various "psychic spy" projects indicate that the CIA has used remote viewing and remote "influencing" operationally for several decades, while simultaneously discounting and belittling the credibility of civilian research and work in this area.[19] Kinesiology (muscle- or energy-testing) is now used widely to assess human allergies and "whole-body" knowledge of remote events.[20] The medical intuitive Caroline Myss has demonstrated a 93% confirmation rate of standard medical diagnosis without the patient even being present - just being given the patent's name and date of birth.[21]

In 1997, Dean Radin published reports on previously classified military-funded experimentation on psychic phenomena along with statistical analysis of experimentation done over the last century in that area.[22] Radin's work should erase any lingering doubts that there is more going on in our universe than meets the rational eye. Several experiments that he reports on showed that the intensity and extent of individual and group focus on *any* particular activity has a corollary effect of imposing an enhanced degree of order or probability on otherwise random and unassociated events. Similar studies at Stanford[23] and Princeton Universities[24] have

The art of almost every culture reflects the existence of chi energy. Glowing auras and heart chakras in Christian mosaics, and the mudras or hand positions in Buddhist statuary shown beaming energy out through hand chakras, reveal equally the conscious use of chi.

[17] Donna Eden's ENERGY MEDICINE, Tarcher/Putnam, 1998 is an excellent resource on these systems and specific healing practices connected with them. See also publications by Caroline Myss, Barbara Brennan, and Myra Knaster, among others. "Soaring Crane" style Qi Gong has, in my experience, a very high success rate with people experiencing chi energy in their bodies.

[18] See Gary Schwartz and Russek, Linda, THE LIVING ENERGY UNIVERSE, Hampton Roads Pub. Co., 1999.

[19] See David A. Morehouse, PSYCHIC WARRIOR, St. Martin's Press, 1998; Dean Radin, THE CONSCIOUS UNIVERSE, HarperSF, 1997; and books by other participants in the projects. Academic studies in this area at Stanford Research Institute are reported in Gerber, above.

[20] Various processes of kinesiology are discussed in Eden's ENERGY MEDICINE, Wright's PERELANDRA GARDEN WORKBOOK, and more conventional books on medical kinesiology. See also Donna Eden, above.

[21] C. Norman Shealy, "Clairvoyant Diagnosis", in T.M. Srinivasan, ed., ENERGY MEDICINE AROUND THE WORLD, Gabriel Press, 1988.

[22] Dean Radin, THE CONSCIOUS UNIVERSE, HarperCollins, 1997.

[23] William A. Tiller, "A Gas Discharge Device for Investigating Focused Human Intention", JOURNAL OF SCIENTIFIC EXPLORATION, 1990; and William Tiller, SCIENCE AND HUMAN TRANSFORMATION: SUBTLE ENERGIES, INTENTIONALITY AND CONSCIOUSNESS, Pavior, 1997.

[24] R. Nelson, G. Bradish, Y. Dobyns, B. Dunne and R. Jahn, "Field REG Anomalies in Group Situations", JOURNAL OF SCIENTIFIC EXPLORATION, 1996.

EXPERIENCING PERSONAL CHI

Start by sitting, comfortably but erect, with legs and arms uncrossed. (Or lie down, if that is more comfortable for you.)

Ground and center (See Plugging-In Exercise, page 30).

Focus your attention fully on your breathing. Feel your body expand as you breathe in through your nose. Feel it relax and settle down as you exhale. Quit holding in your stomach and abdomen. Let them relax and move with your breath. As you breathe in, let your belly expand. Feel your breath fill your entire body cavity down to your hips. Feel it flow out from your chest, belly, and abdomen. Check on any tension you feel in any part of your body, and relax it.

Now bring your attention back to your nose. Feel the air moving in, and out again. Move your attention to the back of your nose, and lightly constrict the nasal passages there, almost as if you were going to blow your nose. Stop and blow your nose a couple of times if you want, to clear your nasal passages and help focus on those muscles. Feel your breath lightly move over those muscles, in and out. Check and see if your other head and body muscles have tensed up, and relax them if they have.

You may start to feel energy start to accumulate in your head, or a tingling sensation, or feel slightly light-headed. If you don't, then change to slightly different muscles in your nose to constrict, moving around until you find a spot that does start to give you a "buzz."

Keep your breath moving slowly and smoothly, and move the focus of your attention to your hands. Now visualize your breath coming in through your fingers, up your arms, and then exhaled out your nose. Keep your attention on your fingers and hands. They may start to feel cool, as if a slight breeze, or breath, is passing over them. Reverse your intention, breathing in through your nose, letting the breath move down through your arms and out your hands and fingers. Your fingers may start to tingle or feel warm.

Now breathe both in and out through your fingers, keep a light attention on your hands, and feel them start to tingle and warm up. Open your heart, feel a strong love for someone, and see if the flow of energy increases. Obviously, this isn't your breath moving in and out of your hands; it is chi energy, which has a connection with our breathing, and focus on our breath seems to trigger our awareness of it and control of its movement. Just focusing on our breathing focuses our minds, turning off the chatter, and sharpening our attention so that when we add intention, such as moving chi, we are focused enough to do it.

Once you've begun to feel chi moving in your hands, start moving it through other parts of your body. Breathe in through your left foot, out through your right. In through your feet, out through your hands. In from all extremities to your heart, out through the crown of your head. In from the heavens through your crown, out through your root chakra to the center of the earth.

Didn't work? Didn't feel anything? Just got dizzy? Try it again another time. Don't try so hard. Your attention and intention IS moving chi - you probably just aren't able to feel it yet. Every person experiences and feels things differently. Next time, try holding your hands about six to eight inches apart, facing each other, slightly tensed, as if you are holding a ball. Move them slightly closer together, then farther apart, then closer. You may get the feeling of a ball of energy between your hands. As with other exercises, doing this in a group, and/or with someone who is experienced in doing it often strengthens the responses and gives us the confidence that lets us loosen up and let things work! For drawings and exercises to learn to sense the various energy systems in you body, see Donna Eden's *Energy Medicine.*

shown that this effect is strongest during periods of strongly focused group attention, high group cohesion, or a shared emotional experience. Research by Rupert Sheldrake has shown similar effects.[25]

Seeing into the future is a mind-boggling and somewhat scary prospect. Psychiatrist Judith Orloff, in her book *Second Sight*, explains the phenomenon, the frequency of its occurrence, its benefits, and how to work with it in a positive way.[26] My own introduction to it occurred twenty years ago, after the house we were building burned down. A friend on the East Coast was visibly shaken to hear of our fire, as she had dreamt – a month before – that it would burn, and had even written the date in her journal. Other friends have had detailed precognitive dreams of disasters such as boats sinking, which later occurred. Not a comfortable skill to have without the proper understanding of its positive use!

The effects of intention, chi energy, and the sacred on our familiar material lives thread into every dimension. Asian martial arts have transformed European-based concepts of personal combat and defense. Many sports now routinely use training concepts based on chi and intention. Even the U.S. Marines now use Aikido training, which is based on chi![27] Walking on beds of burning hot embers without injury, under trance, is common in many cultures and spiritual traditions.[28] Well over 100,000 people in the U.S. alone have experienced firewalking in the last decade. It has even become a cult of corporate bonding.[29] Interaction of the material and spirit worlds fundamentally changes our familiar ground rules about how things behave.

This energy dimension of existence is key to understanding esoteric practices of many cultures that we have found difficult to comprehend. The Australian Aborigines talk of healing broken bones within a few hours. Tibetan Buddhism *lung-gom* and *tum-mo* practitioners can run with extraordinary swiftness over fields of boulders, and keep themselves warm in snow and ice without clothing. Native American tribes use fasting, trance drumming, and other techniques to attain altered states. The !Kung people of the Kalahari Desert in Africa practice a particular dance to "heat up" their *n/um*, or what the Hindus call *kundalini*, so that a state of transcendence can be attained. In those dances, more than half of the tribe can attain such states. In the *!!kia* state, extraordinary feats are possible.[30]

Recent work by anthropologists, linguists, and historians is transforming our awareness of the role that chi energy and the spirit world has played in various cultures throughout history. In Chapter 3, we will discuss some of these from the

---

[25] Rupert Sheldrake, SEVEN EXPERIMENTS THAT COULD CHANGE THE WORLD, Riverhead Books, 1996.

[26] Judith Orloff, SECOND SIGHT, Warner Books, 1996.

[27] Richard Strozzi Heckler, IN SEARCH OF THE WARRIOR SPIRIT, North Atlantic Books, 1992.

[28] See Wade Davis' SHADOWS IN THE SUN, Island Press, 1998, on such practices in Haiti's Vodoun tradition, Richard Katz' BOILING ENERGY on the Kalahari !Kung, Harvard University Press, 1982, or Vilenskaya, below.

[29] See, for example, Larissa Vilenskaya, FIREWALKING, Bramble Co., 1992, or McDermott and Biayak's MASTERING FEAR, Frog & Latte, 1996.

[30] Richard Katz, BOILING ENERGY: Community Healing among the Kalahari Kung, Harvard University Press, 1982.

CHAPTER ONE – Entering the Universe of Chi 23

standpoint of chi energy in place. Linguists' recent translation of the Maya alphabet is now allowing reading of the actual inscriptions on buildings and monuments, which tell amazing stories of the psychic dimensions of their culture. Translation and interpretation of the cuneiform writing found on clay tablet libraries in archeological digs of the ancient Middle East have revealed the historical accuracy of Biblical events and of what were once considered "mythological stories" of many of those cultures. These translations are leading to radical reconstruction of history.[31]

The New York State school system now employs accredited teachers of psychic awareness. The schools in American Samoa now teach about parapsychological perception, including the latest research on telepathy, clairvoyance, and precognition. Students test themselves for various abilities, and learn abilities from their elders.[32]

✦

William Tiller, of Stanford University, outlines some of the characteristics common to various manifestations of this energy:

1. From experiments on telepathy, psychokinesis (PK), manual healers, etc., we seem to be dealing with energy fields completely different from those known to conventional science.

2. From a large variety of experiments, we find indications for a level of substance in nature that exhibits:
  (a) characteristics that are predominantly magnetic, as distinct from electric, in nature;
  (b) an organizing rather than a disorganizing tendency as the temperature increases (in seeming violation of the Second Law of Thermodynamics for the physical universe);
  (c) a radiation pattern or hologram of energy that acts as a force envelope for the organization of substance at the physical level.

3. From experiments on plants, animals, and humans, evidence is mounting that there is an interconnection at some level of substance between all things in the universe.[33]

A technical description of chi – whether it is a form of electromagnetic energy, some "unknown" type of energy, or some sensory expression of other more mundane bodily processes – is not of immediate concern in terms of our consideration for design. Like acupuncture, gravity, or the common cold, lack of a detailed understanding of the process is not necessary for a broad acknowledgment and acceptance that it does happen, and even some refinement in dealing with it. And, like acupuncture, it probably will be some time before a clear and detailed under-

---

[31] For example, see Zacheria Sitchen's THE TWELFTH PLANET, Bear & Co., 1991; Graham Hancock's FINGERPRINTS OF THE GODS, Three Rivers Press, 1995; and John Anthony West's SERPENT IN THE SKY, Harper & Row, 1979.

[32] Jim Swan, SACRED PLACES, Bear & Co., 1990.

[33] Tiller, above.

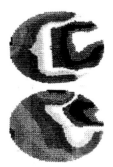

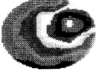

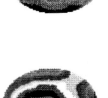

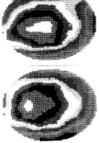

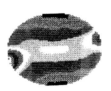

EEG monitoring of dowsers' brainwaves shows unusual simultaneous high levels in theta, alpha and beta waves; unusual coherence levels in theta, alpha and beta; and unusual coherence resulting in high power levels and "smoothness" combined with right brain dominance in both alpha and beta. This implies thoughrts and visions coming directly to the cortex from the limbic brain system.

standing of the underlying science develops – and with it, a welcome refinement of application.

In any case, personal experience of chi is the critical factor in moving it from an intellectual question to an operative principal based on personal knowledge. In this area, recent developments in bodywork and deep tissue therapy[34] have probably done more than generations of yoga and meditation instructors to achieve replicable success. New techniques have been developed which make the experience of chi something that can be easily attained by most people. Chi is no longer an esoteric concept requiring years of monastic training to grasp.

Millions of people in our own culture have now *experienced* this chi energy – through martial arts, meditation, bodywork, acupuncture, or other contexts. It is no longer a theoretical philosophical concept or a foreign spiritual tradition. As we deepen our understanding of how chi operates in various contexts, it is important that we look at its implications for society as a whole, and for our individual lives.

Since World War II, scientists have been absorbed in exploring the material consequences of breakthroughs achieved in a few branches of physics. As a consequence, they have neglected to focus their powerful tools on other unexplored areas. We have given names – like "gravity" or "magnetism" – to blank spaces in our understanding, but then assume we therefore know more about them than we do. Do we really understand magnetism? How does it transmit power through space and vacuum?

Or what about gravity? The mass of the moon is immense. Simple mechanics tells us what incredible forces gravity applies to the moon to keep that mass in orbit instead of shooting off on a tangent into space. But *how* does it work? How are the moon and sun able, through enormous distances, to *pull* the entire oceans of our planet six feet into the air twice a day and pull the Earth around in a circle?

Chi is one of these areas still poorly explored by our current sciences. Unlike the moon hanging over our heads, it has until recently been a subject that we could brush aside and pretend it didn't exist. But experience and success in its use are today forcing its recognition.

It may seem that chi is a simple and peripheral thing, but its central role in the sophisticated philosophies of many cultures should be a hint of its importance. The impact of its acknowledgment is likely to be as foreign and initially inconceivable as the atom bomb. Fortunately, the power of chi is integrative rather than destructive – a power of giving life rather than of taking it. Its acknowledgment will bring changes as great as those achieved by our modern technology, but in vastly different directions.

---

[34] Mirka Knaster's DISCOVERING THE BODY'S WISDOM., Bantam, 1996, gives an outstanding overview of current research on the role of body tissue in memory, the differences and similarities among various bodywork techniques, and criteria for choosing a bodywork therapist.

CHI AND THE SACRED

The pathways by which the sacred affects our lives are many, varied, and sometimes unfamiliar. The sacred gives us the security of support and nurture by others and removes our feelings of solitary responsibility. It affects our hearts by balancing the ever-present negative emotions of life with the healing, supportive emotions of love, caring, and feeling of value. It affects our minds by making known the pathways through which all life cares for us. And it affects our souls through direct connection with the spirits of all Creation.

* The sacred is a measure of our connection with all Creation. When we hold Creation inviolate, we acknowledge our wholeli-ness and inter-importance. That connection and interaction occurs in the realms of chi. Our *internal chi* alters the energy of the places we inhabit; in much the same way, the energy of the places themselves affects us.

* The role played by *intention* is vital in directing and focusing chi and allowing its movement to reflect our goals and values. Intention also gives coherence and focus to our actions when we shape and use our surroundings, increasing their capacity to embody our values and dreams. Any action inspired by love, for example, conveys that love and the importance of it to others.

* *Ritual and our patterns of use* of places bring depth of meaning to our experiences, make our commitments visible, and embody our values and beliefs. They affect our experience, our places themselves, and the energetic interchange between them. They are an important vehicle for invoking change in chi , opening us to the spirit world, and sustaining community health.

* *Energetically empowered symbols and design elements* allow actual spiritual manifestations and provide yet another means by which our surroundings can bring us in contact with the sacred. Unfamiliar to our culture, these have been important tools in virtually all other cultures.

* Our surroundings, by their innate nature, design, or use, can become *portals to the spirit world*, through which we can access the wisdom and support of our ancestors and other spirit entities.

We are clearly not separate from the world in which we move. Influence and awareness move both ways across our skins and entwine us and the rest of the universe into a single organism. Harm we cause to our surroundings returns to cripple and diminish our own lives. With this awareness, there is no excuse for taking from our neighbors and surroundings. There are only infinite reasons for *giving* and enriching life on both sides of our skin. The implications for how we shape and use our surroundings and our lives are immense.

KINESIOLOGY – YOUR BODY KNOWS

Kinesiology is a group of techniques of using muscle-testing to amplify and confirm our whole-body response to the energetic truth or rightness of a question we ask ourselves or are asked. It also is widely used to check on the state of the various energy systems of our bodies, and by chiropractors or wholistic medical practitioners to check on allergies or other bodily information.

With the most common technique, you hold one arm out horizontally, and hold firm when it is pushed down. You can do this with a friend. Start by saying, "My name is . . ." Your arm probably stays strong when pushed down by your friend. Then say, "My name is [your friend's name or some other name]" Usually your arm suddenly gets weak, and is easily pushed down.

Another technique, which you can use less obviously (like while trying to figure out answers on a multiple-choice test) uses the fingers on one hand to spread apart fingers on the other hand (see illustration opposite):

Touch the tips of the thumb and little finger on your non-dominant hand together to form a circle. (Left hand if you are right-handed; right if you are left-handed.) Put the index finger and thumb of your other hand into the circle. Make a yes-no question or statement, and try to force the circle finger/thumb apart with the same strength as you are holding them together. If the statement is true (My name is [. . . your name . . .]) the circle stays strong. If false, the circle-finger/thumb suddenly lose strength and come apart.

Sounds crazy, . . . but try it. Didn't work? Did you remember to ground and center, and focus your intention before starting?

Now ask yourself, or have a friend ask, a series of questions with a "yes" answer. Your circle finger/thumb should stay firm – use the exercise to adjust the pressure and get comfortable with the technique. Then do a series of questions or statements with a "no" answer, and use them to adjust technique and become comfortable with negative responses. Then alternate.

Other tips for better results: be sure your question is very clear, not a double question and can't be misinterpreted; stay alert; be sure you complete asking the question before you start testing; get away from external distractions; let out a deep breath to expel random thoughts; be sure you are willing to accept the results of the test regardless of which answer it is; and focus your intention (not on a particular answer, but on getting valid results).

For most people, this works fine initially, but pretty soon we say, "Well, I'm not really sure about that, let me try again." Then it stops working correctly. Lack of self-trust seems to cause it to lose effectiveness, as does a number of temporary or long-term energy imbalances in the body. Preconceptions and strong emotional attachment to an outcome (I *really* want that chocolate fudge sundae) also affect results.

Because these techniques link the brain more consciously with the subtle energies in the body, mastering them will, over time, allow you to use a tingle in the end of a finger, or "just knowing" to get the same answers. For more details on energy-testing, see Donna Eden's *Energy Medicine*, or Machaelle Small Wright's *Co-Creative Science* or *Perelandra Garden Workbooks*.

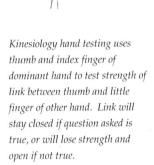

CHI AND PLACE

Chi is intimately connected with and inherent in place and our associations with it. Every culture has emphasized and developed certain aspects of place energy, while virtually ignoring others. Here are a few examples, from the almost universal use of chi in cultures worldwide, of use of chi in the places people live. We will look in more detail at some of them in later chapters. What is exciting is that these are *living* traditions which can be learned from, shared, melded, and forged into a living tradition for our own culture.

Kinesiology hand testing uses thumb and index finger of dominant hand to test strength of link between thumb and little finger of other hand. Link will stay closed if question asked is true, or will lose strength and open if not true.

* The feng shui tradition of China provides a broad and relatively comprehensive philosophical basis for understanding and applying energetics of place, and constitutes one of the most impressive written records dealing with chi in our surroundings. Feng shui's myriad traditions and practices demonstrate various approaches to environmental modification for improving local chi patterns. It has made extensive use of astrological information in siting, and generated culturally specific practices for aligning our buildings with the chi of a site. Yet there are major gaps in the approach and dimensions of feng shui. Fortunately, other traditions have pushed the frontiers of understanding even farther.

* The mapping of energy flows and concentrations in the earth has been well developed in the European geomantic tradition, which has also located buildings relative to that energy. The Australian Aboriginal tradition has developed use of such energy lines in the earth even further, using them for long-distance communication.

* Relative to the built environment, the Japanese have developed the role of *li* or *intention* to great refinement and power. Chi (or *ki* in Japanese) is if anything more central to Japanese culture and design than to Chinese. The Japanese language, for example, has over 600 terms employing the ideogram for *ki*, compared to about 80 in Chinese, and the concept is pivotal to all of their arts and sciences.[35] Their gardens, homes, and temple designs have taken special form as a result.

* In our own culture, contemporary work by architects and designers who work with chi has not reached the refinement of the Japanese or Chinese, but a tradition specific to our own conditions and time is developing.

---

[35] David Kubiak, "Ki and the Arts of Sex, Healing and Corporate Body Building," KYOTO JOURNAL, Winter 1988.

* The Khmer culture in Cambodia shows us immensely powerful roles that our built environment can play in connecting us with energy from the spirit world.

* The Yoruba in Africa can show the emotional power that can be developed afresh in our building drawing directly upon intimate connection with that world.

* African cultures – from the !Kung to the Yoruba and the Dagara, along with the Wiccan tradition in Europe and many other cultures – have worked powerfully with direct community raising of energy, and the roles it holds in cultural survival and health. As a result, surroundings are perceived and used relative to their energetic, rather than material, nature.

* The recent work of contemporary dowsers and energy workers, such as Joey Korn, Sig Lonegren, Michelle Small Wright, and others, has shown that earth energies are not immutable; they move and change. We can ask for balancing of negative energies, and for focusing and relocation of positive ones. We can call upon earth energies, and they respond – almost consciously, it would appear – to our requests for aligning with our lives and activities.

* The Australian Aboriginals have developed to a high level the use of unique and specific connections to the spiritual realm from different natural sites. The Khmers, Maya, and Egyptians have demonstrated dramatically how buildings can enhance such connections.

* Energetics of place also involves information and communication. African cultures have worked strongly with personal interaction with energy of place to access ancestors and other beings in the realms of energy. Native American, Aboriginal, Celtic, Greek, and many other traditions work with direct communication to, and through, the individual elements of nature.

Such communication at the level of chi may be one of the important missing links in our efforts to reconnect with the rest of nature. Alienation arises from our blocking out the eternal sharing and connection with all life which occurs on that level. As Malidoma Somé has said, "Literacy may fill a place in our psyches intended for other purposes." But we are now learning and relearning ways to set aside literacy when needed, and reestablish direct linkage on the level of chi.

The experience of other cultures with chi is important to us. Our culture does not stand alone in the world. Our traditions and needs both differ from and are connected with those of the Chinese, the Zulu, and the Maya. We are *all* exposed today to *all* the different traditions of millennia of different cultures' experience. Today is a time of both gathering in and sharing the wisdom of all ages. All cultures have things to offer, all have limitations and omissions. The more tools we have, the better the chance of good fit.

DESIGN WITH CHI

Design, in a chi-based world, is very different than in our present world.

The energy bodies of our homes and communities are damaged by place-rape and abuse from greed-based activities such as overlogging, overfishing, extractive agriculture, and mining, just as our human energy bodies are damaged by rape and abuse. Healing the energy bodies of our surroundings is both possible and essential if we are to have surroundings that contribute to our own health.

The chi of place and people interact, and our love or anger remain in a place to affect the next users. Gifts of honor and pilgrimage bestowed on a place are passed on to its subsequent visitors. We can generate and direct group energy that sustains the joy and health of our human communities and the natural communities within which they exist. The possibilities for people working with earth energies are expanding in scope, depth, and concrete application.

A chi-centered worldview changes how we design and use places. It requires, obviously, that we give consideration to the chi of a place. It also means, however, that the kinds of institutions and the kinds of personal needs we design for may be very different. It demands integrity of material choice, design, and use. It stresses the importance of paying attention to our tummies – how we feel about a place, the psychology of place, and the role of our minds, fears, and dreams. It requires that we design for the needs and aspirations of all Creation, not just our whims. Our attitudes and values – what we want in a place – change dramatically.

When we work with chi, our *intention* in approaching design is critical. An approach that just considers "job functions" delegates people to "back-room" jobs and "back-room" consideration by others, while an intention to provide rewarding work changes the building configuration and gives respect to each person in their work.

As discussed in *Silence, Song and Shadows*, the role of the sacred becomes central to our relationship with our surroundings. Buildings with soul, gardens for our spirits, and cities of passion become the goal rather than rentable square feet. Accommodating and enhancing ritual and its role in both the making and use of places becomes important, as does being a part of the local ecological community. Low-impact ecological design is taken for granted. Growth, greed, and consumption give way to the goals of sustainability and nurture.

Chi, and the connection and wholeness with which it imbues our lives, underlies the spirit of place. The ways that we can access and nurture it show us also the place of spirit in our lives and our surroundings.

As acknowledgment of chi forms throughout our culture, we are faced with startling implications for the goals and operation of our society and our lives. We'll look at some of these implications in the next chapter.

PLUGGING IN TO THE ENERGETIC UNIVERSE

The most important thing to remember about any work with chi is that we need to be "connected" to it before we do something. An electric light won't work unless it is plugged in. A telephone won't work unless it's turned on and we've dialed up. To reach our chi, we need to set aside the protective barriers each of us have put up to disconnect from feeling what our culture has done to the world.

PLUGGING IN: GROUNDING/CENTERING

Find a comfortable place, and remove yourself from distracting sounds: shut the door, unplug the phone, turn down the thermostat or turn off TV/stereo as needed. Sit, stand, or lie down, and let your body relax. Take several deep breaths . . . clear to the bottom of your belly. Let each out slowly, and send the tension of the day with it. Shrug your shoulders, roll your neck, let go of tensions held in other areas. Let go of all the things you're trying to track – note them on a piece of paper, if necessary, and then put them out of mind.

Focus your attention inward to your heart, breathing chi in and out of it if you are able. Visualize yourself as a tree, with your roots spreading deep in the earth; your branches reaching up to the sky. Breathe in and out through your roots. Extend your taproot deeper into the earth with each breath: through the soil, the rock, the molten magma, down to the crystal core of the planet. Stay there for several breaths, feeling the increasing power of your connection to the earth. Breathe its energy slowly back up to your heart. Then focus on your tree branches overhead, with the stars twinkling between them. Breath your energy upward from your head, through the crown of your head, up through your branches, past the birds flying over head, and up to the stars.

This process breaks our mental connection with past, present and future outside stuff – leftover emotions, mental tracking, tensions, tomorrow's agenda, the rain coming down outside. It lets us focus all of our energy and attention on the present moment and our present tasks, and helps us achieve a strong and clear intention as we proceed.

PICKING UP THE PHONE: MOVING INTO SACRED SPACE

Sacred space exists when we are connected to our chi, have created a physically, emotionally and psychically safe space in which to work, have opened to the spirit world, and have let go of control of what happens. To open ourselves to others, we have to let down our barriers and allow ourselves to be vulnerable. We don't intentionally let that happen unless we feel safe, which is one purpose of moving into sacred space. Some people just visualize a sphere of white light surrounding and protecting them. Others ask for help:

Ground and center. Smudge the space and yourself with sage or incense, light a candle, or otherwise cleanse and focus yourself. Call in the spirits from the seven directions: east, south, west, north, above, below and within. Honor them for the special qualities they give to our lives, and ask that they be present to assist and protect your work in sacred space. Sacred space is a space of truth, and speaking from the heart. Focus your intention, open your chakras, and begin your work.

TURNING ON THE POWER: OPENING THE CHAKRAS

Our chakras are spinning vortices or focal points in our energy bodies, through which energy comes into and leaves our bodies, focused on the specific nature and intention of the different chakras. The seven primary chakras along our spinal axis focus on particular aspects of our relationships: root (survival), womb (creativity), solar plexus (power), heart (love), throat (expression), third eye (transcendence), and crown (unity). See Donna Eden's discussions in *Energy Medicine* for more details on their organization, function, testing, clearing, balancing and strengthening. We open our root and crown chakras in the process of grounding and centering. We intentionally open and extend connection from other chakras depending on what and how we are wishing to make a connection:

Once settled comfortably into sacred space, focus your breathing and attention on the chakra you wish to open. Breathe in and out through it. Visualize it as a flower or a whirling golden cone of energy. As you breathe in and out, let the petals of the flower open out slowly, until its heart is fully open. Let the cone of energy strengthen and unfold, allowing the deep, rich light from the center shine beautifully outward.

DIALING UP A CONNECTION: FOCUSING ATTENTION AND INTENTION

Now you're energetically ready to do whatever you came to the realms of energy for.

Reach out with your awareness and connect with the entity or spirit you wish to contact – an ancestor, a deity, a friend who needs diagnosis for an illness, a spirit guide or helper, an energy pattern that needs to be changed. Send out a golden cord of energy to link to that entity from the appropriate chakras. Use the third eye if you want to "see far." Use the heart if you're wanting to send healing energy and love. Use the solar plexus if you are sending intention to change energy, and so forth.

HANGING UP: MANAGING YOUR PHONE BILL

Staying connected with chakras wide open and the spirit world on the line takes a lot of energy, even if only to keep out unwanted noise and connections. You can become quite drained, if you don't disconnect when you're done. So be sure to close down when finished:

Thank whatever entities you have been in connection with and disconnect from them; close off the outward connections on your chakras so you aren't inundated when you go back into our noisy everyday world; let the petals of your chakra flower fold closed; thank, say good-bye to, and disconnect from the spirits which created and held a safe sacred space for your work. Check and see if you are totally disconnected and back on the ground here – use kinesiology, eat (you'll probably be hungry, and sugar in particular, helps shut down psychic connections); see if you can remember your name and social security number. If you continue to feel spacey, you probably haven't totally disconnected. Reground, focus inward, and ask that all links be fully disconnected. Soak in a tub of hot water with sea salts. Drink a lot of water.

2 BUILDING WITH THE BREATH OF LIFE

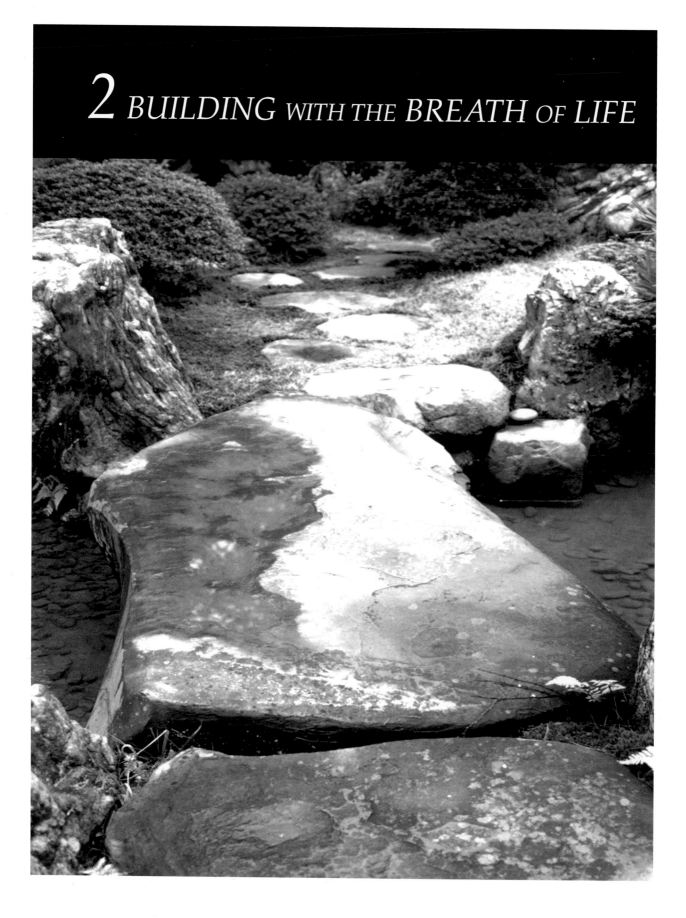

OUR SURROUNDINGS AS MIRRORS

Our surroundings truly *do* act as mirrors, reflecting the values, dreams, fears, and fascinations of the individuals and societies that have shaped them. We can, if we wish, read them like a book, pointing out item by item what was in the minds and hearts of those who created and shaped a place.

An interesting curiosity, but it is more than that. These images in stone and steel, those dreams in faded neon and spalling stucco, deeply affect and shape us. They affect us as strongly as they were affected and shaped by their makers.

* They affect us in part because they convey the true fears behind our painted smiles, the cruelty behind the benign surfaces of actions, the love behind the modest gesture.

* They affect us because they clarify and embody our dreams, marshaling our inner resources to their achievement.

* They affect us as they show – often with a beauty or ugliness that makes their message even more poignant – the confusion of our goals, the inconsistency of our actions, the humanness of our lives.

* They affect us because they do not lie; they stand witness to our lives as they are, in their fullness or emptiness.

The way our surroundings reflect our values usually occurs unconsciously and without direct attention. But in those rare times when society is undergoing fundamental change, we suddenly see the disparity between our beliefs and our actions, and can actively move to establish new touchstones in both.

We are now living in one of those times of change. We are beginning to see through the contradictions in our beliefs to a deeper, clearer basis for our lives. In the process, a new and encompassing sense of the role of the sacred in our surroundings is emerging.

As our society moves from a period of growth into a period of mature sustainability, we need a renewed and deeper touchstone of the forces that vitalize us and our surroundings. This renewed subtle-energy-based vision gives us powerful guidance for transforming our placemaking arts. It gives an inner kernel of

What we value is what appears in our surroundings – reflecting back to us those very values. If we value haste and ease of construction, we end up with concrete with a drainpipe under it. If we value rocks, moss, water, and time, we might end up with the bridge on the opposite page.

power to these arts, out of which a deeper, richer, more meaningful, and more unified expression can unfold. It gives us the means to create more bountiful surroundings in harmony with both our inner vision and our connection with all of Creation.

We have built walls around our hearts to lessen the pain of what our culture dreams into being around us. That isolation, in turn, has created its own inner pain, as well as surroundings of inconceivable emptiness and meaninglessness. The changes that are underway bring with them a healing and an opening in our individual lives, giving rise to a society that can endure and prosper.

Those changes are – and aren't – simple. They need to run deep, not be cosmetic. Sources as ancient as the *I-Ching* specifically warn against superficial attention where major change is needed:

> *Grace – beauty of form – is necessary in any union if it is to be well ordered and pleasing rather than disordered and chaotic. Grace brings success.* ***However, it is not the essential or fundamental thing; it is only the ornament and must therefore be used sparingly and only in little things.***

> *. . . beautiful form suffices to brighten and throw light upon matters of lesser moment,* ***but important questions cannot be decided in this way. They require greater earnestness.***

A CHI-CENTERED UNIVERSE

The basic principles of any design system based on subtle energy are only partially recorded in its manuals or taught by its masters. Perhaps more important for us are the frequently unstated assumptions that underlie a range of specific rules and practices. These assumptions were so integral a part of the culture that no one considered the need for stating them. But to a totally different culture such as ours, they are essential to understanding the differentness and fundamental roots of sustainable design.

There are ten principles that seem to underlie the practice of design in any sustainable society. For a person brought up in the beliefs of our society, some of these may appear strange, or their design significance difficult to grasp. Later chapters will give examples of their application in our world.

The principles underlying sustainable design are:

* *Life force energy underlies all Creation.*

* *The energy fields of the earth are a source of nurture and information to all living matter.*

* *The breath of life – or chi – exists in all people, places, and things, and is vital to their interaction.*

* *The astrology of people and places, and the timing of their interaction, play an*

active role in the outcome of those interactions.

* The health of all Creation is essential to our well-being.

* Our minds and hearts are an integral, powerful part of our interaction with the world on both sides of our skin, and must be addressed in the design and use of place.

* Our relationships with the past and the future – with our ancestors and our descendants, what preceded us and what evolves out of our existence – are important to the outcome of interactions with our surroundings.

* Harmony with a coherent cosmology is important to the guidance of our lives and the surroundings that contain them.

* Sacredness is central to meaningful lives and an enduring society.

* Design and use of our surroundings are spiritual paths, based on love and giving.

PRINCIPLES OF ENERGETIC DESIGN

Let's look in more detail at what these principles entail:

✧ LIFE FORCE ENERGY UNDERLIES ALL CREATION

Current research suggests that our bodies and the physical world around us are particular patterns of matter that have gelled around specific matrices of chi energy. In this sense, our energy bodies are more primal than our physical ones; the processes and relationships there more basic than those in our physical bodies. And our energy bodies are profoundly interconnected with our physical ones.

The aspects of chi that we can experience today fit so exactly into the descriptions given in classical literature and living traditions that few doubts can remain as to its existence or efficacy. It would be wonderful for us to develop a clearer technical understanding. But the leadership role today is in experiencing and acknowledging its existence, its roles, our connections with it, and in discovering how its acceptance and use can transform our lives and culture. Further research will follow close behind.

Experience of this aspect of existence profoundly changes our view of our lives and our world. Energy flows through and nurtures our bodies except when we block it off. In the realm of chi, we experience ourselves as nodes in interconnecting fields of energy rather than as discrete objects. We feel our own chi performing what was long known as spiritual healing. We find ourselves so coherently interlinked with others that our thoughts and memories are one. We walk in the fields of incipient form where things and events take shape. Strange and unexpected new worlds open before us.

Our understanding of the role played by our familiar material world is very different in a chi-based universe than in a universe where we believed that our material world was all that existed. And building design which acknowledges, responds to, and incorporates both of these worlds in their complex interaction is very different from merely creating pleasing spatial designs.

✦ THE ENERGY FIELDS OF THE EARTH ARE A SOURCE OF NURTURE AND INFORMATION TO ALL LIVING MATTER

The visible light that fuels photosynthesis and supports all life on earth constitutes but a minute fraction of the sun's energy intercepted by our planet. The "solar wind" is comprised of plasma radiations as well as electromagnetic waves. When intercepted by the Earth's magnetic field, the solar wind shapes the magnetosphere and the plasmasphere of our planet.

These, in turn, induce much of that energy into the earth's atmosphere and mantle in the form of electromagnetic energy. As those charged particles oscillate along the magnetic lines of the earth between the north and the south poles, their intensity is visible through the ionized gas effects of the northern and southern lights – the *aurora borealis* and the *aurora australialis*.

In turn, electromagnetic fields in the earth's mantle, coupled with variations in topography and geology, create variations in local electromagnetic fields. Like any available energy source, these have been seized upon by the multitude of life forms that have emerged on this planet, to fuel and inform their lives. It remains a question today which of these "earth energies" consist of pulsed electromagnetic fields, and which are other forms of "energy." For now, we have to be satisfied with the knowledge that they have been and are apprehensible and useful.

Chi permeates our surroundings – intensely in what are called sacred places, in helpful or harmful concentrations elsewhere. Traditionally, virtually all cultures considered it in finding favorable locations for temples, shrines, homes, businesses, and tombs. For millennia, "power spots" where these energies are particularly concentrated have been used by animals and humans for birthing places and healing; for shrines and churches; for propitious location of cities, homes, temples, and tombs. Divination, or dowsing, for temple siting is recorded in almost every culture.

Temples of some sects in India were even built of bricks fired in place after the building was built. Constructed that way, the magnetic field orientations of each particle of clay of the bricks would be in full alignment with that of the place at that time. No repairs or changes were permitted in these temples, to preserve that purity of alignment. They were allowed to fall to ruin in their own time, rather than alter the purity of the fields established in their making.

This is use of the chi of place for specific and sensitive situations. Such subtle effects of the natural chi of place may, or may not, have significant effect on our more mundane daily activities.

✦ THE BREATH OF LIFE – OR CHI – EXISTS IN ALL PEOPLE, PLACES, AND THINGS, AND IS VITAL TO THEIR INTERACTION

Disruption of acupuncture meridians moving chi in our bodies has been shown to lead to rapid tissue degeneration and deterioration of neural reflexes.

Our bodily energy fields extend beyond our skin, as do those of other forms of life, and interact with each other and with larger flows of energy in and above the earth.

Of importance here is that the chi of people and place are interactive. Chi is not just something static in the ground or in our bodies. Our chi alters the chi of places we use, and their chi alters our own. The chi of built places and the human chi interacting with them is definitely strong enough to alter the lives of people who use those places. The good or bad energy of users of a place lingers to affect subsequent users. Our interaction with place is additive and cumulative. We need to both design and live our lives aware of this dialog.

✧ *THE ASTROLOGY OF PEOPLE AND PLACES, AND THE TIMING OF THEIR INTERACTION, PLAY AN ACTIVE ROLE IN THE OUTCOME OF THOSE INTERACTIONS*

The energy fields of the earth are influenced by heavenly bodies other than the sun, as well by all life on earth, and possibly by other realms of existence. In turn, the earth's energy fields convey those influences into our lives. The energetic traditions of many cultures alert people to room positions, orientation, colors, and other aspects of their surroundings which could have good or bad effect on them, depending on their astrological needs. How this might affect our own lives through our use of places, or in what ways we can alter those effects is still poorly understood.

✧ *THE HEALTH OF ALL CREATION IS ESSENTIAL TO OUR WELL-BEING*

Our skin is not always a meaningful line of distinction between what is and is not "us." What is inside our skin depends on myriad kinds of food, air, and nurture from outside our skin. The world outside our skins depends equally on us as a source of CO_2 and food. The health and well-being of what lies on either side of our skin cannot be separated from that on the other side.

The ecological interconnectedness of all life means that the well-being of all life must be part of our designing – not just things that influence our individual health and well-being. The health, richness, and latent creativity of our planet's biosystems is central to both our current wealth and our future well-being.

When our numbers and our appetites press too hard on the earth, when our actions deprive other life of its existence, we are increasing our own poverty as well as harming and destroying other life. Other life is more than just a reservoir of unknown pharmaceuticals and DNA. It is a celebration of the richness and beauty of Creation. The fewer the voices, the more diminished the song.

It is also not just our numbers, but the inner sense of connectedness underlying our actions that is affected. We create landscapes with visually appealing ornamental plants, yet the "weeds" we eliminate are the essential food or shelter for birds, butterflies, beetles, and spiders, and might even be useful for our own health.

Our rapid logging cycles destroy the mycorrhizal fungal mats upon which weave together the health and life of coniferous forests. Our freeways and fencing cut migration routes. Our pesticides kill the food of unconsidered species. Our monoculture lawns deplete the genetic bank of wild species. Our houses rarely have nesting places for birds and bats, or food supply for spiders.

A life-based awareness can change how we deal with all these issues. It allows us closeness with other life and the joy of being part of a particular ecological community and place.

Our health is part of the health of all Creation. Getting to know other life – from bats to spiders to slugs to fungus – we begin to see the unique wonder of each lifeform, and we come to respect and protect it.

✧ ***OUR MINDS AND HEARTS ARE AN INTEGRAL, POWERFUL PART OF OUR INTERACTION WITH THE WORLD ON BOTH SIDES OF OUR SKIN, AND MUST BE ADDRESSED IN THE DESIGN AND USE OF PLACE***

Our psychology – our values, beliefs, fears, and memories – directs our actions or blocks them from certain paths, and determines much of the satisfaction or unhappiness we derive from our interaction with places. The surroundings we create inescapably reflect and make manifest these deepest and most hidden values.

Even in a business environment, expenditures on making people happy are worthwhile. A study done for the California State Architect showed that measures which resulted in as little as a 3% increase in productivity would more than pay back even a doubling of the cost of the building![1] Operable windows, daylight, human-scaled spaces, adjustable task lighting, and comfortable furniture are all part of such conditions. Design so that people aren't always worrying about the boss sneaking up behind and checking on them is also part of comfort and productivity. Such "green office" design has now been shown to bring very profitable improvement to workplaces.[2] But the real bottom line is that paying attention to our emotional needs makes us feel better.

How we feel about a place or a pattern of interaction with place is important. Yet we're never encouraged to trust our gut reactions, and the consideration of the psychological dimension of people and place is virtually nonexistent today.

Simply stated, this principle says to listen to your feelings and trust your tummy. If a place doesn't feel good *to* you, it isn't good *for* you. If we can change how we feel about a place through ritual, or through real or symbolic changes in our surroundings, we change some aspect of how the place affects us. If, for instance, we let our surroundings show our honoring of others, it will deepen that honoring and reflect back to us the importance of that value of caring.

It is telling that Christopher Alexander's *A Pattern Language*, the strongest proponent and example of the value of following our noses and tummies in design, is shunned by mainstream design professionals.[3]

[1] Tom Bender, BUILDING VALUE, Office of the California State Architect, 1976.

[2] Rocky Mountain Institute, GREENING THE BUILDING AND THE BOTTOM LINE, 1994.

[3] Christopher Alexander, A PATTERN LANGUAGE, Oxford Univ. Press, 1977.

OUR RELATIONSHIPS WITH THE PAST AND THE FUTURE –
TOWARDS OUR ANCESTORS AND OUR DESCENDANTS, WHAT
✧ *PRECEDED US AND WHAT EVOLVES OUT OF OUR EXISTENCE –*
ARE IMPORTANT TO THE OUTCOME OF INTERACTIONS WITH
OUR SURROUNDINGS

Many traditional cultures ask that the impacts of actions be considered as far as seven generations into the future. They do this both to see the full impacts of those actions, and so as to not restrict the potential of that future. Living with the results of a society that has disregarded the immense long-range costs of its actions, we can see the wisdom of such a perspective. We invariably do receive what we dream of. And when we dream only of the present and ignore the future, we reduce the likelihood of even having a future.

Interestingly, at least one culture speaks of those seven generations differently: as three past, the present, and three future generations. Why consider the past? What is gone is gone . . . or is it?

Perhaps not entirely. Consideration of the gifts from past generations results in humility, acknowledgment of the size of the shoulders upon which we stand, and gratitude for those gifts as a basis for our actions. It provides a realization that our achievements do not belong to us alone, and requires acknowledgment of our obligation to pass equivalent gifts on to *our* descendants. Sustainability requires both of these perspectives on duration and relationship over time.

Many cultures assert that our ancestors are actually with us in the present. This, amazingly, is consistent with what we are learning today of energetics and the existence of non-material realms of our universe. Research in many fields supports the concepts of the non-linearity of time, parallel universes, and the contiguous existence of past, present, and future. More connection seems to be occurring between embodied people and those whose existence currently is not on the material plane. Our understandings and awareness in this area are changing dramatically.[4]

Consider how differently we would feel as a community making decisions, if the actual ashes of a hundred generations of our ancestors were kept in urns under the benches we sit upon as we ponder our actions. We would have a sense of continuity, durability, and responsibility to the future far different from our sense of acting alone in the here and now.

The greatest achievements and most shameful failures of the past would unavoidably be present in our minds as guidance, support, and a measure of our own actions. Aware of how our lives are impacted by past actions, we would realize how greatly the future is impacted by our present behavior. We would instinctively draw upon the wisdom of the past, as well as our own, and at times perhaps feel unequal to the standards they have set. We would think to call on the aid of our ancestors themselves to resolve our problems.

If we consider ourselves to be *a part of* ongoing creation, rather than *apart from* it, we have different attitudes toward the possibilities we foreclose or create

---

[4] The psychic sections of any bookstore are filled with anecdotal accounts of contacts with deceased relatives, etc. Work such as that of Tiller, Gerber, Schwartz and Russek is beginning to develop a deeper understanding of the forces involved.

for the future, as well as how we relate to the entire shape of an ever-evolving history. Having a future implies ongoing Creation.

⬦ *HARMONY WITH A COHERENT COSMOLOGY IS IMPORTANT TO THE GUIDANCE OF OUR LIVES AND THE SURROUNDINGS THAT CONTAIN THEM*

A world built upon contradictions and lacking inner harmony destroys itself in the inner battles between competing values. If our beliefs lack consistency and harmony, how can we put the full power of our will behind them, to say nothing of asking others to believe in them?

If our surroundings do tap the emotional, intellectual, and spiritual core of our beliefs, they gain great dominion, and imbue our lives with that same power of coherent and powerful belief.

Every age and culture has a different view of the universe and our place in it. One role of our surroundings, like the results of all of our actions, is to give form to and represent those unique beliefs. Within them, then, we have the opportunity and support to bring our lives into harmony with the cosmos we perceive.

The hierarchical order of a Chinese city, the sacred geometries of Islamic ornament, or the bold power of a 20th century skyscraper all reflect unique views of the universe, consistent with the beliefs and the world their builders dreamed into being. In doing so, such creations renew and strengthen the universe within which they are founded, and those who inhabit that universe.

Maurice Freedman speaks of the difference in the meaning of their surroundings to Europeans and Chinese enjoying a view. The Europeans think of the combination of hills and sea producing splendid vistas. Their pleasure is aesthetic and objective – the landscape is out there, and they enjoy it. The Chinese appreciation is cosmological. For them the viewer and the viewed are interacting, both being part of some greater system. The cosmos is Heaven, Earth, and Us. We are in it and of it. So while the European reaction is to find it beautiful, the Chinese may remark that they feel content or comfortable. Their philosophy asserts a human response to forces working in the cosmos, and just as landscapes affect us, we may affect them.

Our cosmology has become one of contradiction. We're asked to be rational and efficient in work, yet irrational and inefficient in consumption. We happily consume the very resources that are needed for continued support of our lives. A new sense of the cosmos and our role in it is both needed and emerging. If how we live, work, and govern ourselves is headed in a different direction from our innermost dreams, or fails to incorporate major elements of those dreams, we head for failure and trouble.

Public expression of sacredness is rare in modern society. Interestingly, there *is* one particular place where people publicly and powerfully express a sense of spiritual reverence and awe, of yearning, and of wonder. It is the exhibit in the Smithsonian Institution in Washington DC where we can touch a piece of rock from the moon.

Our urge to embrace, be part of, and reunite with the cosmos is a primal and valid one. It may well not require the massive space program and travel between worlds envisioned in our first outward spasm. Yet how contrary to those dreams it is to live in the cities of our world where incessant electric day shuts out the night and we can't even *see* the stars!

Until our interactions with the stellar world come from a reverence in our hearts, we will not find a harmony between our dreams and our actions. When our vision of our universe has wholeness, we will see all that surrounds us as part of that wholeness. The *aurora borealis* will change from being a strange natural phenomenon into a visible sign of the energy fluxes channeling into our planet through its poles, linking our own existence to the stars.

In the same way, our attitudes towards the sacredness of all Creation and all forms of life must come to a fullness and rightness of expression.

Our world view is turning from one of taking, greed, and violence to one of harmony, sharing, and nurture. As it does so, our surroundings must take on powerful expressions of those new qualities if they are to take part in our nurture and become part of a harmony between us and our universe.

✧ SACREDNESS IS CENTRAL TO MEANINGFUL LIVES AND AN ENDURING SOCIETY

Our society stresses freedom – absence of connectedness, responsibility, or effects of our actions. It is a legalistic society of limited commitments that are easy to break, and with great incentives for those who find new ways to take from others or to destroy the rest of Creation. Fed by its own power of destructiveness, it cannot last, and cannot create a basis for sustainability.

The only true alternative is a basis for our lives which makes harmful action inconceivable rather than the rule. Nothing less than our holding sacred the health of our surroundings and the well-being of others will ensure that we act strongly enough or soon enough to ensure that health and well-being.

✧ DESIGN AND USE OF OUR SURROUNDINGS ARE SPIRITUAL PATHS, BASED ON LOVE AND GIVING

A sacred world requires that all relationships – including our relationship with work – be based on patterns that support the health, well-being, and spiritual growth of those involved. The traditions of energetics of place and sacred building demonstrate how design and building, specifically, can be pursued as a process of spiritual growth, as well as being an integral part of a sacred society. What we design can only reflect what we *are*, so a sacred society requires work processes that nurture our own spiritual health and growth.

This implies work patterns that support and encourage the development and enrichment of skills. It implies design and building processes that honor and encourage the creative contributions of the makers and users; that honor the life of materials given up into our construction and the place on the earth that our buildings occupy; that honor all forms of life.

✧

Together, these principles constitute and reflect a worldview and a basis for design that are profoundly different from what currently exists. Our recent worldview honored material wealth, freedom from responsibility, deceit, mobility, self-centeredness, and being apart from and outside the laws of nature.

The worldview we need to build on today is one which honors sustainability. To ensure a healthy world, it needs to embrace the needs of the ecological systems that support our lives. It must nurture our emotional and spiritual, as well as physical, health. And that requires finding a sense of our universe that gives meaning to our lives. Our worldview needs to ensure the health of our relationships – with our selves, with each other, and with the rest of Creation. And it needs to include a deep understanding of our universe and the ongoing Creation of which we are part. It needs, in sum, to reflect a future worth living for.

3 UNFOLDING THE PAST

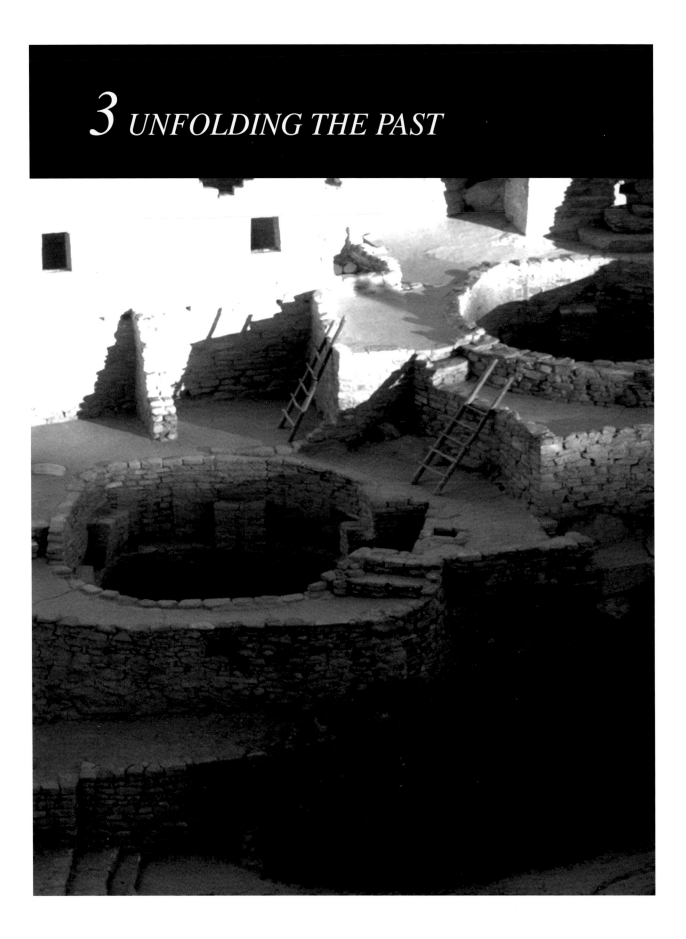

Awakening a new sense of the possible

A wonderful myth has been going around for the last twenty years about the incredible wisdom and solar design sensitivity of the Anasazi builders of the cliff dwellings at Mesa Verde. The myth is usually accompanied by a diagram showing how the overhanging cliff shades the dwellings from the high summer sun, while allowing the low winter sun to warm the dwellings and their inhabitants.

In real life, however, the ravines at Mesa Verde almost all run north and south, with the cliff-dwelling alcoves therefore facing east or west – bad for solar design, not good. The myth, however, has had the effect of successfully inspiring a contemporary generation of architects to attempt more sensitive solar design in their own buildings.

The reasons people built and lived in the cliff dwellings were far more complex. The cliff alcoves were dramatic and inspiring places; who wouldn't want to live there! They provided protection from weather and other tribes, plus a wonderful sense of community.

And, not insignificantly in a region of little rain, the cliff-dwellings had their own sources of water. The cliffs originally formed as huge sand dunes, at one point underwater, where silty runoff later turned to a thin layer of impenetrable shale. Groundwater, draining through the porous overlying sandstone, flowed out on top of the shale causing the alcoves to form. Even today, the springs flowing out of the inner wall of the alcoves wash over the ripples in the lake bottom mud frozen into the surface of the shale.

Opposite: Cliff Palace at Mesa Verde. The past is a living, changing construct of what we believe happened before us which is of value to know. New understandings continually bring us to look at the past, present, and future in new light.

✧

The past has many facets, which are continually lost, rediscovered, or altered in our understanding. They can confuse us or inspire us in many ways. We can learn from:

* What we *imagine* happened (Mesa Verde)
* What people actually intended, and what actually *did* happen

* Other things that really did happen that the people weren't aware of
* Totally new patterns that we are somehow inspired to see
* Various combinations of the above

All can be useful.

✧

The last twenty years have also brought a revolution in our understanding of the energetic dimension of how other cultures have related to their surroundings. Chi energy and access through it to the spirit world have been shown to play central roles in society after society.

The !Kung Bushmen of the Kalahari Desert in Africa achieve a state of awakened chi and connection to the spirit world through dancing. Other cultures achieve the same state through hypnotism, pain, trance drumming, chanting, psychoactive drugs, or sleep deprivation. !Kung descriptions closely mirror those of awakening kundalini energy in yoga and other spiritual practices:

> *You dance, dance, dance, dance. Then num lifts you up in your belly and lifts you in your back, and you start to shiver. Num makes you tremble; it's hot. . . . But when you get into kia, you're looking around because you see everything, because you see what's troubling everybody. Rapid shallow breathing draws num up . . .*
>
> *In your backbone you feel a pointed something and it works its way up. The base of your spine is tingling, tingling, tingling, tingling. Then num makes your thoughts nothing in your head.[1]*

During *kia* (trance state), the !Kung do extraordinary things: performing cures, handling and walking on fire, seeing the insides of people's bodies and scenes at great distances from their camp, or traveling to the home of gods. But most important, they do these things to heal sickness in individuals, to restore community emotional intimacy and spiritual harmony, and to access the wisdom of the spirit world.

✧

The patterns of accessing altered states of consciousness and their functions in community health are amazingly consistent from culture to culture. Native American sundance rituals, South American shamanism, Maya community ritual, tribal practices from Africa and Siberia; and certain practices in Christianity, Islam, Buddhism, and Hinduism share surprisingly similar territory.

Malidoma Somé reports a similar role of ritual and access to the spirit world in the community health of modern tribal Africa:

> *Whenever a gathering of people, under the protection of Spirit, triggers a body of emotional energy aimed at bringing them very tightly together, a ritual of one*

---

[1] Richard Katz, BOILING ENERGY: Community Healing among the Kalahari Kung, Harvard University Press, 1982.

type or another is in effect. People prepare the space for the ritual and its general choreography. The other part of ritual cannot be planned because it is in the realm of Spirit. That part is a spontaneous, almost unpredictable interaction with an energy source, and a response to a call from a nonhuman source to commune with a larger horizon.

A sense of community grows where behavior is based on trust and where nobody has to hide anything. There are certain human powers that cannot be unleashed without such a supportive atmosphere – powers such as the one that enables us to connect with ancestors and to unlock potentials in ourselves and others far beyond what is commonly known. When an individual feels connected to an entire community, this connection can extend far beyond the living world. A healthy connection with one another can spill over into a connection with the ancestors and with nature. In a tribal community, healing of the village happens in ritual.[2]

And Malidoma's wife, Sobonfu, speaks on the role of community and ritual:

The whole concept of the intimate is primarily derived from ritual. Outside of ritual, nothing can be truly intimate. Which is why, in the village, every emotion is ritually understood. So human relationships, when they begin to deepen, enter into the canal of ritual.

In the village, everybody is addicted to ritual. There people experience intimacy not just with their partners, but with the rest of the village, at all times. . . . There's such a high from this. . . . Maybe that's why they don't care about television.[3]

Ritual, community, and the spirit world are essential to both individual and community health. They permit trust, deep opening, emotional melding, giving and support from others and the spirit world – resources that are unavailable to an individual alone.

Community intimacy in harmony with the spirit world involves:

* The community of people, nature, and the spirit world
* The healing and nurturing energy of chi
* Intimacy of ritual
* Cathartic resolution of conflict
* Healing emotions of shared grief, passion, joy, and pain
* The ever-present support and caring of friends
* Experience of intense human connection and attention
* Access to parts of our souls and wisdom from which we are otherwise walled off
* The fullness and freedom from worry coming from abundance of life

All these are parts of the web of community, chi, and health. It is these things which have caused society after society to create unique and powerful places designed to access and enable this community.

[2] Malidoma Somé, THE HEALING WISDOM OF AFRICA, Tarcher/Putnam, 1998.

[3] Sobonfu Somé, THE SPIRIT OF INTIMACY, Berkeley Hill Books, 1997.

✦

Because energetics of place has not been part of our own recent tradition, we' haven't considered looking for its role in the monuments of the past. Archeological and anthropological studies of many different cultures have now uncovered incontrovertible evidence concerning the role of energetics of place in the shaping and use of people's surroundings.

The application of energetics of place in our own culture has reached a point where we now have a broad range of applicable techniques and verifiable achievements of our own which affirm and can build upon the historical record. A few examples of energetic practices from different cultures can show the scope of that foundation. We will examine others in later chapters.

INITIATORY TEMPLES OF EGYPT

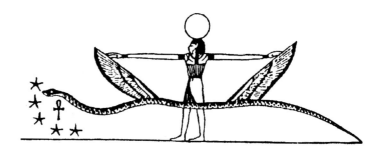

One of the most ubiquitous elements in Egyptian art is a symbolic object called an *ankh*. In bas-reliefs and sculpture in temples and tombs, there are scenes everywhere showing gods, goddesses, pharaohs and other individuals holding ankhs in their hands, usually extended towards another person or deity. The ankh, however, is not just *held* in these scenes, as other symbols often are. It is almost always *actively extended*, a symbol of transmission of something from one person to another.

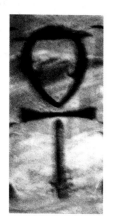

The Egyptian ankh - column carving at Temple of Karnak.

Once we see the ankh carved by itself in hieroglyphics, its symbolism becomes immediately apparent. Three separate elements . . . a symbol of a vagina, and one of a penis; joined by the third, a bar hieroglyph standing for connection or union. The generative power of life - *life-force energy* - is what the ankh symbolizes. This can be confirmed looking at the contexts in which it is used, and the meaning of the accompanying inscriptions. Almost invariably, it is the symbolic element in an act of empowerment, of transmission of life-force energy from one individual to another. Chi energy was central to both Egyptian culture and building, with a variety of terminology attesting to detailed understanding of its roles.[4]

To anyone familiar with the existence and nature of chi or life-force energy, and particularly the process of energy healing, it is immediately visible as the dominant theme in Egyptian sculpture, painting, and funerary objects. Images of energy healers, extending their hands to convey healing energy to another, are everywhere. Images, arms outstretched to create protective fields, surrounded burial sarcophaguses and canopic jars. Statues themselves are shown being empowered

---

[4] See Normandie Ellis, DREAMING ISIS, Quest Books, 1995 and Jeremy Naydler, TEMPLE OF THE COSMOS, Inner Traditions International, 1996.

Granite sarcophagus of Psusennes, with the Goddess of the North Wind making an energetic connection to the remains of the king, allowing it to connect to the spirit world.

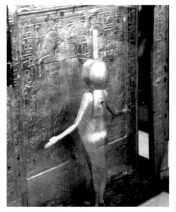

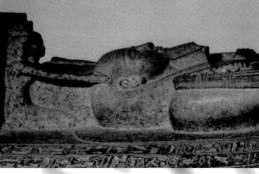

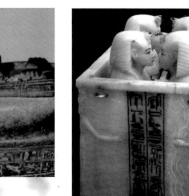

Figures of the goddesses surround the gilded sarcophagus of King Tut, with hands extended creating a protective energy field.

Figures carved in the alabaster container of Tut's canopic jars, emphasized by the striations in the stone itself, represent creation of a protective energy field around the vital organs.

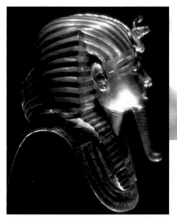

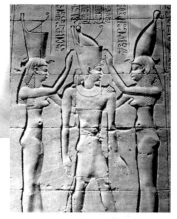

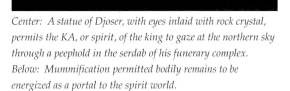

Cobras emerging from the second chakra (Third Eye) are common elements of sculpture and headresses, signifying psychic powers and connectedness to the spirit world.

Typical coronation scene. Note that the crown, not the king, is being invested with energy. Whoever wears it then becomes intermediary between the Heavens and the Earth.

Center: A statue of Djoser, with eyes inlaid with rock crystal, permits the KA, or spirit, of the king to gaze at the northern sky through a peephole in the serdab of his funerary complex. Below: Mummification permitted bodily remains to be energized as a portal to the spirit world.

as portals to a deity. Coronation scenes show the deities extending their hands empowering *the crown* which is being placed on the pharaoh's head, so that whenever it is worn, that individual is connected with and embodies the spirit world.

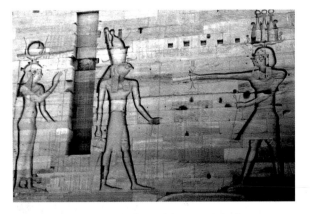

Above: Pylon from Temple of Isis, Philae. Hands holding energy at left, energizing with an ankh at the right.

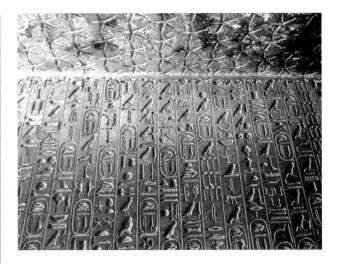

Right: Pyramid Texts from Pyramid of Unas, Sakkara. Like any other creation, words can be energized as icons with total connection to their referent, allowing the reader to obtain greater depth of knowledge through them, or to bring to life the words of a Deity.

Below: A sistrum column from the Hathor Temple at Hatshepsut's tomb, Luxor. Sistrums were ritual rattles used as means of initiating trance or entering sacred space, using sound as a vehicle.

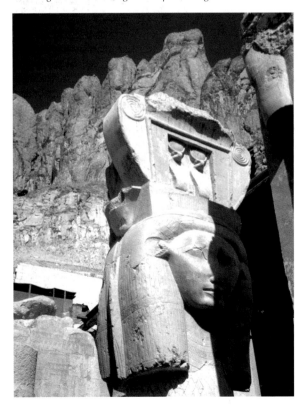

The Egyptian language, itself, was an element of using life-force energy. Like Hebrew and certain other languages, the vowels were never written, as they were considered sacred sounds used for calling on the spirit world.[5] Inscriptions, such as the Pyramid Texts in the Pyramid of Unas, were themselves energized to convey wisdom from that world. Healing temples, such as that associated with the Temple of Hathor at Dendera, contained energized statues with inscriptions on them for calling in healing for different diseases.[6] Water was poured over the statues and inscriptions, and then led to healing basins for immersion of the patients.

Even after several thousand years, the hieroglyphics in the Pyramid of Unas; bas reliefs, sculptures, and chambers in certain temples; and statues removed and transported to museums retain powerful energetic charges which strongly affect people coming in contact with them.[7] "Bindu points" in the rear walls of certain temple sanctuaries may have been used to energetically activate the buildings with sound during

[5] See Brian & Esther Crowley, WORDS OF POWER: Sacred Sounds of East and West, Llewellyn Publications, 1991; "Hieroglyphic Thinking" in Jean Houston, THE PASSION OF ISIS AND OSIRIS, Ballantine, 1995; and Rudolf Steiner, EURYTHMY AS VISIBLE SPEECH, Rudolf Steiner Press, 1984.

[6] See Sylvie Cauville, LE TEMPLE DE DENDERA, Bibliotheque Général, 1990.

[7] Jean Houston, THE PASSION OF ISIS AND OSIRIS, Ballantine, 1995.

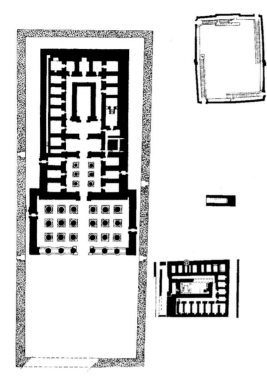

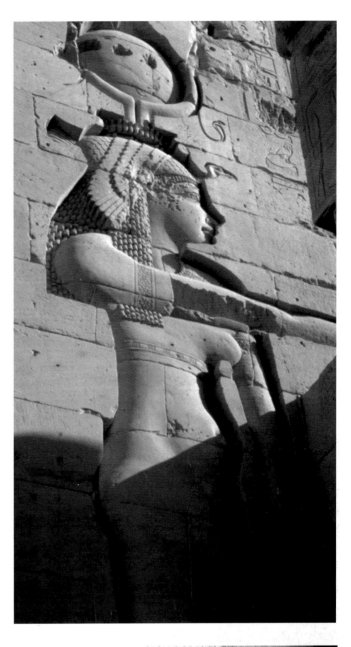

Above: Part of the temple precinct at the Temple of Hathor, Dendera. Main temple is to the left. In the upper right is the sacred lake; below it, steps to the sacred well. The smaller structure to the lower right is the Healing Temple, where ablutions over energized statues and inscriptions were used, somewhat similar to homeopathy, for immersion, washing, or ingesting by patients.

Right: A deeply-incised carving of Isis, from Philae, with her arm powerfully extended investing energy in the king.

Lower right: The seed scarab from the rear wall of the sanctuary at the Temple of Horus at Edfu. Located at chest height in this and other temples, these "bindu points" are said to have been used to activate the temples with the use of sound.

ritual.[8] Excavation at many temples has revealed drainage channels and cisterns to save ablutive waters for healing purposes.[9]

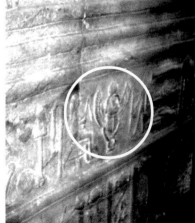

[8] Normandie Ellis, DREAMING ISIS, Quest Books, 1995.

[9] The Chapel of Satis at Elephantine, the Mortuary Temple of Khufu at Giza, and the Temple of Hathor at Dendera, for example.

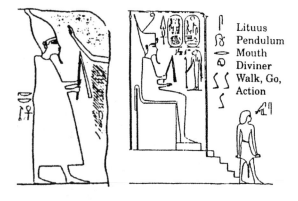

Lituus
Pendulum
Mouth
Diviner
Walk, Go, Action

Above: Use of different kinds of dowsing rods to collect and verify information. This kind of "lie-detector" could put much of our legal profession out of work.

Below: The Stele and Block Statue of Sihathur. Statues such as this, seen alone and out of context, appear curious because of their unusual shape. In context, you can feel their intention of oneness with the monolithic stele, and with that, of the earth itself.

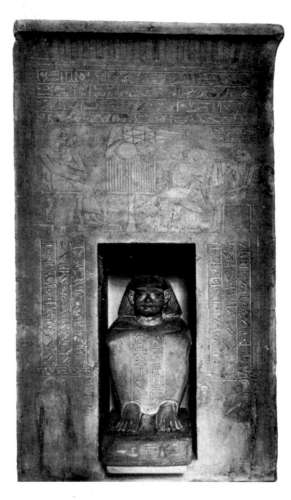

Frescoes and carvings give widespread evidence also that the Egyptians used a variety of dowsing rods for diagnosis of patients needing healing, for obtaining oracular information, and for determining truth or falseness in resolving disputes between individuals, as well as for finding water. Such wands, making visible bodily responses to subtle energy information as done in kinesiology or dowsing today, were both symbol and tool of a pharaoh's use of life-force energy in judgment.

One straight rod was called the "was" wand. Another, made of a pendulous plant, lupinus termis, responded with a shaking or trembling movement. Woven wands, of grass or stalks of grain, became part of the hieroglyphic symbol for "to speak", were shown in The Egyptian Magic Papyrus, and were probably the precursor of the caduceus used by Greek and Roman physicians as a diagnostic tool. Another type of rod, the lotus calyx wands, appears in Etruscan, Minoan, Greek, Algerian and Christian imagery as well.[10]

The temples of Egypt were not used for congregational religious assembly as in Christianity, or merely for homes the Gods/Goddesses or their images. Their religion was a Mystery religion, focusing on individual initiation and communication with the spirit world. Temples were places of psychic training and ritual.[11] Statuary was a means of embodying energy into an image which could communicate on many levels the spirit of the deity concerned, and become a portal of access to that spirit.[12]

Temple construction occurred more fundamentally on the energetic level than on the physical one. Temples were often located on the site of earlier ones, to use the energy accumulated in that place. Such power spots can still be located beneath almost all Egyptian temples.

Massive "temenos" or enclosure walls frequently surrounded the temples themselves along with ancillary structures. Such walls were often thirty to fifty feet thick

[10] Bob Ater, AMERICAN SOCIETY OF DOWSERS QUARTERLY, Spring and Fall, 1997, Spring 1998.

[11] See Barbara Watterson, THE HOUSE OF HORUS AT EDFU, Tempus, 1998 for discussion of outward aspects of typical temple design and ritual; Ellis, Houston, or Naydler for inner aspects.

[12] For a modern translation of the "Opening of the Mouth" ritual, see Chris Tice, "A Ritual for Empowering Statues", SHAMANIC JOURNEYS NEWSLETTER, 1998.

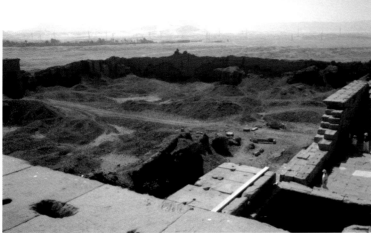

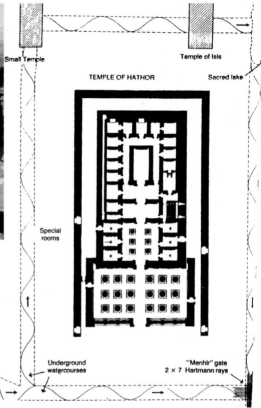

Above: View from the roof of the Temple of Hathor, Dendera. Remains of the massive, five million cubic foot enclosure wall of the complex can be seen in the background. Right: A dowsing map of the Temple of Hathor, by Blanche Merz, showing the energy barrier around the temple, and starred chambers with low energy. High energy points she notes, such as the fresco of Nut (lower right), are powerfully apparent on site.

and up to eighty feet high. Those of the Temple of Hathor at Dendera enclosed an area almost 1000' square, and contained upwards to five million cubic feet of material. As with the pyramids and the megalithic construction of the Osirion at Abydos and Khufu's Mortuary and Valley Temples at Giza, the power of intention which such walls convey, even today, is immense.

Site energies were manipulated for protective barriers around the temples, for creating special environments for working with different energies and spirits, and to make places for calling in specific connections with the spirit world. The pioneering work of Blanche Merz[13] in documenting these energy patterns has been confirmed by other researchers.

When the Temples of Ramses II and Hathor at Abu Simbul and the temples on the Isle of Philae were relocated to new sites in the 1960's to avoid being submerged by the Aswan High Dam project, they at first showed a severing of connection to their power spots. Subsequent performance of ritual in the new locations has been successful in relinking them to their energy sources.[14] Two thousand years later, powerful concentrations of chi can still be felt at particular statues, frescoes, or chambers.[15]

---

[13] Blanche Merz, POINTS OF COSMIC ENERGY, C.W. Daniel Co. Ltd., 1995.

[14] Nicki Scully, Martin Gray, and Joey Korn, personal communications.

[15] The ceiling frescoes of Nut in the Initiatory Chapel and roof chapel at Dendera and the statue of Sekhmet at Karnak are particularly powerful.

The line drawing of the Nut ceiling in the Ouâbet of the Temple of Hathor (below) gives little sense of the immense energy, particularly in the hands, of this ceiling. Even half-obliterated by smoke from centuries of inhabitants after the temples were closed, it – and other chambers of this temple – are among the most powerful in Egypt.

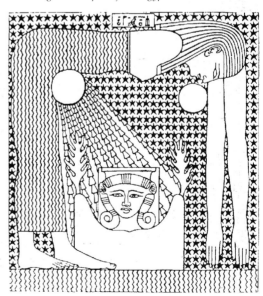

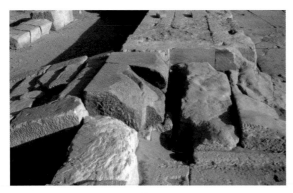

Left: The exterior wall of the Temple of Khnum on Elephantine Island, showing the massive thickness of the walls. Highly crystaline black or red granite is visible in the thresholds of openings in those walls to maintain the energy enclosures. It was also used for sanctuaries, shrines, and statues where the energetic nature of the stone was important.

Temple buildings themselves employed the highly crystalline black and red Aswan granite for inner shrines, sanctuaries, and thresholds at openings in their enclosure walls, because of their ability to focus life-force energy. Crypts in walls and beneath the floors (a total of thirteen at Dendera) and sealed rooms in several temples - with no doors, windows, or other access - contained some of the most sacred images as well as wall sculptures as beautiful as in the main temple areas, and were used for initiations, training, and trance work.

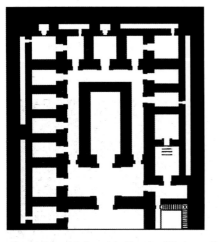

Above: A partial plan of the Temple of Hathor at Dendera, showing one of the three layers of bas-relief filled crypts in the walls behind the various chambers and in the foundations.

Below: The semi-trailer sized individual stones used in constructing the Sphinx Temple, the Valley and Mortuary Temples and lowest courses of the Pyramid of Khafra at Giza. In some cases less work than smaller stones, their massiveness accentuated the chthonian or underworld aspect of these constructions.

Such spaces, as well as the "mortuary temples" connected with the Giza pyramids probably constituted an ongoing ritual base for psychic travel to the spirit world. Psychic journeying is a significant part of spiritual practices connected with chi energy, and access to "sealed" spaces an achievable part of such worlds.[16] With the Giza pyramids, access to the soul of deceased pharaohs using the embodied energy of the adjacent pyramid as a vehicle is a far more

---

[16] Yes, even the CIA has been doing it. See David A. Morehouse, PSYCHIC WARRIOR, St. Martin's Press, 1998, or "Remote Viewing" in Richerd Gerber, VIBRTATIONAL MEDICINE, Bear & Co., 1996.

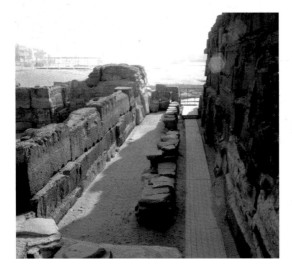

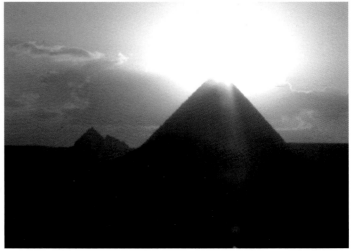

reasonable practice than assuming people would climb a highly polished hundred foot high 51° face of the pyramid to gain entry to interior ritual spaces. The immensely powerful intention which these constructions represent would have vast capability of enabling and enhancing any attempts at joining the powers of the earth and the heavens.

Light levels, particularly in the inner parts of the temples, were carefully regulated to progressively reduce outside stimulus as a person moved farther into the temple, finally arriving at the inner image chambers which were lit by as little as an 8" square hole in the ceiling. This carefully controlled darkness required that perception and connection with the empowered images in the chamber come dominantly from within, with subtle clues from the half-light, rather than "seeing" the images from the outside in customary ways.

In the darkness of inner temple areas, the beautiful bas-reliefs and hieroglyphics were meant less to be seen than as a comforting presence embracing us with meaning and power.

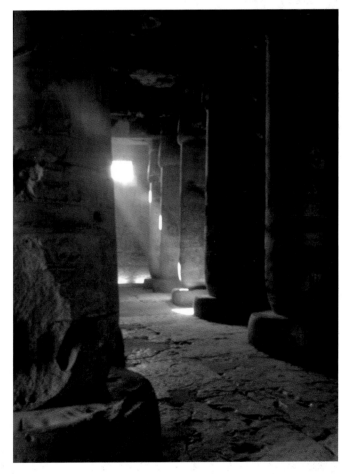

Left: Plans of Khafra's temples at Giza show their unusual design – not "constructed" as much as if hollowed out of the earth itself. This, plus the power of intention inherent in their massiveness and that of the Pyramids themselves (middle left), enhanced the performance of ritual inside them.

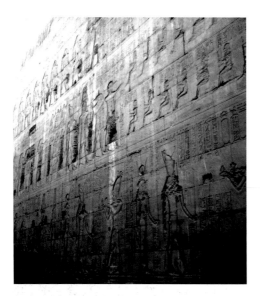

Temple genealogy on the outer enclosure wall of the Temple of Horus at Edfu, bringing into the present temple the energy accumulated through all of its predecessors. Linkage to the energy of other temples and and Neters throughout the country was similar accomplished by incorporating linked chapels into each temple, and by ritual procession from one temple to another throughout the year.

Inscriptions on the enclosure wall of the Temple of Horus at Edfu illustrate another way used to augment the energetic effectiveness of a particular temple. These inscriptions gave the genealogy or ancestry of the temple, connecting it with each of its predecessors back to the first temple of Creation.[17] This was not to show the current temple's "royal blood," but to connect with and draw into it the energy of intention accumulated in the spirit world from each of the preceding temples. Likewise, stones of earlier temples were often ritually included in the construction of new ones, to deepen the connection with the energy of worship and honoring which had built up through the lifetime use of the earlier temple.[18]

✧

Mystery / shamanic / psychic-centered spiritual practices are connected to but the *obverse* of meditational practices common to many spiritual traditions. They are involved in use of the same chakra-based, chi-centered systems. But instead of a focus on individual practice of inner quieting, they concentrate on opening outward to create specific energetic connection with other parts of Creation.

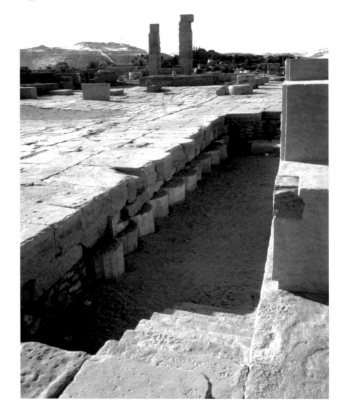

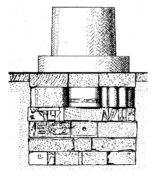

Carefully chosen elements from older temples are often used as "seeds" to connect the energy of a new temple to that of a previous one. Stone blocks or mud bricks from the old temple are used for foundations; elements from old sculpture inserted into new. Temple of Montu at Karnak (left); Temple of Khnum at Elephantine Island (right).

[17] E.A.E. Raymond, THE MYTHICAL ORIGIN OF THE EGYPTIAN TEMPLE, Manchester Univ. Press, 1969.

[18] See R.A. Schwaller de Lubicz, THE TEMPLE IN MAN, Inner Traditions International, 1949/1977; or John Anthony West, SERPENT IN THE SKY, Harper and Row, 1979.

Success of Egyptian sacred architecture is not measurable in terms of magnificence or visual drama, though that was often present to a high degree. It is measurable in terms of success in grounding, in focusing energy, in centering attention and intention of participants in their rituals and to the success of the psychic dimensions of the specific rituals being performed. Evaluation of the overall success of their architecture requires, as well, awareness of the energetic elements of their design and of effectiveness of the experience for both ritual participants and onlookers. As with Maya ceremonial centers, experiential participation in the kinds of occurrences involved is necessary to their understanding and evaluation.

Connection with the spirit world played a vital role in Egyptian culture, as it can in ours today. The energetic world of chi says that we live on in our energy bodies after death. Those souls can see into all of our hearts without the attachments and singular viewpoints we inevitably hold. Their wisdom is invaluable to the many difficult decisions of life and the pivotal events of a society. Past rulers with demonstrated wisdom and love for their community while on earth can be a particularly accessible and valuable resource to their present descendants.

Individuals able to reach through the veil between the worlds to contact these souls and other deities perform a vital role in the health and well-being of society. The techniques available to them are many and varied - oracular readings, out-of-body journeying to the spirit world, dream walking with the spirits, channeling their voices, or bringing their presences into the gatherings of the living are but a few. Places which encourage, enable, and enhance such practices make true contribution to our well-being.

Even today, consistent and unique experiences occur to people at various archeological remains from the Egyptian spiritual tradition. They beg for a reexamination of the role and function of those temples, the spiritual practices which they housed, and what that heritage can contribute to our lives today.

The purpose of sacred space is to enable and enhance the performance of ritual – and through it, the alignment of our lives with our true nature and that of our universe, and the attainment of our highest potentials. Here, the Couryard of the New Year of the Temple of Hathor at Dendera – starting point for the cycle of yearly ritual of the temple.

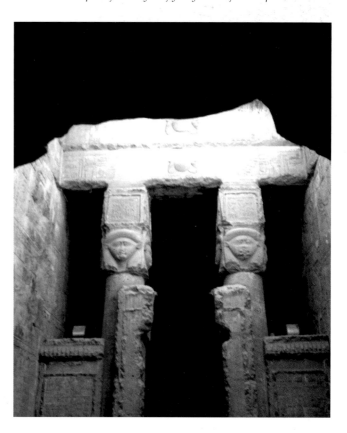

Right: Honden, or main shrine building at Izumo Taisha, in ancient Shinto style.

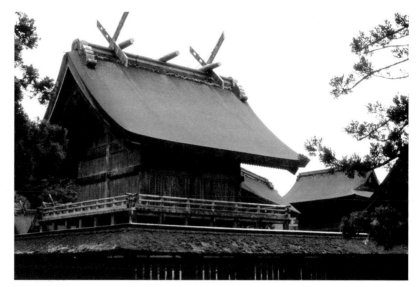

VISITS OF THE KAMI TO THE IZUMO SHRINE, JAPAN

Located near a small bay on the west side of Honshu Island across from Hiroshima is the Izumo Shrine, the most ancient Shinto shrine in Japan. This shrine has been venerated continually for well over a thousand years. Every year in late fall the *kami*, or earth spirits, of Japan leave their normal homes throughout the country and gather for a week at the shrine. During this period, the Shrine is also visited by thousands of pilgrims who have come to celebrate the arrival of the kami. This visit of the spirits even has a special name in the Japanese language – the period of the visit is known as *kami-arizuke* (period with the gods) at Izumo, and *kannazuki* (period without gods) in all other parts of Japan.

At the time of their 1998 visit, we performed an experiment in remote dowsing to see if the visit caused any change in the chi energy of the Shrine's site. Dowsers Sig Lonegrin in Europe; Joey Korn and James Sullivan in North America; and Hitomi Horiuchi in eastern Japan dowsed a map of the shrine precincts before, during, and after the visit of the kami.

All found a major change in the energy of the site during the visit, and a return to the earlier energy state after the departure of the spirits. One dowser registered confusion because his reading first showed an energy node at one shrine building, and rechecking later, found it at a different building. A call to the Shrine produced a schedule of events during the week, which indicated that a welcoming ceremony had been held at the first building at the time of the first reading; and later the spirits moved to the second building for another ceremony!

In spite of the Westernization of Japan, the Japanese still acknowledge the existence of the kami and continue their annual visits to the Shrine to honor them, as they have for probably more than a thousand years. The presence of the spirits is still perceptible to visitors, and people gather from around the world to celebrate and honor them.

Below: Diagrams by dowser Joey Korn showing multiple crossings of energy lines on main shrine buildings while kami were in residence.

Light lines are "echos" of opposite energy resulting from the abrupt shift in energy. Right: Energy lines on site before and after kami visit.

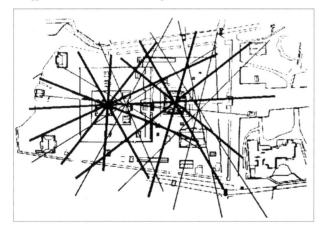

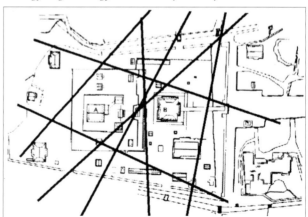

MAYA COMMUNITY PORTALS TO THE SPIRIT WORLD

Breakthroughs in deciphering the Maya written language in the last ten years have brought a transformation in our understanding of both the nature of their ritual centers and the events that transpired there. Emerging is a picture of a society living in amazing intimacy with the spirit world, where the soul and the supernatural were physically present phenomena in all aspects of their lives.

In the Maya world, all things are alive and imbued with sacredness - a sacredness especially concentrated at special places, such as caves, mountains, and ritual centers established by the people. The principal pattern of power spots was established when the cosmos was created. But within it, a complementary human-made matrix of power points is generated by the actions of the community.

Ceremonial centers were considered not so much places for ceremony, but places that *are* centers *because of* ceremonies performed in them which create sacred space and open portals to the Otherworld. Individuals – whether kings, shamans, or warriors who could enter and

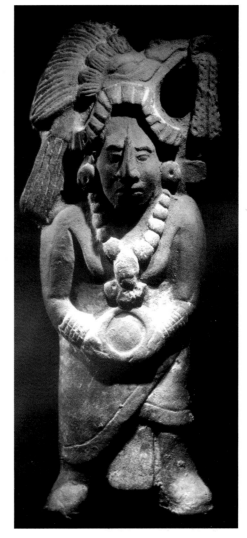

Above: A diviner figurine, holding skrying mirror made of hematite or obsidian. Mirrors created portals by which ancestors, Vision Serpents, and other supernatural beings entered the world, and let diviners see deeper realities than those of the everyday world.

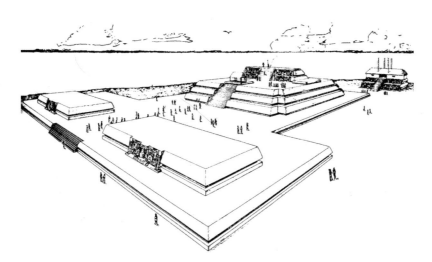

Left: A reconstruction drawing of the Second Temple Complex at Cerros gives a sense of the monumental outdoor spaces established for community ritual in the various Maya centers.

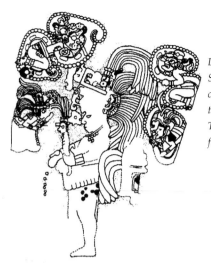

Left: Scene from Ixlu Stele 2, showing conjuring clouds with the Paddler Gods and Tlaloc Warriors floating in them.

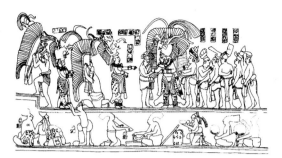

Above: The dressing of three dancers for the ceremony of dedication and ensouling of the temple at Bonampak.

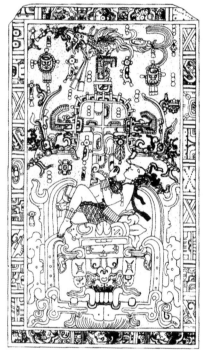

Above: Sarcophagus lid of King Pacal of Palenque, showing him traveling down the Milky Way to the Spirit World.

leave the spirit world at will, manipulate its forces, and bring its wisdom to the rest of the community – held central power in the community.[19]

Visionary rituals involving the whole community – possibly somewhat akin to today's *"raves"* – were a central part of life. Unlike many other cultures, in which trance journeying is done in seclusion, it was performed here by the rulers in public – experienced and affirmed by the entire community. With the use of dance, drumming, song, sleep deprivation, and psychoactive substances, both individuals and large groups went into altered states that allowed personal transformation and communication with the Otherworld.

For the Maya, the most important interactions are not between people and objects, but among the innate souls of persons and material objects. *Ch'ulel*, *itz*, or *k'awil* – all referring in different ways to chi energies – are central to their language and culture. It is hardly surprising that they called their kings *ch'ul ahaw*, or "lords of the life-force."

Warrior deities from the spirit world took major part in military battles. There is a K'iche Maya account of the battle in which thousands of their warriors were defeated by only 720 Spaniards led by Pedro de

[18] See Linda Schele and David Freidel, A FOREST OF KINGS, Wm. Morrow & Company, 1990; Schele and Peter Mathews, THE CODE OF KINGS, Scribner, 1998; and Freidel, Schele, and Parker, MAYA COSMOS, W. Morrow & Co., 1993.

Below: The supernatural dimensions of war conjured by the lords of Chich'en Itza. Left, a battle ranges in a village, while overhead, spirit guides and battle beasts emerge from portals of the Otherworld. Right, another battle scene, with spirit guides in battle overhead.

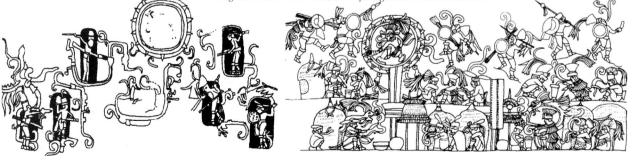

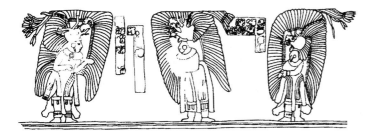

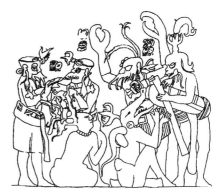

Above: The same three lords performing a feather dance at the Bonampak' temple dedication.
Right: Masked dancers in the same ceremony, portraying the Otherworld beings they have become through trance dancing.

Alvarada. Contrary to Spanish accounts, it reads as a battle of both spirit and earthly worlds – between the Gods as well as between the warriors and their spirit guides.

Below: A Vision Serpent, showing a materialized ancestor emerging from its jaws.

The K'iche leader, Tekum Uman, transformed himself into his *way* (spirit companion) and fought – along with the *wayob* of their gods and ancestors – as a sorcerer and an eagle against the magic of the Spanish supernaturals. He was ultimately unable to kill Alvarado because of the Spaniards' defense by a floating maiden (the Virgin Mary), many footless birds (angels), and an exceedingly white bird (the Holy Spirit), who blinded the K'iche warriors and forced them to fall to the earth.[20]

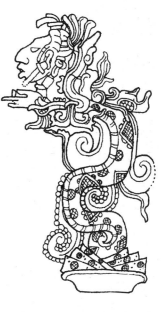

In Maya public architecture, the plazas, courtyards, and exterior spaces were more important than the buildings surrounding them. The buildings acted as ceremonial definers of space for the rituals, dances, and processions at the heart of Maya life. Their small interior spaces held gods, ancestral images, regalia and equipment for ceremonies, and spaces for individual ceremony. Temples were frequently built in the image of mountains or *witz*, the volcano being a powerfully experienced gateway of the vital forces of Creation. Caves, or interior spaces, were often used as places for conjuring ancestors.

20 David Freidel, Linda Schele, and Joy Parker, MAYA COSMOS: Three Thousand Years on the Shaman's Path, Wm. Morrow & Company, 1993.

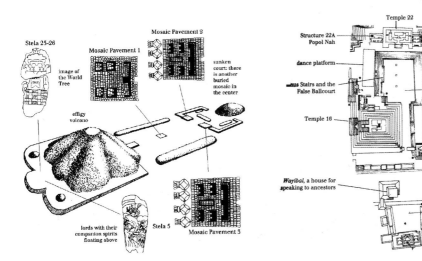

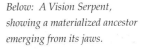

Far left: La Venta, with its fiery volcano portal to the spirit world, and a courtyard with mosaics representing the three stones of Creation and massive deposite of serpentine stone.

Left: Plan of the East Court of the Acropolis at Copan, which provided the interior and exterior sacred, magical space in which pageant and ritual could unfold, joining together the worlds of human and divine experience.

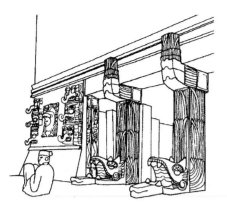

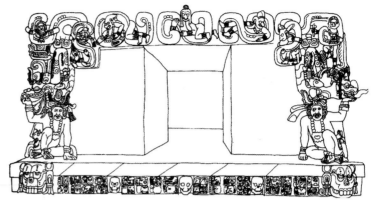

Temple of the Warriors, Chich'en Itza, showing feathered Vision Serpents as door piers, and Itzam-Yeh belching up a "Way" from the Otherworld.

Copan, Inner Door of Temple 22: A Cosmic Monster, representing the Milky Way, frames the doorway. The cloud parts of its body represent spirits conjured up by the bloodletting rituals inside, which the king called upon in the exercise of his power.

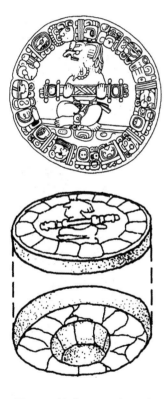

The central ballcourt marker and offering hole beneath it at Tonina, marking the location as a portal to the Otherworld where spirits enter and leave us at birth and death.

Plazas were seen as portals, or Spirit World gateways, opening onto the Primordial Sea. To concentrate energy, special areas were paved with rare stone several meters deep. Maya ceremonial ball courts represented the crack in the earth where humankind emerged. They used this crack to access the inner earth to contact their ancestors and consult oracular deities. Treaties and transfers of power to new rulers took place there in the presence of beings materialized from the spirit world. They negotiated and sealed alliances in the ball court, and captured kings were sacrificed there. Tombs, such as that of Pakal at Uxmal, had "spirit channels" built in so that the spirits of the dead could continue to communicate with the living in the attached temple. Sacred precincts were often entered by a ceremonial path – *sak beh* or "white road" – which corresponded to the Milky Way and gave access across the stellar realm to the spirit world.

The names and sculptural imagery on Maya ceremonial structures leave no doubt as to their nature. Fixed portals to the spirit world were called *pib nah. Kunul* were conjuring or bewitching places. Sorcery houses were *Itzam Nah*, often marked by the winged *Itzam-Ye* birds. *Waybil* were dreaming places, and *kyxan sum* were sculptural representations of the umbilicus connecting individuals on earth to the spirit world.

To the Maya, *"Nothing important is just made. It also has to be born."* All things made by the gods during Creation were imbued with sacred force and an inner soul. Places, buildings, and objects made by human beings, however, had to have their inner souls – their *ch'ulel* – put into them during dedication ceremonies.

Dedication rituals, accompanied by depositing ceremonial plates of sacred objects below the floors, were part of bringing the *k'ulel*, or life-force, into the buildings or ritual spaces. Once the rituals had established energetic linkages to the spirit world, those ceremonial spaces became portals connecting to that world:

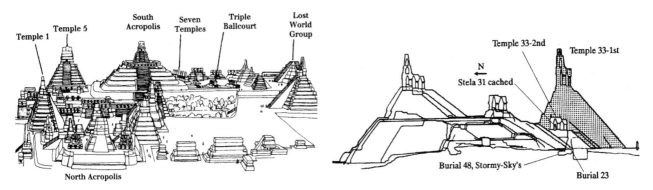

View and section of the central area of Tikal, showing the layering of construction as ritual spaces and structures were deactivated, rebuilt, and reactivated over time as astrological and dynastic changes occurred.

When the Maya materialized their gods and ancestors through these portals, the spiritual beings left residual energy in the buildings and the objects that opened the portals. Thus very old buildings, very sacred rituals, and very powerful people affected this energy in proportionally greater ways, so that the oldest portals contained the most intense k'ulel of all. The Maya kept building over these portals for hundreds of years, so that their buildings were like onions – layer after layer accumulating over the sacred core.[21]

As long as the community used these ritual spaces, that power was safe. But when a ruler died, when a cycle of the calendar finished, when a sacred area was abandoned, the Maya performed special termination rituals to protect the community or put that power "on hold." A new ruler or period of time would bring construction of another layer over the existing one, accompanied by ceremonies to reactivate the portals.[22, 23]

The Maya spirit world was a powerful part of their everyday lives, in ways difficult for us to fully comprehend today. But their ritual centers remain, as testimony that such a world exists and can be brought into our own lives.

The Vision Serpent, here with a materialized ancestor emerging from its mouth, represented the ritual act of opening the axis linking the material and spirit worlds.

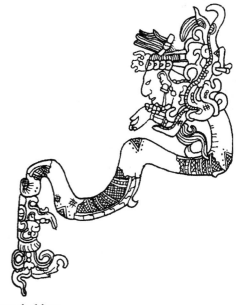

[21] Schele and Mathews, THE CODE OF KINGS. For an incredible visual introduction to the Maya funeary figurines, see Schele and Jorge Pérez de Lara's HIDDEN FACES OF THE MAYA, 1997.

[22] See A FOREST OF KINGS for discussion of dedication and termination rituals.

[23] John Anthony West, in SERPENT IN THE SKY, Julian Press, 1987, documents similar consecration and deconsecration rituals, along with ritual reuse of materials from deconsecrated temples in new ones, in Egypt.

HINDU TEMPLES
AND THE GEOMETRY OF CONSCIOUSNESS

The Hindu spiritual tradition makes strong use of chi (prana) in its spiritual as well as medical practices. *Mantras* (energized sounds), *yantras* (energized geometric figures), and *mudras* (energetic yogic postures linking specific meridians and chakras) are widely employed to develop and train energetic aspects of our inner lives.

Yantras are widely employed during design and construction of temples. Sculpture based on geometries of space and time measurement are part of teaching galleries of temples and monasteries, used to guide and empower student meditations. In some cases, these have been experienced as highly energetically empowered; in other cases there is less evidence.

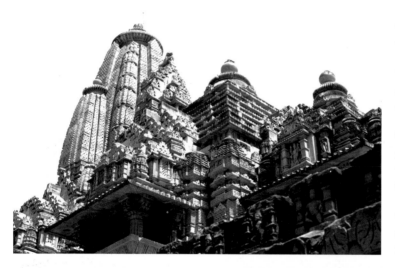

There are several dimensions of energetic empowerment imployed in various temples:[24]

* Intention of honoring the mathematical and geometric interconnectivity and interaction of natural systems.

* The use of specific mathematic/geometric relationships that empower harmonic transfer of energy within physical, biologic, and psychic systems.

* Employment of geometry as a means of demonstrating connectivity back into unity from the diversity of manifested form.

The design of classical Indian temples such as the Kandariya Mahadeo Temple in Khajuraho (above) and the Temple of Konarak in Orissa (right) involved both consideration of them as a diagram of the Cosmos (as seen from above), and mantra-seeded energy centers put in place during their design and construction.

* Conscious investment into a structure or sculpture of energetically-active elements that impact psychic structure and connection to divinities and the spirit world.

Keith Critchlow, though speaking specifically of similar Islamic use of geometry, explains the role of geometry in connection with Unity:

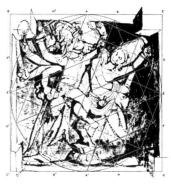

> *In our manifest world, we observe things developing, having a duration, and being reabsorbed. This elementary law can be symbolized geometrically in the way that space is created by unfolding through the dimensions. By reversing the geometry through the folding up of the dimensions, we are led back to the point of Unity or the indivisible. In terms of consciousness, this can be described as the path of reabsorption, indicating the reconciliation between Knower, Knowing and Known.*[25]

Andreas Volwahsen explains how this is manifested in the geometry of centrally-focused temple design – a pattern of organization to be *known*, not necessarily *seen*:

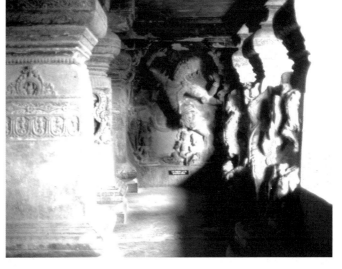

> *Hindu architecture teaches us not to accept some axioms unconditionally. The Orissan temples, for example, have in effect no façades. The vertical sections flow without a break and fuse with the most important of all angles of vision, the view from above. Again, the architectonic system of a temple can best be perceived from an inaccessible viewpoint, namely from the air. The shikhara tapers toward the top, and there are no overlaps or recesses even in the lower part. Thus there would be no better vantage-point from which to view the monument as comprehensively as possible than a point directly above the temple, exactly on its vertical axis. From this perspective all the ornaments which, to those viewing the temple from other angles, appear to be swelling luxuriantly in ever more exaggerated forms, would fall into place as subordinate to a geometric order; this order is only imperfectly reflected in the ground-plan of such buildings, because a ground-plan is after all only an arbitrarily drawn horizontal section. The north Indian temple tower, as an image of the cosmic order, has every side facing outwards into space.*[26]

A sculpture panel in the teaching galleries of the Kailasa Temple at Ellura. Energized in part through use of specific time/space geometries documented by Alice Boner (top), such panels were designed to activate specific parts of our inner energy systems.

---

[24] Andreas Volwahsen, LIVING ARCHITECTURE: INDIAN, Grosset & Dunlap, 1969; Keith Critchlow, ISLAMIC PATTERNS: An Analytical and Cosmological Approach, Schocken Books, 1976; and Alice Boner's PRINCIPLES OF COMPOSITION IN HINDU SCULPTURE, E.J. Brill, 1962, along with Stella Kramrisch's THE HINDU TEMPLE, University of Calcutta, 1946 are probably the easiest and most coherent introductions to these issues and applications. See also the Chapter Six discussion of numbers and geometry.

[25] Keith Critchlow, ISLAMIC PATTERNS: An Analytical and Cosmological Approach, Schocken Books, 1976.

[26] Andreas Volwahsen, LIVING ARCHITECTURE: INDIAN, Grosset & Dunlap, 1969.

SETTING THE INTENTION OF A NATION
IN HAN CHINA

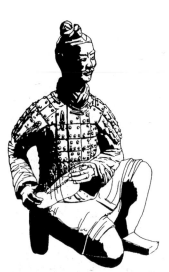

Above: One of the armies of terra-cotta warriors has been excavated. Historical records hint at the existence of others.

Below: Location of Qin Shihuang's tomb and army of terra-cotta warriors correspond with the dimensions and normal geometry expected if the full complex of four armies and palace exist.

The archeological world was set abuzz in 1974 with the chance discovery, near Xi'an in central China, of an underground army of terra-cotta warriors. The terra-cotta army, of extraordinary artistic workmanship, dates from the reign of Qin Shihuang, the "First Emperor," who unified China in 221 B.C. and established the Han Dynasty. The subterranean vault of earth and timber eventually yielded more than 7,000 life-size terra-cotta warriors and their horses in battle formation. Their 10,000 weapons were treated to remain sharp even to this day.

Historical accounts of Qin Shihuang's tomb in ancient texts describe it as containing palaces filled with precious stones, ceilings vaulted with pearls, statues of gold and silver, and rivers of mercury. The walls of the inner sanctum were supposed to be 2.5 km long, and the outer walls 6 km long.[27] The texts also speak of the terra-cotta army, and hint that other ones exist on other sides of his tomb facing the other cardinal directions.

Qin Shihuang is known also for construction of the Great Wall of China, linking separate walls of formerly independent kingdoms to keep out marauding nomads. Most commentators consider the terra-cotta army as a symbolic defense of the ruler's tomb, and make no connection of it with the Great Wall. However, the Chinese feng shui energetics of place tradition suggests a somewhat different interpretation.

Feng shui suggests that the clarity and strength with which an intention is expressed plays a vital role in its success in achieving its aims. Qin Shihuang's aim was a unified China which would endure. The vast effort of time, material and artistry that he marshaled into creation of the Great Wall, his tomb, and the terra-cotta armies represents a massive commitment to a strongly held intention.

The armies are symbolically prepared to defend the kingdom he created against encroachment from any of the four directions, while acknowledging their own success in unifying the country. The tomb, if its configuration follows its position relative to the known terra-cotta army, would embody relationships between the ruler, the people, the country and the Cosmos demonstrated in the archetypal Chinese city plan or Ming Tang ceremonial center.[28] The Wall represents, more than anything, a statement of edge or boundary – a distinction between what is and is not China. Its potential

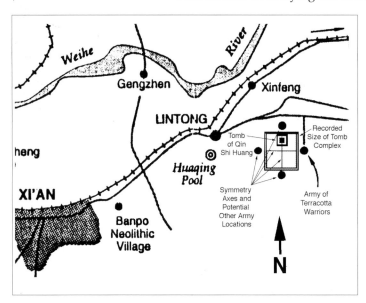

[27] "Basic Annals of Qin," in HISTORICAL RECORDS (Shiji-Qinbenji).

[28] For the Ming Tang, see Nelson Wu, CHINESE AND INDIAN ARCHITECTURE, George Braziller, 1963. For Chinese city formal organization, see Wu (above) or Andrew Boyd, CHINESE ARCHITECTURE AND TOWN PLANNING, University of Chicago Press, 1962.

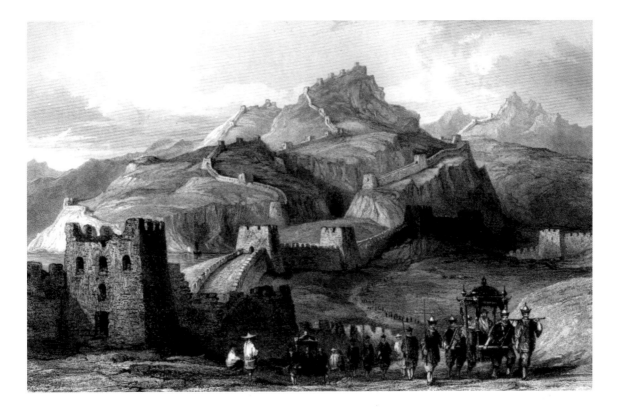

value as a defensive structure, however questionable, is probably far less than its value in defining for the Chinese themselves an image of their collective self.

From an energetic standpoint, Qin Shihuang's tomb and its surrounding armies represent a powerfully protected and held point of continuing access to the ruler, now returned to the spirit world, who sparked the creation of this vast new self of the Chinese. It is an immensely powerful statement, radiating in all directions and infusing the entire country with the energy of unity. It is a unity of image which has held, through vicissitudes and change, for over 2,000 years and remains strong today.

If excavation of the remaining parts of the tomb complex bring to the surface what is suggested in the ancient texts, it will reveal one of the most extraordinary efforts ever undertaken to manifest and project into the future a dream of what a people can become. It will also stand as the most forceful known example of feng shui practiced on the level of an entire country, focusing its energy into the future.

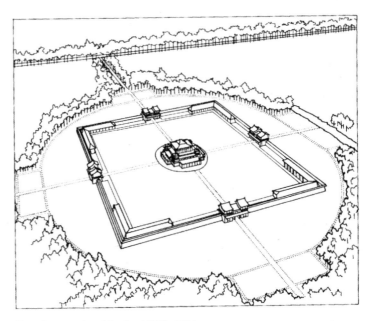

Top: Construction of the Great Wall of China was more a definition of boundary than a vital defensive element.

Above: Reconstruction drawing of a possible Ming Tang from the last years of the Western Han period – a ritual center for the emperor to bring his actions and his country in alignment with the order of Heaven and Earth.

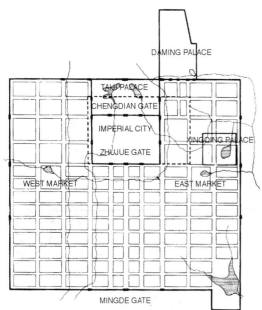

Above: Chang'an of the Tang Dynasty – axial and rectangular layout typical of Chinese administrative cities. Symetrical layout of markets, axial location of the Imperial quarter on the north, facing south, grid street layout; walled, enclosed blocks.

Below: The Western Gate of Beijing in the 19th century – an impressive greeting for visitors.

FENG-SHUI OF CHINESE CITIES: MIRRORS OF THE COSMOS

Feng-shui outlined a process for locating and laying out Chinese cities. The view of the cosmos on which city location was based spoke symbolically of four Gods: one dwelling in a stream to the east, one in a plain to the south, one in a highway to the west, and the fourth in a mountain to the north. A site with these surroundings was felt to be suitable.

A rectangular plan was made in the symbol of the cosmos, reflecting the rhythms of the sun, the stars, and the seasons that most strongly affected the land. The east-west axis is the path of the sun and the stars. The north-south axis is the direction of the still point in the heavens and the yearly path of the sun and the moon through the seasons.

The Emperor was placed in the north of this rectangle, as he always faced the holy south—in alignment to receive the growth-granting forces of the earth and sun. In the northeast, temples were built to a guardian deity, as that direction was felt to be unlucky; devils dwell in the mountains (as well as enemy troops). Buddhist temples were often placed in the west, as it was felt that Buddhism had a tendency to proceed eastward, and their influence would positively affect the city. The entire geometry and detailed layout of the city symbolically reflected and reinforced their understanding of the cosmos.

Thus sites were selected with mountains to protect the city from winter winds, and monasteries were founded in the mountains so that the city could be warned of attack. Southern orientation brought sunlight, warmth, cheer, and sanitation. Fresh water and air were provided for by proximity of the mountains and rivers, and the commerce and food supply of the city assured by the proximity of a river to the east and fields to the south. At the same time, every activity involved in making the city, living in it, and participating in its life reminded a person of the forces that acted upon their world. They became aligned with those forces, and gained nourishment from them.

This Chinese tradition of clearly placing themselves and their places of living within a pattern of the forces of the universe played out in a similar configuration of the *Ming Tang*, or "Bright Hall." In this ritual temple, the Emperor followed a progression of ceremony within the circle of the seasons, with the configuration of the temple complex tied to the same heavenly directions. Similar patterns determined the design of tombs, possibly including that of Qin Shihuang.

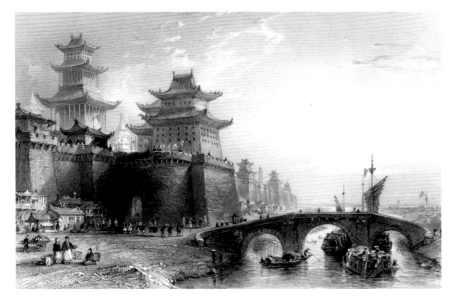

Angkor was interlaced by a network of reservoirs and canals – used both for transportation and for regulating the water supplies to agricultural areas.

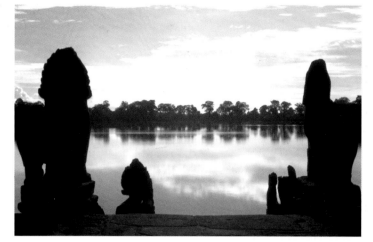

CHI AND THE SPIRIT WORLD IN KHMER WATER TEMPLES

Monuments in the Khmer capital of Angkor in Cambodia demonstrate chi-based design that achieves dimensions of power and function far beyond today's conventional design concepts. The Khmers created a unique and integrated structure of sculpture, temples, royal cities and palaces, reservoirs, irrigation systems, and local shrines that both provided irrigation water for their fields and created a powerful and ubiquitous image congruent with their beliefs. This system also infused the water with chi energy, and permeated their entire physical world with creative power from other, more primal, energetic dimensions of existence.

Agricultural productivity in the Mekong region is impacted by the seasonal nature of the rains. During spring melt and the monsoons, the flow of the Mekong River is so great that it reverses the flow of the Tonle Sap, backing water up into the Great Lake in the central basin of Cambodia. During the wet season, that lake changes from a shallow, muddy chain of pools to a body of water eighty to one hundred miles long, fifteen to thirty miles wide, and as much as forty to fifty feet deep. As the waters recede, they leave millions of fish stranded in the many muddy pools and bayous.

The Khmers worked out sophisticated systems of reservoirs and irrigation canals to distribute the stored water during the dry season, and to function as communication and transportation routes as well. A primary role of the government was to ensure the prosperity of the country through developing and maintaining this system.

Angkor, the Tonle Sap and Mekong Rivers.

Angkor and the nearby agricultural water system between it and the lake.

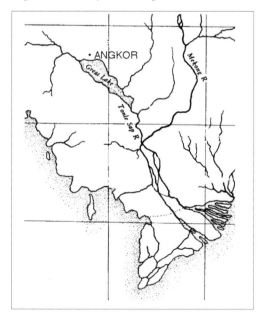

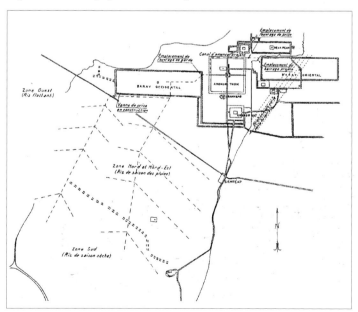

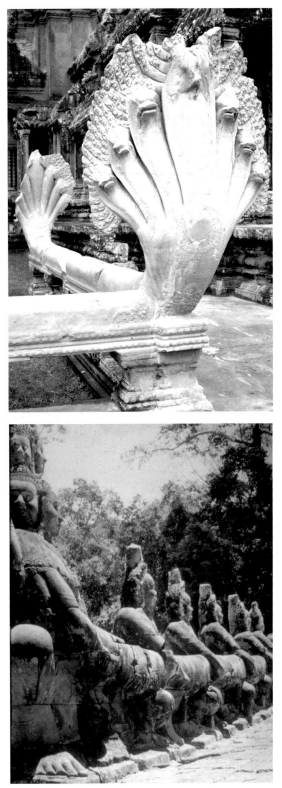

Naga railings at Angkor Wat are based on "serpent energy" life-force. In the Hindu tradition it is called prana. The Chinese call it "chi."

The canals, levees, and waterworks were executed on a scale that dwarfed the monuments and shrines, such as Angkor Wat, which are themselves of impressive size.[29] The temple and royal palaces from which the water systems radiated acted both as celebration of vast achievements and as moral guarantee of success for a deeply religious people.

On another level, chi was considered of central importance to the entire culture of the Khmers. The seven-headed (seven-chakra) hooded cobra, or *naga*, became one of the central themes of their art and mythology. Their creation story was a tug-of-war between the gods and the demons, who alternately pulled on the serpent *Vasuki* encircling Mt. Mandara. This caused the mountain to revolve like a giant churn in the primal void, or Sea of Milk, drawing forth the *amrita* which ensured the welfare of the king's subjects.

In the layout of the Khmer structures and waterworks, the temples and the royal city represented this central mountain, and charged the surrounding waters with chi through their connection with the spirit world. The gods, demons, and snakes formed giant balustrades for the causeways giving

---

[29] Viktor Goloubew's "L'Hydraulique Urbaine et Agricole a l'Epoque des Rois d'Angkor," in BULLETIN ECONOMIQUE DE L'INDOCHINE, 1941 fascicule 1, or abbreviated in CAHIERS DE L'ECOLE FRANCAISE D'EXTREME ORIENT, vol. 24(1940), gives breathtaking aerial views of the extensive network of canals and reservoirs.

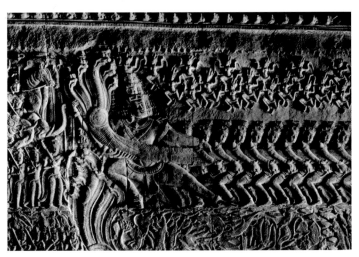

Right: Churning of the Sea of Milk bas-relief at Angkor Wat.

Above: The same theme in stone railings lining causeways entering the city and other monuments. In Angkor, the Bayon Temple acts as the "Central Mountain."

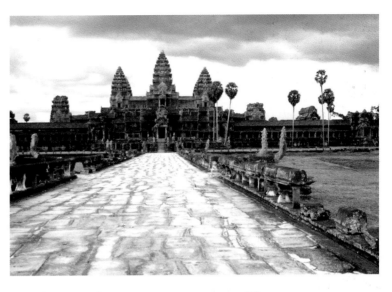

Angkor Wat is the funerary temple of King Suryavarman II, but also a part of the water/chi network of the nation tying it to the ancestors and Gods in the Spirit World.

access to the gates of the city or temple; and the reservoirs and canals distributed the chi-charged water to the fields themselves.

Thus, the Khmers succeeded in creating a powerful symbolic representation of the spiritual beliefs of their society. From the viewpoint of our culture, that was all. But to the degree that *chi* does play a significant role in health, it was a wonderfully practical system also.

However, if we change only one factor in our beliefs, an even more amazing picture emerges.

If it is true that the kings are merely "on the other side" after death, then they remain in touch with and able to help their descendants and their subjects. In this situation, it follows that the rulers' tombs and temples, and honoring of the rulers after death, take on real meaning with substantive effects on the lives and welfare of the people. The effort exerted by the Khmers to make their mortuary temples a part of their "chi-irrigation" system are then far more than symbolic.[30] The dead, and the necessary arrangements for remaining in connection with them, are then an integral part of a functioning support system for the society. They are a valuable means of tapping into the wisdom of the rest of the society living on the "other side."

From this viewpoint, the wonderfully coherent Khmer structure is one of the most powerful and effective examples of cultural or psychic infrastructure ever created. Given the existence of life-force energy and our on-going existence in "energy" bodies punctuated by periodic incarnations on the physical plane,[31] we find a very different meaning and function for buildings emerging. With the vital role of chi in healing and in connection with the rest of life, many of the peculiarities of design in Khmer and other cultures are suddenly explained.

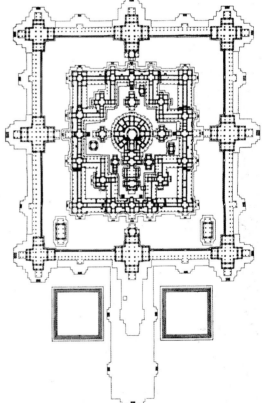

Plan of the Bayon, built with 49 towers, each with giant faces on four sides. The same theme is followed through in the gates of the City.

---

[30] The Chinese practice of locating tombs at places with good chi and using them to honor their ancestors is a clear parallel.

[31] Suzane Northrop, THE SEANCE, Dell Publications, 1994, or Raymond Moodey, LIFE AFTER DEATH, for example, give anecdotal evidence of this. Malidoma Somé's, OF WATER AND THE SPIRIT, Putnam, 1994; and RITUAL: Power, Healing and Community, Swan & Raven, 1993, discuss this from the perspective of contemporary African tribal culture.

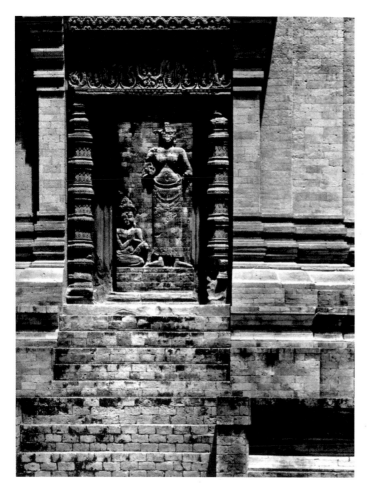

The unusal treatment of doorways to many Khmer monuments – the sophisticated ornamental banding is cut through as with a knife, opening to more delicate and finely ornamented inner layers.

The ornamental organization on Khmer temples, for example, is quite sophisticated and carries unusual meaning. The texture and rhythm of ornament, the positioning of sculptural images, the layering of plinths and entablatures, and the rhythmic vertical and horizontal bands of ornament are handled beautifully and with great refinement.

Yet a peculiar thing happens when we come to a doorway into a Khmer temple. An abrupt and sharp transition occurs – almost like a knife cut. The molding bands at the base of the wall end abruptly, though returned around corners everywhere else. The pilaster capitals and the ornamental entablature over the top of the opening similarly are abruptly sliced off on the side of the opening. And within that opening almost invariably is a second surround of pilaster and entablature, far more richly and finely ornamented with an almost "vibrational" layering and rhythm of ornament.

The same abrupt separation occurs on the terraces and stairways giving access to these doorways. The three-dimensional sculptural surfaces of the terraces are rent apart, with the steps almost always "let in" or recessed behind the surface planes of the terraces. In combination, the effect is of the surface of the temple being cut through and slid apart, revealing a glimpse of an "inner temple" and an "inner access" to that layer.

In most cultures the rooms or spaces inside a sacred structure represent one of two things. In churches, cathedrals, and some temples, we find a congregating space for adherents to gather in worship, meditation, or other religious activity. The other kind of space is a "Holy-of-Holies" – a space belonging to and acting as the home of a God, Goddess, or other representation of spiritual power.

Khmer temples represent a different configuration. The interior of their temples are neither spaces that people walk into, nor the property of some distinct "Higher Being." Instead, they represent a belief that *within* the surfaces of *everything* in the material world there is contained a finer, richer spiritual existence. Entering into the temple is entering into connection with that inner "energy" body which transfuses all of Creation.

Khmer temple design reminds us that the "functional" role of sheltering our activities is often secondary to more vital functions. Important structures have

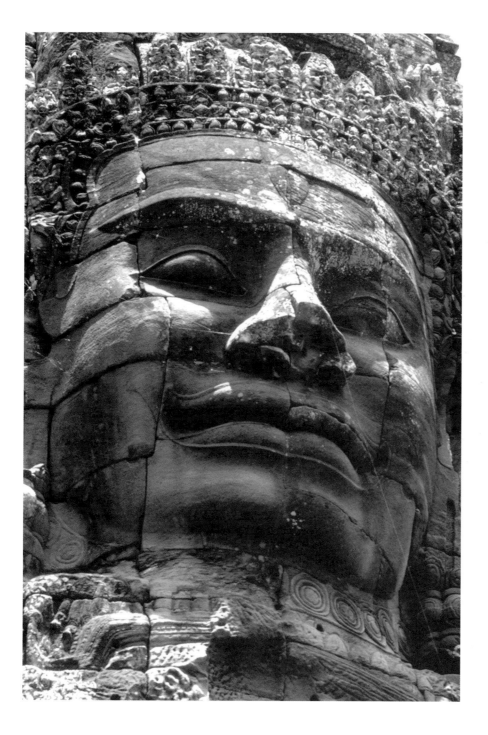

One of the faces of the Bayon – eyes half-closed in meditation, connecting inner and outer worlds; the manifest and unmanifest realms.

a more important role: to access power, to give a clear and potent representation of its efficacy, and to transmit that energy into the surrounding world.

In Khmer culture, funerary temples and sculptures dedicated to an individual were not, as often thought, an egotistical attempt at self-aggrandizement or a desire to better their personal afterlife. The Cambodian images of persons living or dead were intended to contain their "essence," or "vital principle." When consecrated, they acted as a bridge between those on this side of the veil and the person on the other side. King Yasovarman, a Khmer king of the 10th - 11th century once said, "Guard this *dharma*[32] which for me is like a bridge," suggesting its conscious role in connecting the material and non-material world.[19]

The temple, then, acted as a kind of architectural body substituted for the flesh and bones previously inhabited by a now deceased "cosmic person." Through it, that person's soul can continue to be accessed, prolonging their connection with the embodied community.[33] Bodily remains, sculpture, or paintings of the person – if present at the temple – can also be energized to strengthen the connection to them in the spirit world.

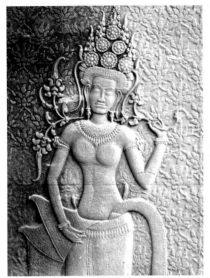

The sculpture detailing as well as the building design, ornament, and sculpture programs continue the theme of vibrating energy central to prana or chi.

The giant sculpted faces of the king facing in the four directions atop the central Bayon temple and the gateways of the royal city were not, as often described, the faces of a "Big Brother" king watching every movement of his subjects. The king's eyes, as those in the vast majority of Khmer sculpture, were actually closed in meditation. These were images manifesting chi or breath of life and conveying it out to all corners of the kingdom. This was chi channeled from the energy dimensions of existence to the material one through the king, in trance, in his sacred role.

In the Bayon we also see these giant faces not as sculptures of independent objects or persons, but as a manifestation of inner consciousness or spirit *within* the stone of the temple. They represent a *human* connection with that source of energy.

This central focus on the breath of life is dominant everywhere in Angkor. Headdresses on sculpture represent "flame emanations of aura energy."   A sculpture with a hooded cobra headdress embodies the kundalini or serpent image of chi energy. Three-headed "Vishnu" sculptures give a sense of male and female, multiple existences, or simultaneous occupation by different manifestations or dimensions of existence.

The temples themselves are covered with fine-grained banded profiles and layers of ornament. Particularly when looked at with the "soft eyes" of meditation, this gives a feeling of the temple being manifested by sound or vibration – a sense of time-lapse emergence, of emerging from or transforming into something else.

The bas-relief Creation story of the Churning of the Sea of Milk at Angkor Wat (page 70) contains a unique sense of chi energy manifested in its design and its story. The top figures seem to vibrate, almost like a plucked string. The central composition of rows of gods and demons tugging on the sacred snake again produce a graphic sound-vibration rhythm pouring out to both sides from the center.

The sacred traditions in India used yantras (specific geometric compositions) or sculpture based on space and time divisions of geometry to entrain a person's mind into the energy of the non-material world.[34] In the Khmer world of Angkor, this was not necessary. Being within the web of its "chi-irrigation" system of temples, sculpture, causeways, water temples, and canals created an equal en-

---

[32] In this case, connoting "sacred establishment" to ensure the perpetuity of linkage between the person in afterlife and the society on earth. See George Coedes, "La destination funeraire des grands monuments khmers," BULLETIN DE L'ECOLE FRANCAISE D'EXTREME-ORIENT, 1940.

[33] See George Coedes, ANGKOR, AN INTRODUCTION, Oxford Univ. Press, 1963.

[34] See Alice Boner, PRINCIPLES OF COMPOSITION IN HINDU SCULPTURE, E.J. Brill, 1962.

velopment and permeation by the flows and the power accessed through its configuration and meaning.

With that, we see another facet of the entire Khmer society. With no meaningful distinction between secular and sacred roles, *every* part of a Khmer's surroundings connected and empowered them through their spiritual/governmental system. A temple is not an isolated, separate "spiritual" place to go to. Instead, it is part of a complex environment imbued with spiritual power that reaches everywhere within the kingdom.

What the Khmers created was a framework encompassing, enfolding, and transforming the entire material world of the kingdom. Wherever one was – on roadways, canals, levees, in fields, towns, between temples and reservoirs – one was surrounded by, one was *within*, a framework or connection system manifesting the spiritual world within the material one and bringing the material one into full congruence with the energetic/spiritual one.

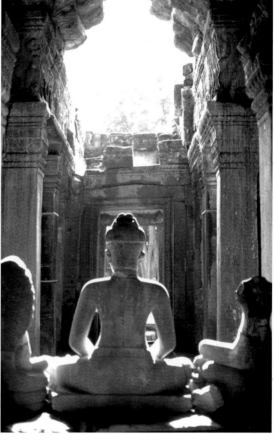

John Stephen Lansing's work in Bali provides an interesting insight on the role of the spirit world in the Khmer water temple system. A similar system was still in operation in Bali in the 1970s when introduction of Green Revolution agriculture created chaos. When the Green Revolution demanded that the farmers practice continuous cropping, they quickly found that the traditional practices of letting the paddy fields dry up was as essential for pest control as for maximizing productivity throughout the region. Lansing's field work and computer studies done there in the 1980s demonstrated that the water temples were essential and highly successful elements in balancing the wants and needs of different water users and determining water use practices throughout the island.

The water temples' decision of which farm areas got water at what time was not a human/political decision. Irrigation water came from an immense freshwater lake in the caldera of Mount Batur in central Baliasking. Allocation decisions involved contacting the spirit world, asking the "Goddess of the Lake" and the ancestors to meld the needs and situations throughout the island with knowledge not available in our realm, to sort out the intricately complex patterns of soils, rainfall, pest cycles, unexpected climate variations, etc. for the good of all. As Lansing showed, it worked – far better than our computer systems.[35]

Temples and shrines, the sacred and the spirit world, pervade all corners of the kingdom and all aspects of life in Khmer culture.

All things – buildings, sculpture, ornament and yantras in particular – *can* contain and be imbued with the energy to jump-start our personal and community access to that deep font of creative power. They can twist that boundary between worlds to create a cusp, to bring the matrix of the other dimensions into reach within our physical dimension. At a minimum, they can act as mementos or testimonials that, like the crutches on the walls at Lourdes, confirm the existence and efficacy of what lies behind the veils.

[35]   John Stephen Lansing, PRIESTS & PROGRAMMERS: Technologies of Power in the Engineered Landscape of Bali, Princeton University Press, 1991.

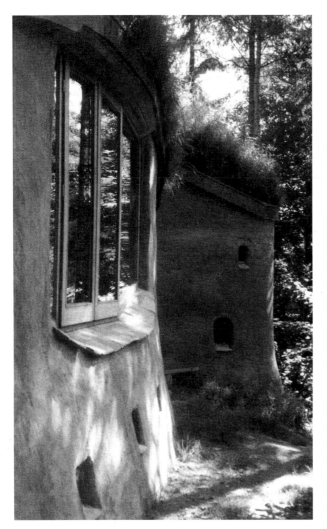

Above: Chris Day's wonderful Nant-y-Cwm Steiner Kindergarden in Wales shows the gentleness attainable by avoiding the use of straight lines.

STEINER SCHOOLS: LEARNING IN SPIRIT

After WWI, Austrian philosopher, artist, and scientist Rudolf Steiner was asked to design an educational system that would ensure that the horrors of the Hitler years would not recur. The resultant Waldorf School system focused on the nurture of children's senses, kinetic activity, community, and honoring connection with the spirit world. There are now over 640 Waldorf Schools in 46 countries, providing a solid integration of physical, emotional, intellectual, and spiritual learning tied to the developmental phases of a child's growth.

Waldorf is one of the few educational systems that acknowledge the diversity of the spirit world and our ability to access it individually. They have developed unique environments for learning, with emphasis on the energetic as well as the physical surroundings. Architects such as Christopher Day in Wales and the late Eric Asmussen in Sweden have created singular structures in the Western tradition that attempt to connect our children's development with the sacred.[36]

The structures place heavy emphasis on color, light, luminosity, the "thought-forms" associated with different activities, ecological fitness, and special age-related needs that support growth. Ceiling height, spatial geometry, craft-work, and elements which connect with nature and the spirit world are all given special attention.

[36] See Gary Coates, ERIK ASMUSSEN, ARCHITECT, Byggfolaget, 1997 and Christopher Day, PLACES OF THE SOUL, Aquarian, 1993.

Erik Asmussen's Culture House at Järna, Sweden uses subtle, rich colors on the interior, glowing in natural daylight, and expression of different forms for different elements of the building.

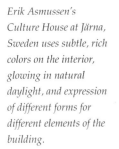

LEARNING FROM THE DAGARA
HOW TO HEAL OUR ANCESTORS

Our individual root intentions come from the spirit world. And that world contains all of the ancestors that have come before us. Energetics connects us with that world, and allows us to draw upon its wisdom either by gift or by practice. Thus, care and consideration are given to places that are gateways to those worlds. Ernest Eitel says, in reference to Chinese energetics:

When, through exhaustion of the vital breath, the body is broken up, the animus returns to heaven, the anima to earth; that is to say, each is dissolved again into those general elements of nature whence each derived its origin and the temporary embodiment of which each was within the sphere of individual life. The souls of deceased ancestors therefore are as omnipresent as the elements of nature, as heaven and earth themselves.[37]

When we consider relationship with ancestors from an energetics standpoint, we move into what is to our culture a totally foreign realm. Energetics (whether from a Buddhist, Taoist, Vedic, Yoruba, Hopi, or other philosophical or religious context) says that an incarnate person begins as an intention in the eternal energy body of that soul. That intention joins with chi to create an etheric template or auric body, around which material structure gravitates and coalesces into our physical form.

When we die, that energy body or soul remains in the energy realms, altered by its recent material life. So we rejoin our ancestors on death. But these cultures also claim, and willingly demonstrate, that the doors are not closed between these earthly and heavenly realms. Through specific techniques, the veils can be parted; we can communicate, journey, and work together between the worlds.

To feel that directly from a living culture, listen to the words of Malidoma Somé from the Dagara tribe of Burkina Faso in West Africa:

For the Dagara, every person is an incarnation, that is, a spirit who has taken on a body. So our true nature is spiritual. This world is where one comes to carry out specific projects. A birth is therefore the arrival of someone, usually an ancestor that somebody already knows, who has important tasks to do here. The ancestors are the real school of the living. They are the keepers of the very wisdom the people need to live by. The life energy of ancestors who have not yet been reborn is expressed in the life of nature, in trees, mountains, rivers and still water. . . .[38]

---

[37] Ernest Eitel, FENG-SHUI: The Rudiments of Natural Science in China, 1873. Reprinted Synergetic Press, 1993.

[38] Malidoma Somé, OF WATER AND THE SPIRIT, Tarcher/Putnam, 1994.

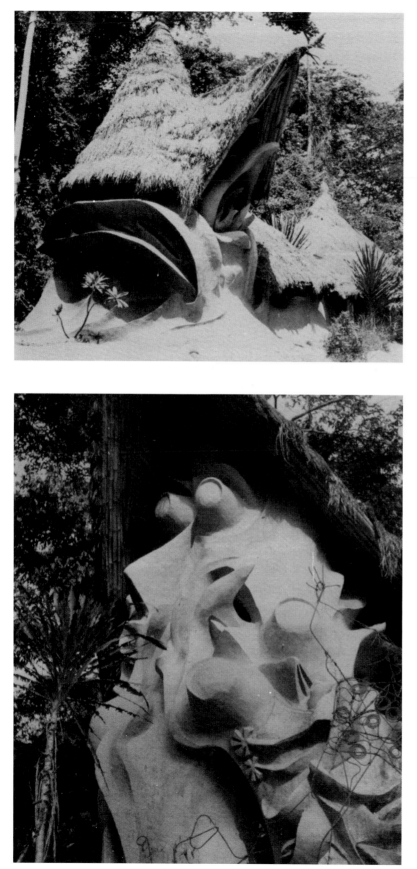

Out of this, Somé also provides an interesting perspective on our relation to our own ancestors:

In many non-Western cultures, the ancestors have an intimate and absolutely vital connection with the world of the living. They are always available to guide, to teach, and to nurture. They represent one of the pathways between the knowledge of this world and the next. Most importantly – and paradoxically – they embody the guidelines for successful living – all that is most valuable about life. Unless the relationship between the living and the dead is in balance, chaos results.

When a person from my culture looks at the descendants of the Westerners who invaded their culture, they see a people who are ashamed of their ancestors because they were killers and marauders masquerading as artisans of progress. The fact that these people have a sick culture comes as no surprise to them. The Dagara believe that, if such an imbalance exists, it is

Suzanne Wenger, an Austrian artist who moved to western Nigeria in 1950, sparked a vital new expression of the Yoruba religion through reconstruction of a series of shrines in Oshogbo. Trance-inspired by the orishas, she manifested a new vision of sacred place for the community. Above, the first Aiyedakun shrine, embodying the mouth and trunk of the elephant, the symbol of Obatala. Destroyed by fanatics, it was rebuilt in a yet different fashion, below.

the duty of the living to heal their ancestors. If these ancestors are not healed, their sick energy will haunt the souls and psyches of those who are responsible for helping them. Not all people in the West have such an unhealthy relationship with their ancestors, but for those who do, the Dagara can offer a model for healing the ancestors, and by doing so, healing oneself.[39]

With variations in different cultures, this is the universe that is acknowledged and inhabited by energetics. We will look in Chapter 12 at the fundamentally different role that religious buildings, tombs, and homes play in such a world.

But here we need to acknowledge only that ancestors and the spirit worlds exist, that we can communicate with and be nurtured by them, and that this connection is part of the philosophical and scientific framework of energetics. This framework is shared by Chinese geomancy, Celtic magic, and the Japanese Emperors *speaking with* (not praying to) their ancestors as part of their inauguration. It underlies the heart of Maya culture and Egyptian society. It is part of shamanic initiation rituals worldwide, and part of our own dream worlds. It underlies the care given by the Chinese and others in locating tombs for good chi, and the attention given to "celestial" influences in many forms of geomancy.[40]

Interestingly, the English-language literature on China (Joseph Needham's *Science and Civilization in China* included) gives a somewhat subdued picture of the Chinese relation to ancestors. Mention is made of speaking with them, considerable energy goes into tomb siting, household rituals are performed. But there is nothing of the emotional intensity, power of experience, immediacy, and involvement in everyday life that one feels from Somé, or from the emotionally compelling Yoruba shrines created by Suzanne Wenger in neighboring Nigeria.[41] And there is none of the vitality of nature spirits inherent in Aboriginal, Japanese, Native American, Celtic and other traditions.

The role of communication with ancestors in energetics of place gives at least an inkling of the spiritual domains tapped into by an energy-based universe and the kind of sustenance gained by those within cultures built upon that basis.

[39] Ibid.

[40] Feuchtwang gives a more detailed discussion of ancestors, the spirit world, relative to Chinese geomancy in AN ANTHROPOLOGICAL ANALYSIS OF CHINESE GEOMANCY, Editions Vithagna, Laos, 1974.

[41] Ulli Beier, THE RETURN OF THE GODS, Cambridge University Press, 1975.

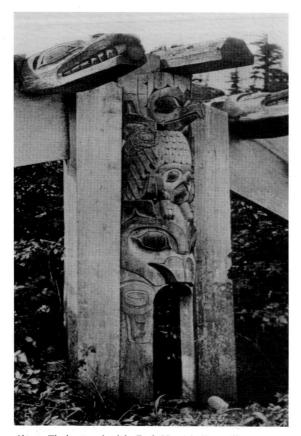

Above: The beam ends of the Eagle House in Tanu village were carved into sea lion heads. Its carved doorpost contains an eagle and baleen whale.

Below: A Raven House at Gwayasdums village. On ceremonial occasions, the beak would drop and people would enter the house through the mouth of the bird.

LIVING IN THE BELLY OF A BIRD IN A KAWAKIUTL VILLAGE

Every form of life, from birds to trees to sunlight to whales, is a different facet of the jewel of Creation and has particular characteristics which distinguish it from other life forms. Those attributes give it unique perceptions, powers, and relationships with the rest of existence.

Through trance, mimicry, and psychic opening to these different life forms, we can enter into and experience their unique nexus of the universe and even assume some of their powers. This ability to connect with all Creation on the energetic level and in the spirit world deepens our resonance and harmony with the song of life, and enriches the wisdom with which we move through life.

Other cultures live intimately with and commune continually with this world and these powers. Some of these cultures, such as the Aborigines in Australia, rarely build; they commune directly with the spirits within the special natural places they inhabit. Others, such as the Mayas or Egyptians, have occupied whole regions of the earth where human action dominates the nature of the physical world.

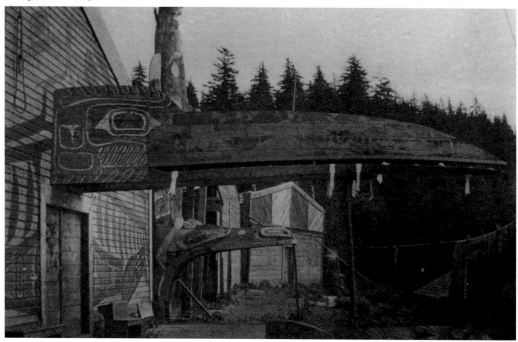

Yet they have been able to retain and even to make more accessible and powerful the connection to the spirit world of their surroundings. This depth of experience and relationship with other life transforms everyday existence, giving immense richness of meaning to every action and a community of support for every situation.

Native Americans in the Pacific Northwest work and live closely with spirit totems in all of their art, experiencing and bringing the nature of those life forms into their community. With compelling masks, dance, and the imbuing of dwellings with the power and imagery of family totems, a family's association with the spirit of certain animals, birds, fish, or other life forms extends tens of generations into the past, creating a depth of support inconceivable to our world.

Massive cedar posts supporting roof beams of traditional Northwest dwellings were carved in the likeness of the spirit totems, and embodied with their energy to shelter, nurture, and empower the family and community. Doorways into clan houses in Kawakiutl villages in British Columbia were frequently carved in the image of a raven, which is associated with their Creation story. In ceremony, the dwelling was entered through the mouth of the raven, using the pivoting lower beak as a ramp. As a person crossed a pivot point, the beak swung shut and the person was "swallowed" into the belly of the raven. A person coming out of the dwelling was similarly "born from the belly of the raven," emerging through its mouth into the village.

Knowing their role and what they embody energetically, we now realize that the fierce figures located in the gateways to Japanese temples are not intended to frighten visitors but to embody shielding protection of those within the complex connecting with the spirit world. And even in the European Christian tradition, a place of sanctuary and shelter is promised by the sculpted images greeting us at the gateway to a cathedral.

Masks used in ritual and ceremony separate us from our conventional world and help us open to the spirit of the life forms we assume. That new awareness carries into our subsequent actions. Incorporation of spirit guides and guardians into our own homes and community places can today give connection to the same fonts of life.

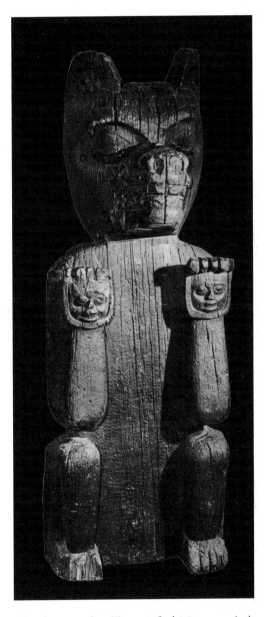

A bear house post from Kitamaat. Such totems, energized with song and prayer in their making and installation, infuse the entire home with the energy and life-force of that particular family animal.

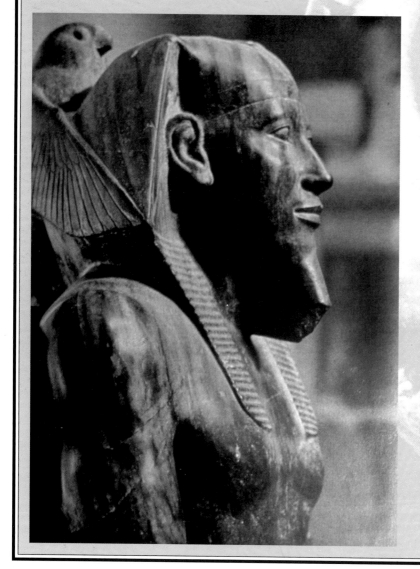

From the front, this diorite statue of Pharaoh Khafre appears to be just of the pharaoh. From the side, however, Horus appears, protecting and channeling wisdom through the pharaoh to his people.

EMPOWERING IMAGES

Energetic linkages can be invested in any object to act as a connector to specific entities in the spirit world or to affect individuals coming in contact with the objects. We've all heard stories of women buying beautiful African bracelets, only to become very sick through voodoo spells placed on the bracelet to affect a former owner. Statues in churches and temples have been used throughout the ages to connect to entities in the spirit world – deities, totems, ancestors, and other spirits. Of course, if it's someone else's religion, we call such objects "Idols". If it is our own, we would be incensed by someone calling them that – it's a statue of Saint Francis, a Pieta, a Crucifix, or Holy Words from the Koran.

Such "living statues" are found in almost every culture. On the material level, they act as a focus for our attention, a clarifier of our intentions, and a way to bring attributes the entity represents to our consciousness. They remind us that unseen spiritual energies beyond our ordinary realities are as much part of our world as fixing breakfast and going to work.

The process of empowering an image – painting, sculpture, or other object – is simple. You merely ask the deity or entity to inhabit the object:

Cleanse and smudge the object and the space it is in. Honor it with offerings of flowers, incense, food, or candles.

Ground and center. Enter sacred space, and expand that space to include the object and the room or place it is located. Open your chakras.

Clear out all old, negative energy and spirits from the object and space.

Connect to the spirit world, to the entity you wish connection with, and extend a cord of golden energy from your heart chakra to that entity.

Focus your intention, and invite the entity to take up abode in the image, stating why you wish its presence. Repeat the invitation three times, and wait a minute for the action to occur, before opening its eyes and senses.

Bring some lighted incense to the image, and offer it a delightful fragrance to smell. Gently open the image's eyes and ears with your finger moistened with water, and ask that it see and hear the needs of our world. Touch the image's heart, third-eye, and crown chakras with a small amount of sweet smelling oil, connecting each to your own. If the image has hands or feet, you can open the chakras on the hands and feet with the oil also, as a means of moving healing energy into your space. Touch its mouth with oil, and state how you wish it to communicate with you. Ask its assistance in bringing harmony between our lives, our world, and the spirit world. Thank the entity for entering the image. Pause, relax, and let chi flow between your chakras and the image.

When finished, release the energy cord, thank the spirits, close the sacred space, and blow out the candle. Make sure you are regrounded in this world.

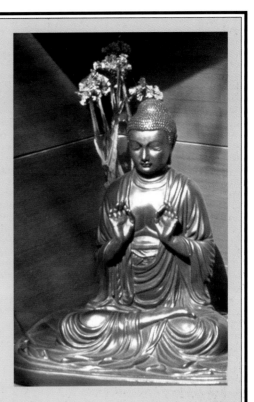

The energy radiating from the hands of this Buddhist statue was strong enough to be felt through a catalog photograph of a copy of the statue.

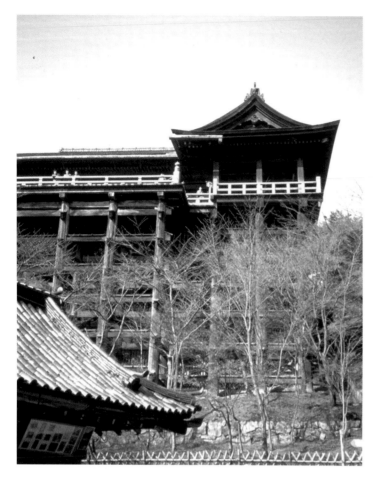

Above: The immense substructure necessary to locate the main building of the Kiyomizu Shrine in Kyoto exactly on a node of positive chi.

Below: Birthing stones in Hawaii are located on nodes of positive chi energy in the earth.

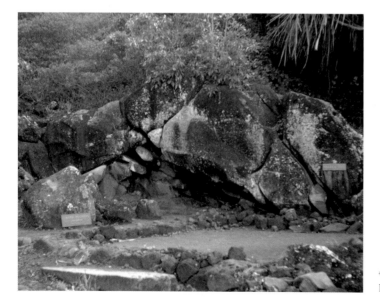

DIVINATION IN LOCATING RELIGIOUS STRUCTURES

Temple records in Japan and other countries describe the use of divination or dowsing in selecting the location of temples and other religious structures. The goal was to locate them on favorable power spots of earth energy or chi. The Kiyomizu Temple in Kyoto is possibly one of the most dramatic examples of the results. The temple location on the edge of a steep hillside necessitated construction of a massive timber substructure to support the building. The results indicate its worth; over the generations, the popularity and fortunes of the temple have remained strong, while those of other temples and shrines throughout the region have fluctuated with the times. All who visit this temple leave with their spirits uplifted, peaceful, and with a full heart.

Dowsing measurements of churches and cathedrals in Europe show that they also were typically located at power spots; often on the site of previous religious structures. Traditional sites used by Hawaiian villagers for giving birth are located on nodes of healing energy in the earth, and Neolithic religious sites around the world have retained their strong energetic power over thousands of years.

An extensive study was performed by Blanche Merz of the energetics of religious structures in different cultures.[42] She made the

---

[42] Blanche Merz, POINTS OF COSMIC ENERGY, C.W. Daniel Co. Ltd., 1983, 1995.

interesting discovery that there is more variation between the energy levels of churches or temples of one religion and those in another tradition than there is between different structures in the same tradition. Energetically strong Christian churches measured consistently around 11,000 units, while Islamic mosques (regardless of geographic situation) gave a reading of 12,000, and Hindu temples most frequently registered around 14,000. Unique specific spots, such as the labyrinth at Chartres cathedral and the pharaonic initiation points in Egyptian temples, measured as high as 18,000 units. Interestingly, certain prestigious places such as Florence, Westminster, Cologne, and Rheims Cathedrals lacked this siting on an energetic node or "power spot."

✧

This sampling of energetic practices from different cultures suggests the intense attention that has been given throughout history to the role of our energetic surroundings in our nurture and health. It tells us that there is sound basis to our developing similar practices in our own culture, and gives both specific approaches that can be adopted to our needs and inspiration to develop new and even more moving ways to deepen connections to our inner and outer worlds.

Our unique opportunity today is one of gathering in, sorting out, and amalgamating this richness of techniques and adding our own unique achievements to develop a comprehensive science of the sacred in our surroundings.

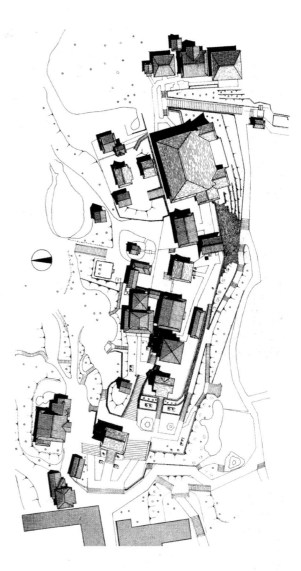

Plan of the Kiyomizu Shrine in Koyto, showing alignment of the temple structures along the edge of a ridge. The steps next to the main shrine building go down to a sacred spring at the bottom of the hill. A gentle "yin" return walkway from the spring balances the strongly "yang" main structure.

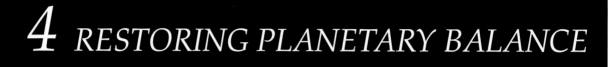

4 *RESTORING PLANETARY BALANCE*

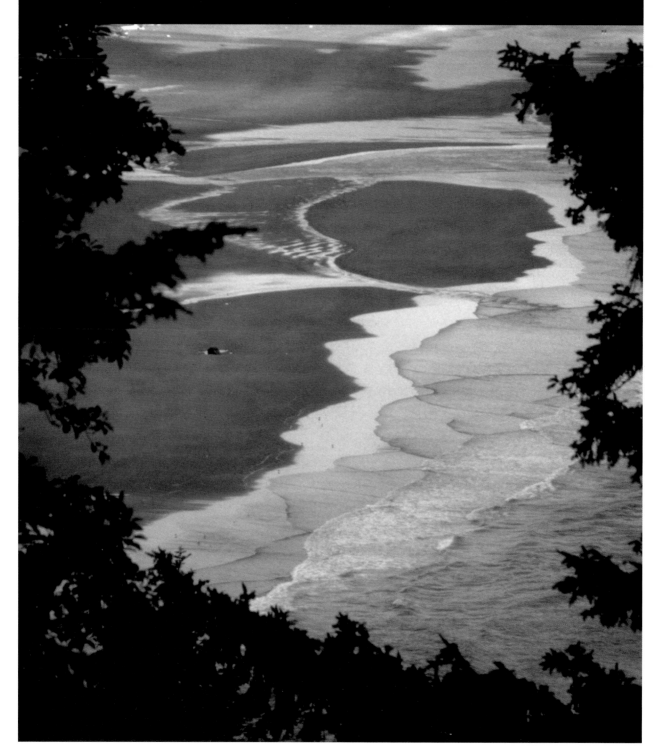

AN EVOLUTIONARY PERSPECTIVE ON CHANGE

Chi opens vital missing perspectives on the nature and operation of our world. Not surprisingly, those perspectives are the very ones needed to restore balance to our society and bring it into alignment with principles that are sustainable and nurturing to our selves, our society, and our planet. A brief look at our present evolutionary status suggests that the universe of chi may offer needed and valuable resolution to many of our present problems.

Boredom, frustration, a feeling that what we're doing doesn't matter – that we don't seem to be capable of doing something, that everything is going to hell anyway . . . by the time we get older, we've experienced these symptoms enough times to recognize them as the precursors of major change – of a leap into a new dimension of being. We've seen it in ourselves and in others. We've seen that frustration in children – learning to crawl, walk, talk, do algebra. Something new is fomenting, is almost together; we know we *should* be able to do it, but the spark hasn't caught yet. Being cranky and hard to live with usually accompanies this stage. As the old saying goes, "It's always darkest just before dawn."

It's worth considering the possibility that our whole culture is in one of those "labor pains" periods. Evolution *hasn't* stopped. Our present condition is unlikely to be the final and immutable endpoint at which all evolution has arrived. If this kind of major change were happening on a societal level, what symptoms might we look for?

One sure sign of change is dissatisfaction with the way things are. Implicit in that is a conscious or unconscious sense of something *better* to which we are already comparing the present. Another sign is when people adamantly and emotionally take divergent positions about how to deal with present "problems." That reflects a strong consensus of the need for change, without having yet achieved consensus on a viewpoint to direct that change. Yet another sign is the fragmented emergence of elements of that "new something" around us.

We know we have reached the nexus of change when a clear vision of how and why things could be better coalesces, and consensus starts to form around it. That may well be the case today with chi or life-force energy, as piece after piece of its role in generating a new perspective of life appears, offering us a higher level of

When we see the interconnected ebb and flow of relationships between things, we begin to pay attention to the fullness of both the costs and benefits of our own interactions. This "whole-systems" view (though it transcends the measurable and material) gives birth to a whole new perspective on economics, and order-of-magnitude improvements in the effectiveness of our actions.

integration of the new information we are discovering on how things connect and operate.

Our "now" seems to be in such a nexus! Viewed from a "cultural break-down" perspective, our divorce rates are frightening, leading to punitive attempts to stuff Jack (or Jackie) back into the Box. But from an evolutionary perspective, we are demanding far *more* out of marriage. Caroline Myss says it well in *Anatomy of the Spirit*:

> . . . *most contemporary marriages require a strong sense of "self" for success, rather than the abdication of "self" that was required in traditional marriages. . . Many people ascribe the breakdown of their marriage to the fact that their spouse had given them no support for their emotional, psychological, and intellectual needs, and as a result they had to seek out a true partnership.*[1]

Robert Gilman, editor of *In Context* magazine, sees us in evolutionary transition from empire to a planetary cultural period. He describes changes – in geographic organization, hierarchy, economic base, and beliefs – as great as those that occurred during the change between our tribal and empire periods. He talks about why our old institutions can't handle the "juice" of new levels of operation. The significant changes are occurring totally outside of existing institutions, which are therefore unable to grasp or track the transformation. Today, for example, while we busily track gross production in the monetary economy, we manage to ignore what is happening to our natural, human, and social capital.

Our beliefs, dreams, and fears, and the actual governance of society, are changing even more rapidly than our technology. It is these lead changes that are already coalescing around new organizing views of our world.[2]

Energetics – application of chi-based perspectives in different aspects of our lives – plays a key role in this evolutionary shift now underway, appearing to fulfill the pivotal role of providing a better model of how our universe operates and what our role is in it. Energetics of place has an important role to play in healing us and reconnecting us with other life. Take it as an old vision or a new one. Take it as clarified, confirmed, reforged. Take it merged with, reintegrating, and giving new meaning to the rational/individualistic developments that have given strength to our present culture. However we view it, it is providing an operative vision with far more power, inclusiveness, and success than other viewpoints we have held for a long while.

CHANGING DIMENSIONS OF GROWTH

Several factors are nudging our more rapid adoption of energetics. It provides a vehicle for resolving intractable problems we have developed, while bringing us a far more desirable quality of life in the process. These factors bringing forth the need for energetics are the Four Horsemen of Our Material Apocalypse: *Oil Depletion, Resource Exhaustion, Ecological Damage,* and *Growth in Population and Material Demands. The spirits they ride are Hopelessness, Hate, Intolerance,* and *Aggression.*

[1] Caroline Myss, ANATOMY OF THE SPIRIT, Harmony Books, 1996.

[2] Robert Gilman, Plenary Talk, HOPES '97 Conference, University of Oregon School of Architecture and Allied Arts.

Simply put, the days *of our present patterns are numbered.*[3] We currently put more than 50% of the net products of photosynthesis on the planet to human use.[4] All that energy goes to only *one* of the millions of species whose complex interactions are essential to the stability of our supporting ecosystems. Within the next 35 years, if nothing were to change, population and consumption growth[5] would push that to over 100%. The likelihood of even approaching this without total ecological collapse is somewhat slim.

The "ecological footprint" of the land area necessary to supply our urban areas with food, forestry products, and energy already exceeds what can sustainably be maintained without our current subsidy from fossil fuel reserves. The Netherlands, for example, requires 14 times the nation's entire land area to provide and import produce to meet their consumption, while the U.S. consumes 80% more than could possibly be produced without fossil fuels by converting *all* ecologically productive land to human use.[6]

Continuation of present growth patterns is expected to exhaust worldwide oil reserves in the next 25 to 50 years.[7] Petroleum economists and geophysicists now solidly project that worldwide petroleum production will peak in the next five to ten years and be virtually exhausted in the next 50 years.[8] *When* we finally run out of oil – that very last drop – turns out not to be an important issue. What is important is what happens *when* and after *oil production peaks*, which is happening right now.

"Peaking" is the point where population and demand for oil continue to increase, while oil production can no longer be increased for technical and political reasons. It is where a permanent and dramatic shift occurs from the buyer's market we have enjoyed (as cheap as you can pump it) to a seller's market (as expensive as you can push it). It brings a permanent skyrocketing of oil prices. It is the point where the oil available per capita (the twenty "energy slaves" each of us have that have constituted much of our material wealth[9]) begins a rapid shift from a flood to a trickle as demand escalates and production dwindles. Actual "exhaustion" of our oil reserves, in contrast, occurs long after the trickle becomes so small that the timing of that "last drop" is irrelevant.

[3] For more detail, see my "It's Oil Right, Folks! There's Good Times Ahead," www.oikos.com/seao/tbender.

[4] Extrapolated from Vitousek, Erlichs, and Matson, "Human Appropriation of the Products of Photosynthesis", BIOSCIENCE 36: 368-74,1986.

[5] Population growth is not someone else's problem. See my *"Their* Population, *Our* Problem," Nov. 1996.

[6] Wackernagel and Rees, OUR ECOLOGICAL FOOTPRINT, New Society Books, 1995.

[7] See, for example, L. F. Ivanhoe's important article, "Future world oil supplies: there is a finite limit," WORLD OIL, Oct. 1995. Also Ivanhoe, "Oil Reserves and Semantics," NEWSLETTER OF THE M. KING HUBBERT CENTER FOR PETROLEUM SUPPLY STUDIES, Colorado School of Mines, Aug. 1996; and James MacKenzie, "Oil as a Finite Resource," WORLD RESOURCES INSTITUTE, March 1996.

[8] Oil production would have peaked in 1992-93, except that the 1974 "Oil Crisis" brought significant restriction in Mideast production and initiated development of energy-efficient technologies.

[9] The easily available oil we have been using can do about twenty times the work it takes us to obtain it. Someone farming without oil fertilizers and fuels, for example, has to compete with a work source that gets wages only 1/20 of what we need!

As we use up high grade ores of mineral resources, the energy needed to obtain and process lower grade ores skyrockets. Several studies indicate that U.S. resource demands would have to be reduced approximately 80% to achieve sustainability without our current fossil fuel subsidies.[10] Meanwhile, the ecologically productive land area available per capita is dramatically decreasing as we convert farmland to cities and other uses. With less fossil fuels, more land is needed to produce fuels, fertilizers, and replace industrial feedstocks now made from oil. Our population thus already exceeds what can be supported at our present consumption levels as oil depletes.

The Limits to Growth model projected that world grain production would peak in 1994. But *per-capita* grain production actually peaked in 1984, and has been steadily declining since.[11] Ocean fishery production peaked in 1989 and is declining rapidly. Similar limits are be being reached in ore-grade metals, water, and other resources.[12]

Increased virulence, resistance, and mutability of human disease vectors is being reported at the same time that population density, mobility and potential susceptibility are increasing.[13] Extreme weather fluctuations and consequent damage to crops and buildings are already occurring, corresponding with predictions of early impacts of global warming trends. Larger impact of these trends is expected over the next decades. Last year, for the first time, all five of the most respected global climate warming models – both public and private – agreed. The insurance industry, faced with record payouts, is quickly becoming one of the more urgent voices for change.

Together, these indices suggest that significant change is imminent and unavoidable. *The good news is that we are now discovering that the changes involved can be significantly for the better.* Every study done on energy efficiency indicates that it makes economic sense regardless of social goals. *Immense economic savings are possible when we do shift from growth to sustainability.*

What we've grown used to and have forgotten is that *growth itself is incredibly expensive:*

> *INFRASTRUCTURE COSTS:* We currently spend 33% to 40% of our time and resources on creating the infrastructure to accommodate more people and things.[14] Stabilizing growth totally avoids these current expenditures. A population doubling means duplicating our entire stock of houses, water systems, power plants, cities, roads - as well as prematurely demolishing existing ones. It also means spending more on feeding and educating those additional people to adulthood.

---

[10] Personal communications from Friends of the Earth, Washington, D.C. See also FOE- Europe data on European needs.

[11] Gilman, above, and Worldwatch Institute

[12] Conference presentations by Prof. Al Bartlett, Univ. of Colorado, and others.

[13] See, for example, Jeffrey A. Fisher's THE PLAGUE MAKERS, Simon & Schuster, 1994.

[14] At this time we can estimate that a doubling to tripling of society's total capital expenditures occurs (plus a 50% increase in consumptive expenditures) for *population* doubling alone, without counting expansion in consumption.

COSTS OF INEQUITY: Growth has been touted as necessary "to help the poor." In actuality, growth over the last twenty years has dramatically worsened the condition of the poor and increased the concentration of our wealth among the rich.[15] Conscious government policy has concentrated wealth to the point where one percent of the population now owns 50% of all our wealth. The median U.S. household income for wage-earners is currently $31,000, with more than 13% of households under the monetary poverty level of $15,000. In contrast, an *equal* distribution of personal income would amount to $59,000 per household.[16]

If we accepted the current median income level of $31,000 per household instead of the $59,000/household which would come from sharing wealth equally, we could *both* eliminate poverty and reduce resource demands. Because of the immense current imbalance in wealth, a $31,000 income for all households would surprisingly need 47% *less* work, and equivalently fewer resources than we now use to maintain poverty and inequality!

DEBT FINANCING COSTS: To achieve growth, we have also developed the habit of paying for personal expenditures, corporate expansion, and governmental infrastructure through debt purchasing (credit cards, government bonds, and bank loans). That debt purchasing has resulted in an across-the-board 20% surcharge on our cost of living, without any substantive benefit.[17]

Together, stabilizing growth and dealing directly with the inequality in our society can permanently release us from almost 75% of our present energy, material, financial, and human costs of living, without lowering our material living standard and without a need for any "technical fixes."[18]

Said another way, greed and growth alone currently *quadruple* our cost of living.[19] These already immense costs will skyrocket as we approach the limits of growth.

---

[15] See, for example, Keith Bradsher's "Gulf widens between wealthy and poor," NEW YORK TIMES NEWS SERVICE, April 20, 1995; also Ravi Batra's THE GREAT DEPRESSION OF 1990, (1987), and Edward Wolff's Twentieth Century Fund report, TOP HEAVY, (1995).

[16] $5,702 billion total personal income; 248,710,000 population; 2.63-person household size. Similar figures occur using national income.

[17] For example, interest paid on national debt in 1994 equaled 20.3% of federal outlays (with no capital repayment). Consumer credit outstanding in 1994 equaled $985 billion – 19.9% of disposable personal income and 17% of national income – roughly equally distributed between auto, home, and revolving credit. Finance, and related fields constituted 22% of national income. For more detail on the illusory benefits of these financial shell-games, see my 1993 "Borrowing Trouble," 1990 "Endgames, and my 1984 "Hidden Costs of Housing."

[18] For further discussion of *how* to achieve these benefits, see my 1996 "Some Questions We Haven't Asked."

[19] Without growth, our needed expenditures would be 60% (present expenditures less growth infrastructure costs) x 53% (subtracting costs of inequity) x 80% (subtracting costs of debt financing) = only 25% of current expenditures needed.

SYSTEM INEFFICIENCY COSTS: Our belief in an endless cornucopia of resources and wealth has also caused us to ignore care and efficiency in all of our institutional structures, production processes, and living patterns. The result is that they have developed almost inconceivable waste – which now represents an equally great opportunity for improved effectiveness and efficiency.

Well-documented research over the last twenty years has shown, and is beginning to produce, a 90% reduction in energy and resources needed in almost every sector of society.[20, 21]

When we put these four opportunities together, they add up to ways to reduce our resource consumption, ecological impact, and use of our time considerably more than appears needed to achieve sustainability.[22, 23]

This overview has looked at these issues briefly and in isolation. In reality, they are interactive. Some provide resource savings but not financial or employment ones. Others, as in any ecological system, involve multiple, interactive effects and savings.[24]

Most importantly, the possible savings are far more than enough to totally transform a once-frightening prospect of change into an opportunity for significant betterment of our lives.[25]

Curiously, just making efficiency improvements – without dealing with the underlying values of greed, growth, and violence – can only worsen the problems. Twenty-five years down the road, it would result in our having twice the

---

[20] It's now more than 27 years since I first showed that these order-of-magnitude changes were possible in "Living Lightly: Energy Conservation in Housing," 1973. See Lovins and von Weizsäcker, FACTOR FOUR: Doubling Productivity, Halving Resource Use, Earthscan, 1997 and Lovins and Hawken's NATURAL CAPITALISM, 1999, for current work by others. These principles have now received public commitment from the governments of Austria, the Netherlands, and Norway, as well as endorsement by the European Union, the World Business Council for Sustainable Development, and UNEP.   My "Living Lightly," 1973; "Hidden Costs of Housing," 1984; "Amazon Married Student Housing," 1994; "Economic Value of Coastal Forest Lands," 1994; "Bamberton," 1993; "Vitality and Affordability of Higher Education," 1993; and "Transforming Tourism," 1993, showing potentials in several sectors, are available at <http://users.knsi.com/~tbender>. In regard to buildings, see also the many progress reports of the Rocky Mountain Institute, 1739 Snowmass Creek Rd., Snowmass, CO 81654; work of the Center for Maximum Potential Building Systems, 8604 F.M. 969, Austin, TX 78724; and John Todd's work with biological water purification at Center for the Restoration of Waters, One Locust Street, Falmouth, MA 02540.

[21] For corporate and insurance-industry responses to these conditions, contact The Natural Step, <www.emis.com/tns> or (415)332-9394, or Rocky Mountain Institute <www.rmi.org> or (970) 927-3851.

[22] Based on preliminary Friends of the Earth studies on European and U.S. economies. See also Bill Rees' excellent "Ecological Footprints and Appropriated Carrying Capacity . . ." in INVESTING IN NATURAL CAPITAL, Island Press, 1994, or "Revising Carrying Capacity . . ." in POPULATION AND ENVIRONMENT: A JOURNAL OF INTERDISCIPLINARY STUDIES, Jan, 1996.

[23] For some of the other non-technical, big-jump opportunities, see my "Some Questions," above.

[24] See Amory Lovins, "The Super-Efficient Passive Building Frontier," ASHRAE JOURNAL, June, 1995 for an outstanding example of the interactive and cumulative benefits of energy efficiency in minimizing building operating costs.

[25] See "Building Real Wealth," above; and "Shedding A Skin . . ."

population, fewer resources, and a lost opportunity for re-leasing resources out of our operating patterns to finance a transition to sustainability.[26]

THE NON-ECONOMIC BENEFITS OF SUSTAINABILITY

The real rewards of sustainable communities, how-ever, go far beyond the material ones inherent in resource-efficient buildings, transit-oriented land use, and renewable energy sources. The true benefits of a sustainable society lie in the totally different dimensions of meaning, and con-nection that give such a society its cohesion, meaning and enduring value.[27] From those dimensions, we quickly be-gin to see the true costs of current cultural practices.

Our *true* wealth does not lie in the monetary realm. The source of our real wealth is not depletion of our re-sources, increase in our numbers, or taking from others. As I indicated in *Building Real Wealth*:

> *A truly wealthy individual* is one who has the love and respect of others and the ability to give; equitable opportunity for the physical, emotional, and spiritual health which the natural world can sustain; and opportunity to develop and employ their abilities and to be of real value to the community.

> *A truly wealthy community* is one with a meaningful sense of its place in the universe; a healthy and growing diversity of capabilities, individuals, and life forms; and a satisfying spiritual, emotional, and material heritage, life, and prospect.

> *A truly wealthy world* is one with a healthy and growing diversity of life forms, communities, and capabilities. With this awareness, we can find far more direct and effective ways of maintaining and nurturing our wealth.[28]

None of this wealth requires *taking* from other people or other life. It, in fact, requires the opposite: our *giving to* and sustaining others. A community, for example, which decides to make itself beautiful and interesting, and "make where

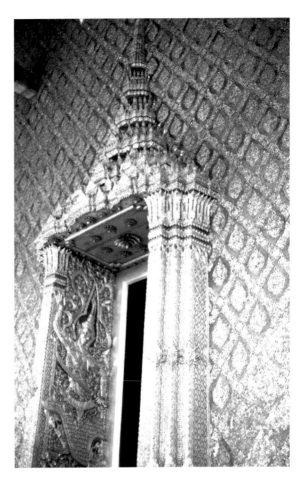

Gifts that come from a fullness of heart and life deplete nobody, and enrich the life of all.

---

[26] There *is* an urgency to this issue. See, for example, L.F. Ivanhoe's "Future World Oil Supplies; there is a finite limit," WORLD OIL, Oct., 1995 on global oil and population trends, and Richard Duncan's 1995 "The Energy Depletion Arch . . ." on U.S. and global oil depletion. Ivanhoe also touches on the falsification beginning to occur in government statistical studies as our denial of resource depletion becomes more acute. Duncan also projects nearly 100% control of petroleum exports by Muslim countries by 2010, with significant political implications.

[27] See, for example, "Shedding A Skin . . ." above; and "Transforming Tourism," EARTH ETHICS, Summer 1993. For values, see my "Sharing Smaller Pies," NEW AGE JOURNAL, Nov. 1975; THE FUTURIST, 1976; RESETTLING AMERICA, Gary Coates, ed. 1981; and UTNE READER, Fall ,1987. Also Lovins and von Weizsächer's FACTOR FOUR, and Lovins and Hawken's NATURAL CAPITALISM, 1999.

[28] Tom Bender, "Building Real Wealth," 1993. Reprinted in IN CONTEXT, July 1996.

we ARE paradise," can easily make major reductions in the need for both daily and vacation travel while making everyone happier in the process.

Not only our wealth, but also our well-being, lies outside the world of dollars. Some dimensions of that well-being affected by a move to sustainability are:

CURING DISEASES OF THE SPIRIT
As mentioned earlier, our most daunting and seemingly unconnected social problems today stem directly from following the beacons of greed and growth. Unemployment, drug addiction, abuse, crime, obesity, and mental and psychological illness – all are symptoms of a single cultural *disease of the spirit*. They are all temptations present in every society. We fall prey to them through the lack of self-esteem, mutual respect, and being of value to each other and our community inherent in our material, greed, and power-centered culture.

The number of people unable to function in our society is growing rapidly: people destroyed by lack of love, not being valued, absence of opportunity; and by the resultant abuse and drug and alcohol addiction. They, in turn, create non-functional families, compounding the damage. To our great danger, we neglect the human, psychological, emotional, spiritual, and communal dimensions of life.

To be sustainable, a community must nurture – not neglect – the emotional and spiritual well-being of all. The nature of its work, institutions, and all interactions must nurture self-esteem, mutual respect, and being of value to each other and the community. The principles of equity, security, sustainability, responsibility, giving, and sacredness are the healing path for these central diseases of the spirit, and living from the heart the way to act upon them.[29]

LIFE WITHOUT FEAR
Within a world of apparent material plenty, it is curious the degree to which life is filled with fear and worry: fear of abuse, mugging, rape, murder; fear of job loss, age, death; fear of auto accidents, plane crashes, hurricanes, floods; fear of inadequacy, failure, nuclear war, crippling disease; worry about what the future may hold, or what it may not.

In a community where we each care about, honor, and ensure the well-being of all life – where life is based on equity rather than greed, where we don't have to hide our fears and struggle alone – life gains a security and fullness unknown in a society of greed and growth. When the primary causes of violence and the reasons to fear others are minimized, and violence itself is not valued, positive relations are possible. Where we identify with the well-being of all creation, the larger climatic, geologic, and evolutionary patterns of nature are seen and honored from within a different understanding. True security comes from equitable access to non-depletable resources, a stable supporting ecosystem, and a real community to provide for our needs and ensure the emotional health of all.

The life-nurturing values and principles upon which sustainable communities are based result in freedom from the most emotionally crippling dimensions of a society based on greed and growth.

---

[29] See my HEART OF PLACE, Dec., 1993, for how these manifest in one aspect of society.

AN ECONOMY OF GIVING, NOT TAKING

The economics of a sustainable community is far different from that of a greed- and growth-centered one. It employs full accounting of social and ecological costs, and restricts its resource use to renewable ones in sustainable quantities. Instead of single-focus engineering analyses, it employs a multi-focused ecological one, keeping intact the connectedness of things and knowing that a real solution to a problem doesn't exist unless it also helps resolve other problems.

Sustainable economics embodies the true value of *sharing* – of allowing multiple beneficiaries of a single action or product. It accounts for the gifts of the rest of creation that provide for our needs, and for our need to provide for the well-being of others in return. It eliminates the false distinction between work and leisure, to restore freedom and giving to our work. It looks at meaningful rewards for all we do with all our time.[30]

Even more centrally, a sustainable community has an economics of *giving*, not of *taking*. Giving is an integral part of loving, and loving is the root of holding the sacred as essential to sustainability. It enriches both the giver and the receiver, and creates multiple value out of every exchange. If "What can I give in this situation?" is in our hearts every time we interact with someone, we not only leave a legacy of gifts, but we generate an enduring climate of trust, mutual caring, thankfulness, and happiness which moves outward like ripples.[31]

The gift economy of a community based on love and honoring provides multiple benefits: it fulfills our emotional as well as material needs, while supplying the glue of trust essential to any enduring relationship.

LIVING FROM THE HEART

Excess material wealth, inequity, and lack of concern for the rest of life poison our souls. Taking from rather than *caring for* others closes off our hearts. Closing ourselves off from the pain we cause obscures the connectedness that gives life meaning. It sentences us to a meaningless existence of psychological and emotional barrenness. The only thing that can alleviate this pain is love – and opening ourselves to the vulnerability and pain of allowing love even in the face of our unloving behavior.[32]

A world where everyone wears masks, hides their feelings, and closes off connection with what lies outside their skin leads quickly to collective insanity. We grow up thinking we're odd because we're not happy, when all we are seeing is the masks that hide the feelings of inadequacy, unhappiness, anger, and confusion of others. We close ourselves off from the flow of energy that generates, pervades, and nurtures all life, with resulting illness and atrophy of our own lives.

---

[30] See "Characteristics of a Sustainable Society," below, for more detail, and my HEART OF PLACE, or E.F. Schumacher's "Buddhist Economics" in SMALL IS BEAUTIFUL, 1974; or in my ENVIRONMENTAL DESIGN PRIMER, 1973.

[31] See my "Sewage is Art —The Healing of Place with Chi," June 1995, for what happens when we apply this to a building project.

[32] See my "Shedding a Skin That No Longer Fits," March, 1996, for a deeper discussion.

As energetics reminds us, the truth is that *we can't lie*. Our super-conscious interconnectedness knows the difference between what comes from the heart and what comes from the head. In the absence of experiencing living from the heart, we mistake our own masks and those of others for the underlying reality.

The actions necessary to move from a world of greed and violence to one of generosity and giving are simple and can be initiated by any of us: speak from the heart; let down our masks; be willing to be vulnerable; open our hearts to others; honor and hold all life sacred; deal with the roots of our fears; learn to give; seek wisdom and joy, not power.

These changes involve humility, trust, and vulnerability; facing and dealing with pain and its causes; dealing directly with hard questions of equity and fairness; and a 180-degree shift in the goals and operation of every aspect of our society.

When we speak from the heart, we speak truth – our own truth. It may not be a universal truth, but it is a real truth grown out of the unique life and experience of each of us. I can take your truth and add it to mine, and find a greater one. You can do the same with me. Your fear of losing a job if we cut back on overlogging or wasteful oil use is as real as my fear of a bigger collapse if we don't. In the open, we can take each of these truths and bring them together into more inclusive solutions that encompass both.

Speaking from the heart, we can touch real issues, fight real demons, and make real progress. We can achieve true consensus and group support for all actions. With that, we lose all patience with the invisible walls created by our conventional patterns and rituals of conferences and meetings and confrontations that prevent real progress.

Living from the heart is the essence of true connection needed for sustainable and effective interpersonal relationships. It yields both the opportunity for others to understand and give to us, and for us to find right action in our interaction with others. It helps us gain the true rewards of self-esteem, mutual respect, and being of value to the community for our efforts – not just the material substitutes we settle for today.

SACRED SURROUNDINGS

Living in a sacred way transforms our surroundings as well as our lives. Not promoting consumption removes advertising from busses, billboards, and the public eye. Living from the heart transforms our cities to reflect the wealth of passions, not inner poverty. Putting our effort into *better* rather than *more*, our cities can – like Prague or Paris – come to reflect the culmination of a thousand years of love poured into the places where we live.[33]

Learning to honor all of Creation gives all of Creation an honored place in our surroundings – trees for *trees*, not trees for shade or cooling or recreation parks. Shrines and places of silence provide space to express thanks, to connect deeply with the rest of creation, to honor the special power and energy of a place; they allow our surroundings to express the sacredness with which we hold them.

---

[33] See my "Sacred Roots of Sustainable Design," Sept. 1995.

Living in a sacred way, our surroundings become sacred to us, and reflect the sacred values underlying our lives. They take on layer after layer of meaning and value, and become loved and inviolate in their own right. At the same time, they give power and strength to our lives and direct our actions into healthy paths. There is no way, as Chief Seattle said, that we can treat our surroundings without reverence when the earth itself is composed of the ashes of our ancestors.

CHANGE FROM A LEGAL TO A SACRED SOCIETY

Our society has been based on a legalistic structure – of limited commitments easy to break. In that kind of system, those who embrace greed receive tremendous rewards. As a result, endless regulations are inevitable to even partly control the damage. The only true alternative is to find a basis for our lives and actions that makes harmful action inconceivable and rare, rather than the rule. Only simple regulations are then needed to embody and convey consensus on right action. That basis for our lives must be a sacred one.

Why a sacred basis of society? As mentioned in the first chapter, nothing less than that – our holding sacred the health of our surroundings and the well-being of all life – will ensure that we act strongly enough or soon enough to ensure that health and well-being.

When we spend time with someone we love, we quickly realize that our happiness is affected if the person we love is dissatisfied or unhappy. Their happiness is our delight, and their lack of happiness quickly shadows our own. That is the glue of life and the essence of holding something sacred – not laws and government regulations. All follows from that love.

Honor ourselves. Honor others. Honor all life.

When we honor life, the absurdity of an agriculture based on violent and futile pesticides becomes obvious, as does that of a medical system based on primary use of biocides to attempt to kill parts of the web of life that sustains us. We learn, rather, to deal with *causes* of the imbalances that allow uncontrolled growth of one part of life.

A basis for social interaction that nurtures rather than drains, tied to creating happiness rather than fighting, creates good and creates wealth for society through its process as well as its products. Its greater effectiveness in managing society's resources is merely a bonus.

LIFE WITHOUT FAILURE

Improvisational drumming is different from traditional western music in a particularly interesting way. Traditional Western music has a *right* sequence of notes and a *right* way of playing. Improvisational drumming has *no* right sequence. Once entrained by the beat, drumming leads us without conscious effort to be part of the shared rhythm, and blesses us with the inability to do "wrong." With any improvisational music, variations we make within it only enrich the music and make it respond to the immediacy of time and place within which it is occurring.

The music breaks only when we fail to incorporate whatever happens into it. One "wrong note" is an error; it stands out that we didn't mean it. But if we repeat it, however odd it may have been – embrace it and draw it in, acknowledge

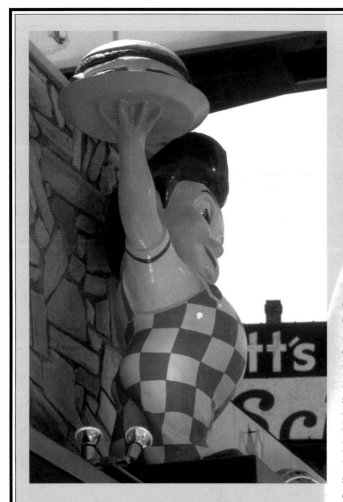

LETTING GO OF A GREEDY WORLD

What we can do with the energy of a place depends on our own personal energy. Change us, change our world. I remember trying and trying to "get out of" our greedy culture. I felt I was at the edge of a gaping chasm I had to jump across to get to a world based on love and giving. Then one morning I woke up giggling. In my sleep I had seen myself standing on the broken and patched-together pedestal of our culture. I felt it crumble and give way, and started to fill with fear. . . . But nothing happened. I looked down, puzzled. There, amidst the broken remnants of our culture, stood the rock-solid foundation of nature and life which had underlain and actually supported us all along. All I had needed to do was *let go!* Here are a couple of exercises you can try:

Sit comfortably, ground and center. Close your eyes. Visualize yourself working at a rewarding job, which is giving you self-esteem, a chance to develop and apply your gifts, and to contribute to your community. Focus on how that feels inside. Then visualize yourself sick, or needing some kind of help, and people in your community appearing and lovingly giving you that help. Then visualize yourself giving in that way to others. Focus on how it feels.

Now, keeping that feeling inside you, visualize yourself in some part of our culture that feels wrong or makes you very uncomfortable. See yourself sitting in a forest as it is being clear-cut; on a mountain being ripped open to strip-mine coal; in a jail; in a school; in a traffic jam on a freeway. Touch base with the feelings that arise in you. Then go back to the touchstone of rightness, fullness, and well-being from visualizing the rewarding job. Let the other anger, frustration, emptiness, sense of wrongness slide off of you, not sticking or leaving any residue. See it melt into the earth, soaked up by the life of the soil, broken down and transformed into new potentials. Keep that sense of rootedness in a rewarding world with you, as you start – piece by piece – to affirm it in your life. Keep that separateness and untouchability from the greedy culture with you, too. When we feed anger or other emotions into an institution, we acknowledge and give it power over us. Without our response, it withers.

Or: Visualize yourself walking down a street. Looking around as you walk, visualize what random acts of kindness and senseless acts of beauty you could perform there. Open your heart and smile at that person who looks like they need a ray of sunshine? Pick up that trash? Plant a tree there, where some shade would be welcome? Make a simple bench for people to sit on? Leave a pot of flowers at the door of some lonely person? Pay attention to how you feel as you act through each of these in your mind. Try one in real life.

Or: Visualize yourself going into a store to do some shopping. Look at the price tags. Do you see things like $19.95; or 3.6oz. for 97¢; or "On Sale;" or "Real Juice Flavor?" Our whole pricing system is based on deceit – confusing buyers, implying that $19.95 is significantly less than $20; giving prices and quantities that make real cost calculation difficult; pretending that everyday prices are really special deals; making you think that a product contains more of something than it really does. Every time we shop or make a purchase, we are literally buying into a world based on deceit.

Now visualize shopping where: the real contents are obvious; prices are round numbers, full dollars – $20 ea. or 10# for $2; where there isn't limitless duplication of irrelevantly-differentiated products to have to choose between. Where a customer is honored, their choices made easy, and their purchases worth making. How do you feel? Keep these feelings inside you as a touchstone and foundation as you expand that new world, from which you can act to make real change in the energy of our surroundings.

it and incorporate it – it becomes part of the path of the music. It sets the participants a new challenge, and sets the music off in a new direction – a good way to approach life, too, perhaps.

All participatory music makes it clear that paying to hear the best performer in the world cannot match the joy of *being part* of making the music, or the dance, or the song. Taking part gives pleasure – to us and to others at the same time. It gives us full-body experience, learning, and catharsis. It leaves us with self-esteem rather than a feeling of inferiority and of never being able to equal the professional. It gives us the value of enjoyment, beauty, and pleasure inherent in the rhythms of life, without money, skill, or fancy equipment. What a wonderful model for life: a way of living designed for *success*, not failure!

"Fail-proof" patterns of work and relationships are inherent parts of achieving sustainability. They restore self-esteem, heal emotional damage, and teach us to honor and know ourselves as a vital part of life and of the goals we pursue.

THE PRIMACY OF INNER RESOURCES

Limited material resources make us aware of the power and value of our inner resources. We've forgotten what many of them are: *will, courage, giving, endurance, anger, fear, love, curiosity, passion, intuition, resolution, resistance, wisdom, cunning, compulsion, restraint, joy, wit, hopefulness, rashness, caution, wonder, pride, humility, gratitude, forgiveness* – to name but a few.

Use of these resources involves us *personally* in the act of creating. It gives the tangible rewards of self-esteem, confidence, and community respect for our accomplishments. In many fields, the wise use of inner resources is far more vital to accomplishment than any material resources.

These resources acknowledge that our emotions are vital dimensions of living from our hearts – dimensions to be respected and used as guides and sources of energy, not brushed aside in favor of what comes only from our heads. They acknowledge the power and value of our inherent ties with others and with all life. They connect us with magic and the power that lies outside the limits of the rational.

*The patterns of life and interaction in a sustainable community give continual reminder that **we,** and the strengths within each of us, are one of the most vital resources of our society and planet. Our challenge is to develop them rather than ignoring them in preference for limited material resources.*

✦

These non-monetary dimensions of change alter our inner beings. They also resonate with a comment made in a book about South African Archbishop Desmund TuTu:

> *We Africans speak about a concept difficult to render in English. We speak of "ubuntu" or "botho." You know when it is there, and it is obvious when it is absent. It has to do with what it means to be truly human. It refers to gentleness, to compassion, to hospitality, to openness to others, to vulnerability,*

to being available for others and to knowing that you are bound up with them in the bundle of life, for a person is only a person through other persons.[34]

These same characteristics distinguish what it is like to live as part of a sacred and empowering world, in absolute contrast to the characteristics of life in a world of greed and self-centeredness.

CHARACTERISTICS OF AN ENDURING SOCIETY

There is a web of actions necessary to ensure that our society is rooted in and fully embodies such qualities:

EQUITY:
* To ensure that all people have equitable access to – and share of – wealth, health, income, security, education, opportunity, respect, political power, and fulfilling work.
* To ensure that all life has scope to ensure well-being and development of its innate capabilities.

SECURITY:
* To remove the inequities of power, self-esteem, opportunity, resource access, and emotional health that engender fear and insecurity.
* To affirm that biosystem health, a lasting supply of world resources, and the capabilities of human and global systems – not material consumption rates – constitute our real wealth. To act to ensure and improve the health and capabilities of these resources.

SUSTAINABILITY:
* To stabilize and restore population to supportable levels commensurate with the well-being of all life.
* To draw materials and energy only from renewable sources and at rates which can be maintained without loss or harm.
* To work within those energy- and material-use levels to both improve our non-material quality of life and more effectively provide for our material needs.

RESPONSIBILITY:
* To enact full ecological analysis to ensure public knowledge of the true costs of our actions.
* To live within our maintainable incomes; not take from future generations and other life, and to ensure them undiminished opportunity for fulfillment.
* To ensure that all industrial producers assume eternal responsibility for the products and byproducts they create.
* To protect, preserve, and prevent destruction of farm, forest, aquatic, and other natural resources.
* To protect local natural, cultural, and spiritual resources until all jurisdictions restore and enhance their own to levels that meet the needs of their populations.

---

[34] Shirley DuBoulay, TUTU, ARCHBISHOP WITHOUT FRONTIERS, Hodder & Stoughton, 1996.

GIVING:
> * To acknowledge the primacy of immaterial rewards in personal and community health, and to develop giving-based principles of interaction which honor the contributions of all life.
> * To replace our violent forms of obtaining food, health, and resources with methods based on consensus and fulfilling the needs of all parties.
> * To ensure that all have roles in the community which offer self-esteem, mutual respect, and value to all of life.

SACREDNESS:
> * To acknowledge that our greatest cultural problems are, at root, diseases of the spirit. To act to improve the spiritual, mental, psychological, and community dimensions of our real wealth and their expression in our communities.
> * To seek the wisdom and connectedness to restore well-being to all of creation, and purpose and meaning to our lives.[35]

MULTICULTURAL SYNTHESIS

Both pressed and nurtured by the forces of change, we live in a time of immense opportunity. Exposure to new people, new cultures, and new ways of seeing and being gives us new mirrors in which to see our own lives – to compare, to question, and to choose the best resources to create new designs for our lives. It is a time of new vigor and new possibilities. It is also, however, a time for finding what fits the uniqueness of the land, the place, and the people – what will take root and flourish with a new, strengthened, and enduring, sense of rightness.

Each new world we encounter brings us in touch with new cultural beliefs and living traditions. On the surface, each is foreign. We can look to places such as Indonesia or Australia, where diverse cultures have blended together, to get a sense of the possible – and a sense of the problems to avoid. There is a world of wisdom and opportunity to build upon and select from to derive our own new, distinctly fitting cultures.

Peter Rich, talking about his work with the Ndebele tribe in South Africa, describes a people who have tried on all the strange and crazy "modern" things that have flooded their country, from top hats to tin whistles.[36] The surfaces of their mud-plastered homes have exploded with dramatic and subtle geometric design with the advent of European paints, whitewash, and other colored materials. Instead of leaving just "the desert" around their houses, they have created mud-plaster-floored ceremonial "porches" defined by sitting-height walls around the houses, investing those spaces with powerful cultural meaning and function. They have chosen what fits into their culture and their lives – with humor and passion, no matter how incongruous it may appear at first – while ultimately rejecting what doesn't fit. That is what we all have to do.

---

[35] See my THE IZU PRINCIPLES, 1994.

[36] Peter Rich, presentation, DESIGN HAS NO BOUNDARIES CONFERENCE, Brisbane, AU, 1995.

✧

Evolutionary forces are thus both closing off and opening out new options for us. Such forces give impetus to the energetics of place, drawing strength from them, and are interwoven in their application. Li, or clarity of intention, gives rise to more nurturing surroundings. But it also helps us clarify our real goals and needs, sorting out what contributes most powerfully and directly to their attainment.

Sacredness, self-esteem, honoring, living from the heart, giving – the aspects of energetics of place – are the same principles inherent in attaining sustainability in our culture. We are nudged into change by the limits to growth; the infinite benefits of sustainability provide the incentive; and energetics constitutes the framework.

5 *THE THREE "I"S:*

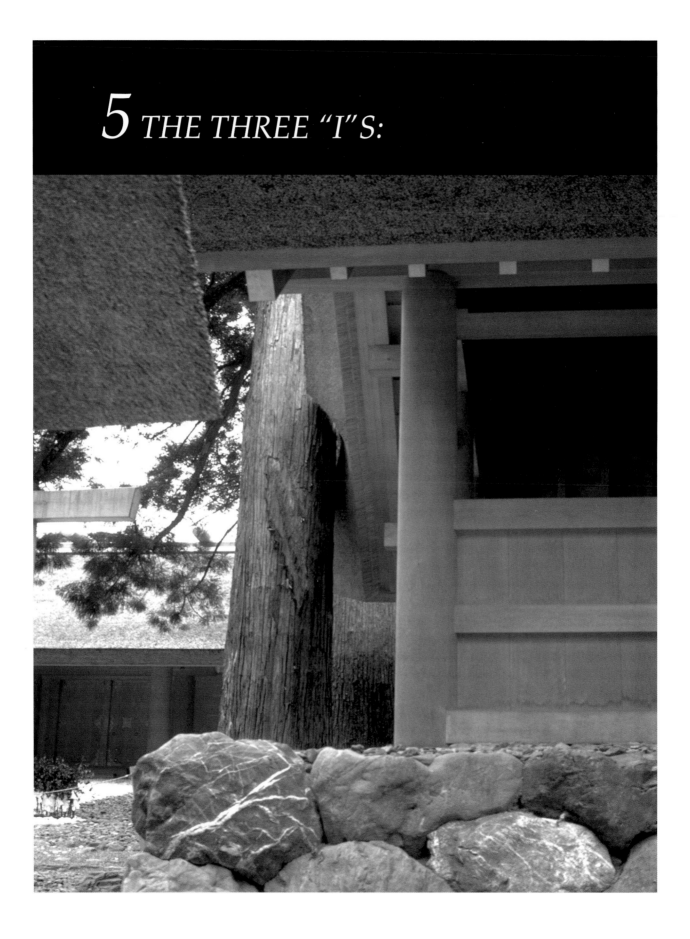

CORE ELEMENTS OF ENERGETIC DESIGN

What I consider the three most important elements of energetics of place can be thought of as The Three "I"s. They are *CHI*, or life-force energy; *LI*, or intention; and *TUMMI*, or paying attention to our own tummies – our personal gut-level intuition about what is right for us.

CHI : LIFE FORCE ENERGY IN OUR SURROUNDINGS

As mentioned in Chapter One, chi in our bodies, its connection with our emotions and those of others, and its role in our health and well-being are now comfortable concepts to a growing number of people. What, then, about chi in our surroundings? When we are dealing with chi in a ghetto of Los Angeles, what are we talking about – and how do we deal with it?

Chi is the fuel of energetics of place, while intention is the blueprint. Health, disease, change, and constancy manifest from the realm of chi into the realm of matter. Chi is vital to supporting our physical, emotional, and spiritual health. It forms the glue that keeps a community healthy. Chi is blocked by emotional barriers, artificial building materials, intensive use of electromagnetic devices, and cultural practices based on taking from others.

As we shape and use places from our hearts, they transform our surroundings and fill us with joy, rightness, and meaning. They reach out and make us at home again in a wonderful world of which we are an integral part.

The word "chi," in Chinese literature, seems to have a variety of meanings. "Earth energy," or "geomancy," in the European traditions, have a similarly confusing ambiguity of meaning. At times, chi is defined as a type of energy - perhaps a type of electromagnetic energy. At other times it would better be called information. Sometimes it's broken into good and bad energy - or perhaps just out of phase energy. There is heavenly or cosmic chi - the influences from other places and dimensions of existence. There is earthly chi - the variations of natural energy in a

Stones that fit together as if they grew around each other. Timbers planed to a silken perfection of finish. Connections that have a feel of inevitable rightness. An absence of the superfluous. A palpable taste in the air of the presence of spirits. The product of a thousand years of honoring the sacred in the process of building – the Ise Shrine.

physical setting. There is personal chi that we bring to our surroundings - our heritage, intentions, and dreams. This disparity of definitions may arise from our lack of proper vocabulary for a number of related phenomena that occupy the same realm.

As energetics emerges today, it is clear that this is a complex and multidimensional realm. Until we can clarify our understanding and terminology, we will have to live with the vagueness of a single term.

People in many cultures have knowingly sought and experienced chi in special places. A late third century classic work of Chinese geomancy by Kuo-p'u states:

At a true [geomantic] Cave there is a touch of magic light. How so, magic? It can be understood intuitively, but not conveyed in words. The hills are fair, the waters fine, the sun handsome, the breeze mild; and the sky has another light; another world. Amid confusion, peace; amid peace, a festive air. Upon coming into its presence, one's eyes are opened; if one sits or lies, one's heart is joyful. Here the chi gathers, and the essence collects. Light shines in the middle and magic goes out on all sides. Above or below, to right or left, it is not thus. No greater than a finger, no more than a spoonful; like a dewdrop, like a pearl, like the moon through a crack, like the reflection in a mirror. Play with it, and it is as if you can catch it; put it off, and it cannot be rid of. Try to understand! It is hard to describe.[1]

The close-in elements of the earth's magnetosphere, which forms from the plasma particles of the solar wind interacting with the earth's magnetic field. The intersection of the magnetic torus with the earth creates the "auroral oval" where it heats atmospheric particles into the luminousity of the Northern and Southern Lights.

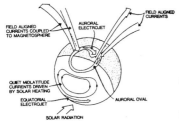

Gyres of flow in the atmosphere, the seas, and the earth's mantle, combined with discontinuities in the mantle, generate local energetic conditions.

CHI AND ELECTROMAGNETIC FIELDS

One aspect of place-related chi appears connected with the electromagnetic fields in the earth's mantle and atmosphere[2]. Much of this energy circles the earth between the earth's surface and the ionosphere. It creates a resonant frequency at about 10 Hertz – the reciprocal of the time required for a beam of electromagnetic radiation to go around the earth. This is the same as one of the base resonant frequencies of our brain waves that controls human circadian rhythms, deep relaxation, and creative imagery. Those electromagnetic fields vary with solar activity, from night to day, and on daily, monthly, annual, and an 11-year solar activity cycle. Field strengths vary from .2 to .7 gauss, about 500 times the minimum a person can sense.

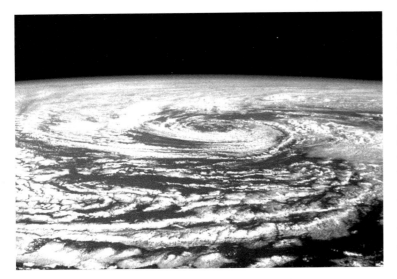

Within the earth's crust, the intensity of electromagnetic fields are affected by conductivity, discontinuities, and the shapes and location of different materials that constitute the crust, as well as circulatory patterns in the magma below. Overall field intensity changes both cyclically and with apparent randomness. Global patterns of energy concentration in the crust shift over time. Magnetic poles wander and fields reverse.

[1] Zangshu, the BURIAL BOOK OF QUO-PU (AD 276-324), quoted in PARABOLA 3, issue 1, 1978.

[2] See Jonathan Wiener's PLANET EARTH, Bantam, 1986, for a non-technical overview.

From a chi perspective, the electromagnetic element of chi in the earth thus changes over time, both predictably and without known cause. This creates "power spots" which appear to be favorable or unfavorable for various activities. Land-forms, waterways, and groundwater flows within the earth focus, disperse, or divert these energies and their concentrations. Human activities seem able to attract or repel these energies. Power lines, radio and TV towers, electrified railroad lines, steel structures, or reinforcing steel in concrete buildings affect and alter the specific energies at any particular point on the Earth's surface.[3]

The influence of such fields on living matter, including people, now is also well documented.[4] Correspondence with the traditional dowser's "ley lines" and "blind springs" have also been studied.[5] Paul Devereaux and others have made a preliminary instrumented study of British Neolithic monuments which suggests such correspondence. They also identified other apparent influences, such as the presence of radioactivity in some of the rocks in Neolithic monuments.[6] Natural radioactivity has also been indicated as an active influence in some of the healing springs in Texas and other locations.[7]

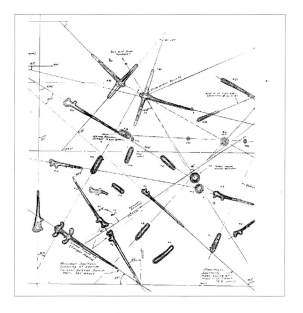

At a Spirit of Place Conference in 1993, a physics professor gave a presentation on his use of aerial remote sensing. He had correlated magnetic anomalies in the earth with the location of Indian Mounds in Wisconsin. As he showed maps of the mounds and the alignment of magnetic anomalies with them, one of the Native Americans in the audience suddenly rose to his feet and stormed out the door. A few minutes later, he quietly returned to the room and asked if he could speak. He apologized for his obvious upset, and said,

You mentioned one really big anomaly where no known mounds were located, which you hadn't had time to investigate yet. Well, that is our tribe's most secret and most holy place, of which no one else knows!

RECIPROCAL EFFECTS BETWEEN PEOPLE AND CHI OF PLACE

The chi in our bodies radiates out and affects things outside us, from where it can in turn affect other people. Such chi can be felt in the energy of pilgrimage shrines generated by the presence of visitors over the ages. By the same token, people, when visiting the sites of W.W.II extermination camps, almost universally report a palpable feeling of horror emanating from the places, even fifty years later.

Lizard Mounds, in Wisconsin, are located on the drainage divide between river systems that drain into the Atlantic and the Gulf of Mexico. The theme of duality is important in both the mounds and local traditions. Seasonal and astronomical alignments are prevalent, as in other mound systems.

[3] See Robert O. Becker, CROSS CURRENTS: The Perils of Electropollution, The Promise of Electromedicine, Tarcher, 1990.

[4] See, for example, Davis and Rawls, MAGNETISM AND ITS EFFECTS ON THE LIVING SYSTEM, Exposition Press, 1974. or Victor Beasley's YOUR ELECTRO-VIBRATORY BODY, University of the Trees, 1978.

[5] See Guy Underwood's THE PATTERN OF THE PAST, Pitman Publishing, 1969, for a good discussion of these phenomena.

[6] PLACES OF POWER, Paul Devereux, Blanford Books, London, 1990, or (less detailed) EARTH MEMORY, Paul Devereux, Llewellyn Books, 1992.

[7] Jim Swan, ed., THE POWER OF PLACE, Quest Books, 1991.

There are holy places in almost every country where the spiritual practices of individuals and groups have left an undeniable imprint on the place, unexplainable by its physical attributes. In places where we habitually sleep or work, power spots appear to form and remain as traces of portals where we bring chi into the material world through our bodies and actions.[8] There are many layers of causes, effects, and interactions through which chi of place is generated and altered.

Though some people can "see" it directly, the actual chi of place is apprehensible largely through secondary intuitive means, such as meditation, kinesiology, or dowsing. At this time, these are far from exact or replicable arts. So we are left with that inexactness and with other means, such as a sense of how landforms, waterways, road cuts, buildings, or bridges affect the chi of a place as tools of chi perception. We can use such tools, however, to supplement our own intuitive reaction to a place.

We need not be concerned, however, if we are unable to personally sense chi. Our cultural beliefs have, literally, blinded us and blocked that ability in many of us. Many of the means of working with chi are simple enough, and their results perceptible enough, that it's okay if we just consider chi as a "black box" and work only with what it *does*, even if we don't know how it works. We do this every day, driving a car without knowing all the detailed combustion mechanics and control-system electronics involved in its actual operation.

Anything that communicates values of love, trust, community, intimacy, or respect sets into motion the effects of those values. Those effects cascade throughout the interactive web that constitutes the collective energy, or chi, of a place. We can change the chi of a place by direct channeling of chi; by changing landforms, waterways, or vegetation; or by erecting, tearing down, or altering buildings or roads. Those mechanisms are important and not to be disregarded.

But all sorts of other actions – a smile, singing a happy song, sweeping up trash, a pot of flowers on a window sill, people doing things together – have effects far beyond the immediate. By influencing other people's perceptions, actions, and energy, they collectively affect the energy of the place itself. They work through the vehicle of chi and on the material level to initiate changes that affect all dimensions of our lives.

Any act of caring about other people or places – allowing ourselves to be open to them, respecting them, or causing them to feel good – generates good chi. And any act of disregard for others – greed, violent thoughts or deeds, taking or lack of caring – generates bad chi.

LI: INTENTION AND PURPOSE

The second important aspect of energetics of place is *li, hara,* or *intention,* which focuses and directs energy to attain life's purposes.

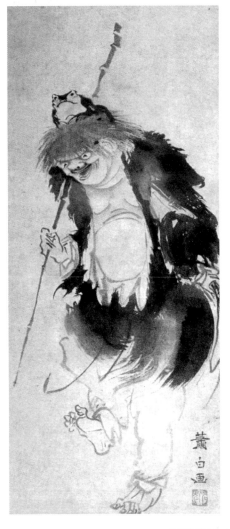

In both China and Japan, chi-based "spontaneous" painting styles developed, where variation in a single brush-stroke, with no retouching, conveyed a deep and clear sense of the object being painted. In both painting and calligraphy, this was based on a process of connecting the hand and brush to the object being painted, without intervention of the mind.

---

8   See Joey Korn, DOWSING, A PATH TO ENLIGHTENMENT, Kornucopia Press, 1998.

All of our surroundings reflect the intention that has gone into their making and use – the values of their makers. If made from greed, if made to deceive, they convey that. If they come from a meanness of soul or smallness of spirit, they surround us with that essence. If made with love, with generosity, with honoring of all life, they support and evoke the same intentions in our own lives.

Clarity, strength, and rightness of intention channel life-force energy, or chi, into a place, with its ability to nurture our lives. The nature of our intention – whether in making or using a place – reflects that same energy back into our own lives, enhancing or weakening our own energy.

There can be many different levels to our intention. A builder may express an intention to build a good house for someone, but a deeper intention to make a lot of money may alter the results. A person may state a desire to build a place with a soul, but deeper values of greed and deceit may lead them to spend their resources on the empty shells of many things rather than one fully satisfying place. Clarity of intention requires that we carefully examine our core values and root intentions, and alter them to ones supporting love and life.

Focused attention on each act in building gives us the opportunity to intensify our connection with the materials, the site, our work, and the spirits of the place. Every step – from planting and harvesting trees, to making and sharpening tools, to every part of construction itself – becomes an opportunity for action, intention, and ritual that implant ever more deeply in our lives the powerful relationships we have with all of Creation. The finely honed attention and intention involved in the construction of the Ise Shrine in Japan has resulted in every post, every board, every joint resonating with the power of the sacred.

The intentions surrounding us are so much a part of our lives that we are often unaware of them until we lose them. Many of the wonderful tree-shaded streets of fifty years ago in Midwestern towns are gone now due to Dutch Elm disease. Those that remain remind us that those shady avenues didn't just happen but were created from the intention and efforts of our ancestors.

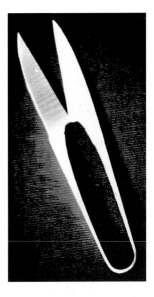

A pair of Japanese scissiors show the powerful sense of rightness and effectiveness resulting from clarity of intention. The cross-section transforms imperceptably to reflect the change in stresses from the blade to the spring hinge.

LI IN CHINESE PHILOSOPHY

Li, or intention, was an integral part of Chinese natural philosophy associated with chi and was considered an equally essential component of the power of place. Curiously, li rarely received emphasis in most traditional Chinese feng-shui practice. Yet in Chinese cosmology, existence emerges out of the seminal void of "T'ai-i", the Great Absolute; or "Wu Chi", Primal Energy. It emerges through two paired concepts: Yin and Yang, and Li and Chi.

Chu Hsi, a Sung Dynasty philosopher (1130-1200) and the main Chinese proponent of the concept of chi in feng-shui, always spoke of chi and li inseparably:

> *Throughout heaven and earth there is Li and there is Ch'i. Li is the Tao (organizing) all forms from above, and the root from which all things are produced. Ch'i is the instrument (composing) all forms from below, and the tools and raw material with which all things are made. Thus men and all other things must receive this Li at the moment of their coming into being, and thus get their specific nature; so also they must receive this Ch'i and thus get their form.[9]*

Stephan Feuchtwang comments that:

> . . . Ch'i is then the animator of Li, capable of condensing into physical being. Li, in turn, is that which makes Ch'i intelligible because Ch'i on its own is just pure being. There is no Li without Ch'i, and no Ch'i without Li; one of Chu Hsi's aphorisms. Everything has both Li and Ch'i in it.[10]

Unlike yin and yang, li and chi are not "mirror" dualities, but are distinctly different concepts, dealing with different interrelated aspects of emergence into the material world. Li is the intention which brings into being a particular chi-based etheric template on the auric levels. It is the purpose we bring to an incarnation, the intention in any creative act, the aspiration underlying any materialization, the goals of any action.

LI IN OUR PERSONAL ENERGY FIELD

Barbara Brennan discusses this from the energy-healing perspective:

> Wherever in our lives we have trouble creating what we want, we discover that we have mixed intentions or crossed purposes. To create what we want, it is essential to sort out our mixed intentions. We must clarify our true intentions so we can realign the ones that are not in keeping with what we truly want. What we truly want is always aligned with our highest spiritual longings. When our personal wants and desires are aligned with our spiritual longing or higher desires, our purposes are aligned and the creative principle in the universe can function unhindered.[11]

Intention or purpose, she indicates, is held in our bodies on the *hara* level – a separate level from the chi, or auric field, level. The hara level forms the foundation for generating the auric field. Hara is Japanese for the lower belly, referring not only to that location but to a quality of having energy, strength, and focused power in that area. It is a center of spiritual power used for centuries by warriors as a source to draw upon in combat. Within the hara is a central point called the *dan tien*, the center of gravity and movement in the body.[12] In people who practice martial arts, this spot becomes a bright ball of gold light, often with a strong gold line of light running through their bodies from head to foot.

On the hara level, the hara point (*"dan tien"* in Chinese) is connected by this energy line upward through the body to a point in the upper chest which Brennan calls the "soul seat," then upward to a point about 3-1/2 feet above our heads, ending in a small inverted funnel shape representing our first individuation out of the void. The hara line continues down from the dan tien deep into the

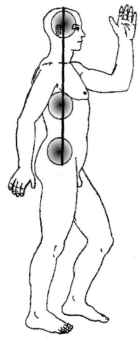

The three chi energy reservoirs in the body (upper, middle, and lower dan tien), with the central channel that connects with the energy fields in the earth and heavens.

[9]   Chapter 49 of *Chu Tzu Chhüan Shu*, from Joseph Needham, SCIENCE AND CIVILIZATION IN CHINA, Vol. 2, pp. 479-80, Cambridge University Press, 1956; also in his THE SHORTER SCIENCE AND CIVILIZATION IN CHINA, Vol. 1, Colin Ronan, ed., pp. 239-40, Cambridge University Press, 1978.

[10]   Stephan D.R. Feuchtwang, AN ANTHROPOLOGICAL ANALYSIS OF CHINESE GEOMANCY, Editions Vithagna, Laos, 1974.

[11]   Barbara Brennan, LIGHT EMERGING, Bantam Books, 1993.

[12]   For a Taoist perspective, see Mantak and Maneewan Chia, AWAKEN HEALING LIGHT OF THE TAO, Healing Tao Books, 1993.

earth's core where we synchronize our field pulsations with those of the earth and entrain energy from the earth's field.[13]

Li, hara, or intentionality, then, is the means by which we focus chi energy to achieve our life's purposes. Clarity of purpose or intentionality magnifies the energy available and our ability to achieve our purposes. Thus the success of the intense "Zen" focus.

Clarity of intention in groups emerges similarly from alignment of individual hara energy into a group hara line. Brennan indicates that:

> *The true individual purpose of any member of a group is holographically connected to the purpose of the group as a whole. Once all have aligned their haras, all have aligned their purpose in the moment with their greater purpose as individuals and as a group. Everyone's greater purpose is part of the great evolutionary plan of the earth. . . . And as was said before, within this framework of reality no adversarial position is possible. The synchronicity can be felt in the room. The room fills with the power of the task at hand.[14]*

LI OF PLACE

Li comes into play in buildings, gardens, or other surroundings because clarity of purpose in a place enables the success of the activity it houses. By removing extraneous matters, our attention is focused totally on issues at hand, better ensuring their resolution. In terms of gardens, such as the famous Zen gardens of Japan, the greater the li and the deeper the intention of the designer, the greater the "emptiness" of the garden and the less distraction in clarifying the purposes of visitors. In a home, when the li is strong and clear, we say that the place has a soul. We relax immediately on entering, finding relief from our confusing cross-purposes in the clarity and power of a far greater source of energy than our own body to draw upon.

There is a wonderful symmetry in finding the frontiers of modern learning fitting exactly into the words of a Chinese sage of 800 years ago! Why did most feng shui traditions embrace yin, yang, and chi, but not li? We can only speculate that li required

The interconnection between the garden and the house at the Tatsamura Silk Mansion in Kyoto is an outstanding example of designing from an intention to connect us with nature, and to remove extraneous elements that might distract us from that connection.

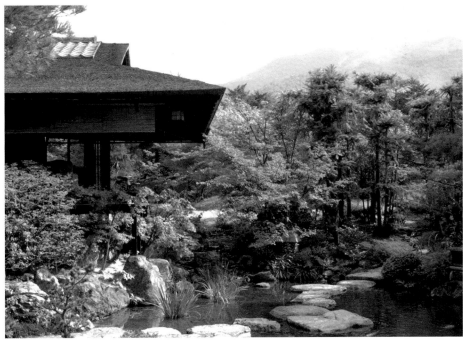

---

[13] See Brennan, above, for more details on this energy system.

[14] Barbara Brennan, LIGHT EMERGING. A similar "drop and open" process is used for clarity of group intention in the modern Wiccan tradition. See RECLAIMING QUARTERLY, Fall, 1998.

more rigorous personal spiritual development, and therefore was much harder to put into practice than chi. Chi, in contrast, was something external and easily apprehensible. It had a real tie to place which could be exploited. Its concentrations could be found and used to advantage, apparently by anyone.

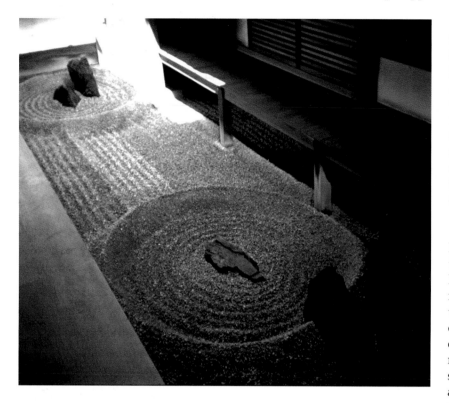

While chi held ascendancy in the Chinese energetics of place, this was not so in other cultures. Egyptian, Mayan, Native American, and African cultures, along with the Old Religions in Europe, were highly skilled in work with energy, and also with hara. Intention is considered today by most energy-working traditions to be the most essential element of change available.

There is one culture that has excelled in working with li in the power of place: the Japanese. It has turned out that the Japanese, rather than the Chinese, followed this particular thread in the weave of an energetic universe to its fullest development. Japan inherited much Chinese culture, including site divination for temple siting and a simplified version of feng-shui (*kaso*) used in house design.

Over the years, gardeners have changed the gravel patterns in this small garden at the Ryogen-in Kyoto. The changes are neither good nor bad - just indication that learning and gardening are living processes here and not just the dead repetition of old patterns.

In Japan, however, hara work or clarity of intention became a central goal of Zen practice. Out of it came a tradition of martial arts, *sumi-e* ink brush paintings, meditation gardens, carpentry, flower arrangement, house and teahouse design, and arts of everyday living that honed clarity of intention to its finest edge. They discovered something obvious: the more we are surrounded by clarity of purpose, the less noise and confusion surround our own existence, and the more clearly we can focus our own intentions!

In those temples, brush strokes, rock placements, or flower arrangements there is an absolute spareness, a total hewing away of extraneous material, purpose, and attention. In *No* drama, every movement and action arises endowed with primal energy directly from the point of stillness and silence. In all these arts, every move, every effort, is essential – filled with power, and coalescing with all others to an inevitable fullness and achievement of purpose. Each action arises clearly and deeply from the silent core of its birth into potent expression. With that purity of intent, a single brush stroke faultlessly conveys the full intention of the artist.

This same spareness, clarity, elimination of the unnecessary, and sureness of purpose can be seen in Shaker furniture and in some of the last sculptures of Michelangelo. The effect it has on us, conveying a feeling of unequaled effortlessness and sense of freedom, is identical.

TUMMI: GUT LEVEL INTUITION

The last of the three main principles of energetics of place deals with the immense importance our minds and hearts play in our energetic relationship with our surroundings. The psychological, emotional, and spiritual aspects of our relationship with place are important, complex and beautiful, but virtually ignored in our design and use of place.

The complexity of our hearts and minds makes it often wisest to ignore the details of their interaction and pay attention directly to the end result: how our tummies feel. Our "gut" feelings *are* important; they reflect manifold cultural and personal beliefs. It usually matters less what someone else thinks is right for you than what *you* know you need or want. Listen to and *trust your tummi.*

Specific cultural beliefs affect what feels good and bad to us. The conventional sitting arrangement of family members and guests in a tipi, a Japanese room, or the home of a French Count are utterly different. If a Chinese family *believes* they or someone else has the most favorable feng shui site, that belief will strongly influence their happiness and success. It probably doesn't matter if you sleep with your feet toward the door, unless your culture has a practice of taking a corpse out of a room feet-first and believes you shouldn't sleep that way.

Acknowledging the importance of our gut feelings gives us personal affirmation. It achieves a degree of success merely by paying attention to and acknowledging the importance of our own selves and our own feelings. Because of the importance of our minds and hearts, many successful chi-related practices don't deal directly with the chi of place but with opening our hearts so that our energy influences the energy of the place. If we are disturbed by something from our surroundings or elsewhere, it colors all of our perceptions and actions. This energetic level of action also accounts for the unexpected success of many actions that are based purely on our individual psychology.

Although we are sometimes unable to alter things in our surroundings that bother us, it may still be possible to take advantage of the importance of our minds to create improvement. Merely giving us something positive to associate with can counter negative energy. The Chinese, for example, might hang a flute on a heavy beam they feel pressing down on them to counter that energy with the association with the lightness associated with music. Native Americans might hang a feather below the beam. Even our culture has its talismans that can lighten our minds.

When we dig into what makes our tummies uncomfortable in a situation, we often find subtle clues that warn us of real

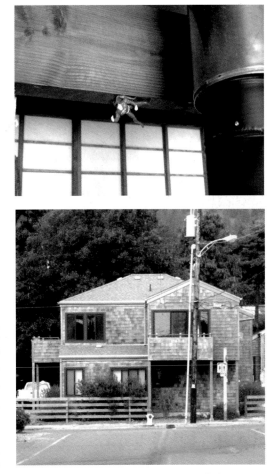

Top: Superman lets us know that holding up the beam is but a small task.

Above: A house at a T-intersection of streets and adjacent to power transformers. Headlights, near-collisions, and disruptive energy flows.

Below: In many spiritual traditions, the house is visibly identified as sacred space

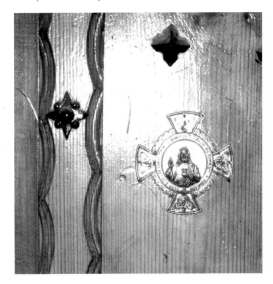

but not immediate hazards. For example, there are energetic hazards in living at the end of a "T" intersection, but there are also distractions from headlights and noise, and the very real potential of a vehicle failing to turn the corner in hazardous conditions.

Purely symbolic actions towards our surroundings, such as the Chinese use of the bagua, Jewish placement of a mezuza at the door of a home, or using colors symbolic of prosperity or happiness, can achieve a degree of success through affirming in us an intention to pay closer attention to a certain aspect of our lives.

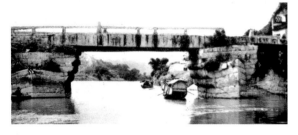

RIGHT DURATION

In addition to the initial effectiveness of an action, we need equally to consider the *duration* of its impact. Duration is an aspect of place-energetics rarely given proper attention. Some chi-influencing actions are long-lasting, some need frequent repetition. Some long-lasting actions need periodic monitoring, others don't. So it is important to be clear about *all* that is required both to develop and to sustain good chi in our relations with place over time. Then we can more accurately choose from the widening range of possible actions ones which best assist us in reaching that goal.

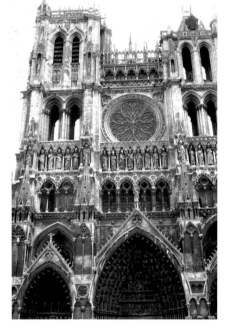

Right duration is an important consideration in all we do. Because it is loved, a building with a soul may often endure beyond the needs of its makers to become a gift to future generations. A cathedral lasting twenty generations, or a bridge lasting twenty centuries, can give back far more than the effort put in their making. Such endurance immeasurably reduces the per-generation cost of the resources that go into creating our communities. Durability thus grants a generosity to the places we make that can be obtained in few other ways. And long- and short-lasting actions have different qualities – there is a hoary strength and a nourishing peacefulness in the timeless qualities of a building that truly fits our hearts and spirits, generation after generation.

Yet not everything benefits from lasting longer than its nature. A generation from now, we may wish that some of the things we have recently created had not lasted beyond their time. It may be good that our homes or vehicles are durable. It may not be desirable that our foods or some of our building materials are preserved with poisons that linger and harm. In India, walking along a single country road we can

Top: A stone bridge in China almost 1000 years old. Below: Amiens Cathedral has been serving its community for 30 generations. The cost-per-year of either is infinitesimal compared to our poorest construction. Their durability provides freedom and generosity to the community.

be surrounded by the ghosts and ruins of untold centuries and dynasties of building. A builder or an artist might be inspired by the accumulation of centuries of the greatest achievements of their society. Or they might find those achievements too lofty a yardstick against to measure their own work, and not even begin to discover what they themselves could create anew. Things that endure can be both a gift and a burden.

It is good, therefore, that some things last and that some things do not, making room for each generation and individual to forge anew the understandings and relationships of a meaningful life. The Inuit who throws away a scrimshaw carving once the empowering act of creating it is finished, or the Balinese village or Indian pueblo that returns imperceptibly to the earth when its use is finished, holds a rightness of duration and of material choice. Finding the right duration for each of our creations is one of the roots of wisdom needed for being a true part of the ever-evolving creation of life.

SIGNIFICANCE

Energetics of place is concerned with the relationship between our personal chi energy and the chi energy in places. It calls our attention to the cycles of change in energy that move through both our outer world and our own lives, and suggests ways to bring our lives into harmony with those changes. It helps us find nurture in natural places and to make and use our own homes and work places so that they also sustain our lives and the rest of Creation. It shows how clear intention, giving welcome, honoring others, making places that have a soul, and bringing our ancestors and the spirit world into our everyday life can give richness and meaning to both our places and our lives.

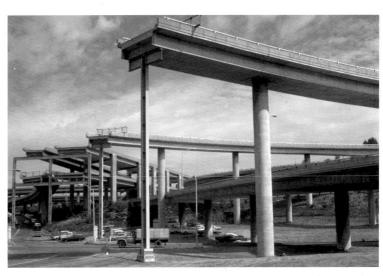

Top: Adobe and thatch construction in Java – low investment, short life, bio-degradable.
Below: Our children may wish that some of the things we've created were less durable.

With the diversity and unfamiliarity of chi-related actions that we can learn from various traditions, it is important to understand the relative significance and effectiveness of the different elements. Different situations have different needs. Different individuals and communities have different skills and traditions. Most people don't know a *Nine Star Ki* from a *Yellow River Chart*, and have little reason to find out. But they may very well know whether they need old chi cleared out of a space, a balancing or enhancing of existing earth energy, or a gateway for them to connect with their ancestors in the spirit world.

The philosophical view of the universe expressed by the Neo-Confucian philosophers is amazingly congruent with what we are confirming today, experimentally and experientially. Yet the dynamics of our materialistic culture are so unprecedented that the truly significant actions needed today to align and improve the energy of place lie outside the normal areas of practice of any tradition of energy work.

The table that follows is *my own* list of elements of energetics of place, and my sense of their relative significance, *today*. Every one of us will have our own, different, list. All will change as we understand these elements more deeply. And all these elements interact with and affect each other. Our energy is best put where we sense it will be most effective, and different situations benefit from different actions.

ELEMENTS OF ENERGETICS OF PLACE

ELEMENT By Importance	ITS NATURE	ACTIONS	DURATION
1 *MOVING BEYOND A GREED- CENTERED CULTURE*	To avoid and heal root energetic damage from greed-based patterns, which is far greater than energetic "cures" can heal. Beside this, all other actions pale.	* *Participatory rather than passive recreation and entertainment* * *Work, learning, family, and institutional patterns that support our sense of doing valued work, contributing to our community, and our worth being acknowledged* * *All actions affirming a love- and life-centered world*	Finding alternatives to cultural values and patterns such as TV, tourism, and bureaucratic work patterns may offer the greatest and most enduring energetic benefit of any actions we can take.
2 *DIRECT RAISING AND NURTURE OF CHI*	To directly heal and augment energy of community and place – even more vital for community than for individual health. A practice almost totally neglected today.	* *Group spiritual practice* * *Community ritual and energy raising, "shamanic" practices* * *Cathartic conflict resolution* * *Internal or external chi adjustments, blessings* * *Use of mantras, mudras, yantras and visualization* * *Simple actions by individuals and communities involving love and giving*	Sustaining direct raising of community chi is an on-going process. Repetition builds long-lasting patterns.
3 *THE PERSONAL ENERGY OF USERS*	To affect our personal energy flows – which are, with few exceptions, the largest energy flows in our homes and communities.	* *Individual spiritual practice* * *Actions that enhance emotional health, self-esteem, or sense of being of value to our community* * *Practices that open us to deeper energetic flows in our surroundings* * *Places that give shelter, nurture, challenge, and harmony to our lives* * *Symbolic actions that affect our emotional and mental interface with our surroundings*	Successful individual changes can last a lifetime. Symbolic actions rarely survive the tenancy of a single user of a place or have the power of actions that actually alter underlying patterns.

ELEMENT By Importance	ITS NATURE	ACTIONS	DURATION
4 *GOOD NATURAL CHI IN LAND AND PLACE*	To find, enhance, and create resonance with, natural flows and patterns of chi in place – not for advantage over others, but to communicate and interact more fully. Some chi of place comes from topography, some from geophysical anomalies, some from how we have attuned the places we build to channel and enhance those energies.	* *"Tangible" feng shui practices: form and compass school; adjustment to interior and exterior factors such as roads, trees, hillsides or waterways; location of doors, beds, bathrooms or workplaces* * *Dowsing to locate and move chi* * *Calling in of energy balancing and enhancement* * *Design of homes, gardens, and communities to focus and sustain place energy*	Good natural chi in land and place may endure for millennia, or change tomorrow due to new road cuts, underground water movement, dams, power lines, ground water withdrawal, etc. Requires monitoring to verify continuation.
5 *ATTENTION TO INTENTION (LI)*	To express clarity of intention and purpose in the soul of a place *can* be the most accessible way to change the energy of a place and its users.	* *Consensus on placemaking goals and their alignment with goals of the rest of Creation* * *Clarity in the specifics of our actions, with those goals as touchstones* * *"Hara"-based practices of individual action and group decision-making* * *Ritual in the building process* * *Honoring work, materials, and the spirit world*	Intention can rapidly change energy of a place, but it can be countered by intention of others or existing energy patterns. Deep intention embodied in physical actions gives greatest impact and duration.
6 *DESIGN : HARMONY OF INNER PATTERNS AND ATTRIBUTES*	To achieve wholeness, a harmony of intention with inner patterns and attributes is essential. This is very much the opposite of conventional design, which focuses on outward appearances.	* *Creating place as invisible servants* * *Tying to the cycles of nature* * *Honoring* * *Gardens that nurture our spirits* * *Connecting to the community of nature* * *Eliminating mirrors* * *Celebrating night, rain, and death* * *Durability* * *Building as rewarding work* * *Putting love, giving, and silence into the places we make*	Design changes may last as long as the facility, or be negated by other changes or use patterns.

ELEMENT By Importance	ITS NATURE	ACTIONS	DURATION
7 **RELATION TO ANCESTORS AND THE SPIRIT WORLD**	To achieve wholeness by reopening the doors to our ancestors, to the spirits, and to the non-material worlds – to honor and work together to manifest the great unfolding of Creation.	* *Establishing temples, shrines, home altars, and sacred places* * *Learning design of "gateways" to the spirit world* * *Rituals and places that maintain ongoing connection between the material and spirit world* * *Design and placement of tombs as in traditional feng shui; scattering of ashes; honoring of ancestors*	Acknowledging and restoring connection to the spirit world can result in enduring energy shifts. Individual actions will have different impacts.
8 **CLEARING, CLEANSING, AND CLUTTER**	To focus intention and energy by simplifying and eliminating distractions. Clearing intention often preceeds direct raising of chi, enhancing the energy of individual users or specific actions. In our materialistic lives, this is valuable for letting go of the past, or for its own benefits of achieving clarity.	* *Dealing with the inheritance of good or bad chi from prior use of a place, such as death, bankruptcy, anger, divorce, or illness* * *Internal clearing, such as fasting, meditation, or Zen training* * *External purification, dealing with accumulated material "stuff," cleaning, and honoring* * *Balancing, freeing, or relocating bad chi and li; exorcism of ghosts*	Dealing with clutter may last minutes or years, depending on how deeply inner patterns are changed. Internal clearing can create life-long change. Clearing inherited chi of a place can have enduring results.
9 **SPECIFIC PRACTICES AND RULES**	To attend to specific psychological, cultural, and ecological problems of people and place. This is as important and effective as a grand theoretical approach to a situation.	* *Taking care of lighting, sanitation, ventilation, structural adequacy, and setting needed for rituals* * *Applying traditional feng shui remedies for such classic problems as "T" intersections, heavy beams, or bad bed locations* * *Verifying applicability of rules by following your tummi– paying attention to what feels right*	Varies with individual situations and actions.

ELEMENT By Importance	ITS NATURE	ACTIONS	DURATION
10 *ALIGNING WITH THE COSMOS*	To symbolically embody philosophical, social, and cosmological principles; astrology, numerology, five elements, and the feng shui bagua. Beyond any direct connections, aligning with the cosmos strengthens our will and sense of the context of our beliefs and actions. Major significance, very different from existing beliefs and practices, may await discovery here.	* *Applying symbolism in house or city design* * *Working with astrology of place. [this takes two main forms – birth-influenced desires and needs for surroundings (Chinese Nine-Star Ki); and time-specific compatibility with places depending upon position in our personal time cycles (Chinese Eight Words or Four Pillars)* * *Using the Elements (Earth, Air, Water, Fire, and Metal in Chinese tradition) to alert us to the qualities of change cycles, particularly chi-related, to which we must relate* * *Honoring traditions of cosmic connection from different cultures for elements of homes, villages, and ritual*	Individual birth needs are lifelong. Position in time cycles change periodically. Symbolism in design and layout has impact as long as aligned with beliefs of society and affirmed in fresh and clear ways.
11 *ATTENTION TO OUTWARD APPEARANCE (HSING)*	To see, through appearances, what inner intentions are being manifested. Harmony, beauty, and balancing *yin* and *yang* in how things look are only "fine-tuning," yet outer appearances *do* affect us and our perception of meaning.	* *Fine-tuning the esthetics, the physical expression, and the patterns of a place to enrich its ability to resonate with our hearts and our lives.* * *Maintaining inner intention as a touchstone so as to not fabricate appearances at odds with what lies within*	Affected by rate of change in society and how much "fashions" change our sense of beauty or harmony. The best work has enduring value. The worst loses value immediately.
12 *OTHER...?*	To look for what unanticipated elements might apply to your individual case. Every situation provides unique avenues of action that resist codification.	* *Varies with situation*	Duration varies with individual action and context.

6 ORDER AND CHANGE

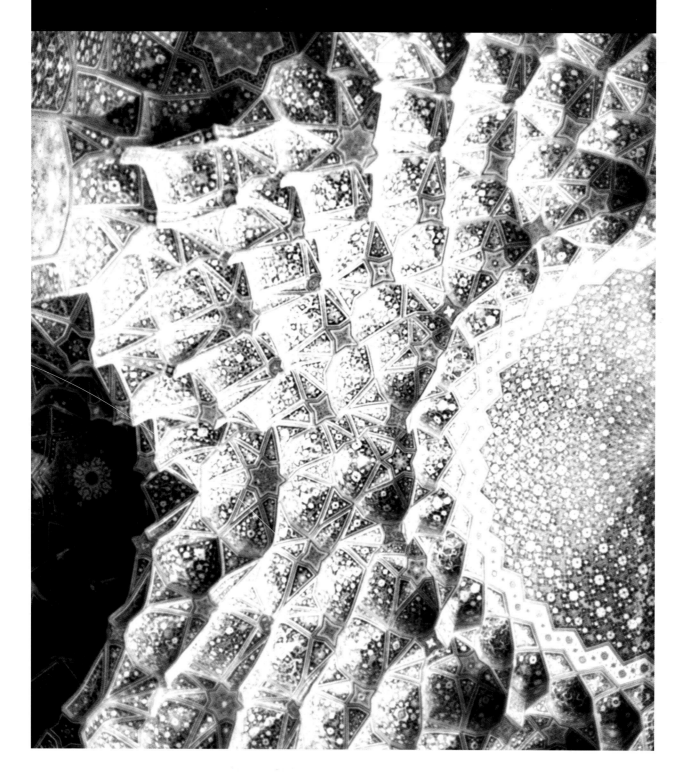

CHI IN A MATERIAL WORLD

The Chinese philosopher Chu Hsi, in the early 1200s, developed one of the clearest articulations we have of the concepts involved with energetics of place. It begins with *"T'ai-i,* the Great Absolute, the primordial cause of all existence. Out of it emerge various aspects which in turn bring about material existence:

> *In the beginning, before any being existed, there was only Li, then when it moved it generated the Yang and when it rested it generated the Yin. Upon reaching the extremest point of rest it began to move once more, and at the extremest point of motion it began to return to rest once more . . .*[1]

This brought about, of course:

> *YIN and YANG: inhaling and exhaling, rest and movement, female and male, contracting and expanding, darkness and light, unifying and manifesting, death and life.*

In that movement, the intention or underlying purpose:

> *LI: the laws or order of nature, universal principle of organization, principle of order; pattern, harmonious cooperation; intention, purpose; the fixed, immutable, and inscrutable laws of nature.*

organized the primordial energy:

> *CHI: the breath of life, the energy animating yin and yang; vital force, subtle energy.*

according to mathematical principles of relationship:

> *SO: the mathematical principles of nature, the numerical proportion of the universe.*

to generate the outward forms of nature:

The faceted vaulting of the Masjid-i-Shah in Isfahan is more than "decoration." It is the direct expression of the mathematical interrelatedness of all Creation, and of the cyclic unfolding of richness of life from its origin and then its folding back into Oneness.

---

[1] Chapter 49 of Chu Tzu Chhüan Shu, from Joseph Needham, SCIENCE AND CIVILIZATION IN CHINA, Vol. 2, pp. 479-80, Cambridge University Press, 1956.

HSING: the outward forms of appearance of nature.

through:

CHIH CHUNG: the invisible attraction between things at a distance.

We've looked at chi and li in previous chapters. Now let's look at how these other principles influence the energetics of people and place, and ultimately affect how we design and use our homes, workplaces, and public places.

YIN AND YANG:
RELATIONSHIPS and TRANSFORMATION

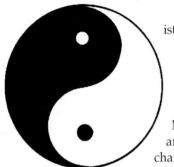

Yin and yang are a relatively familiar concept – of qualities of existence emerging as *complementary dualities*, essential polarizations of unity.

In their oppositeness and cross-definition, yin and yang are inseparable. Inherent in the concaveness of a spoon is the convexity of its backside. Darkness exists only in reference to its complement, light. Quiescence and motion are perceptible only in reference to the other. Male and female, high and low, open and closed, emptiness and fullness are all aspects of this emergence into polarized characteristics of time, change, and existence.

As every thing comes to fullness, its relationship to all else which is still waxing or waning inevitably changes, and those things which are not-it move into ascendancy. Relationships are in constant transformation, and what appears in one moment dominant and unassailable becomes in the next moment eclipsed by some form of its opposite. Balance is dynamic.

Everything holds the seed of its opposite, and each gives way in turn to the other. Their distinctions mirror each other, their primal commonness enfolds them into unity. Both are inherent in completeness.

The yin and yang duality establishes a basic view of the cosmos based on relatedness and change, which is common to both ancient Chinese natural philosophy and modern physics. It introduces the concept of harmony – of coherent relatedness between different and mirroring characteristics. It also develops, as we will see, into specific qualitative characteristics of various positions in cyclic rhythms of change.

Out of yin and yang, exhaling and inhaling, movement and change comes another vital concept for our surroundings: that of rhythm or vibration. Repetition of cyclic movement over time – the ebb and flow of chi – bring form into our material world. As Thomas Lee says:

Time here is neither an independent object nor a measurement subject to human interpretation. Time only exists in the changing strength and direction of chi flow. In other words, if chi is stable, time seems to stand still.[2]

Vibration of material systems organizes them into dynamic geometric structures. These are configured by the frequency and power spectra of the energy vibration and the nature of the materials involved. Change in the underlying vi-

[2] Thomas Lee, "Kan Yu -the Book of Change Concept in Environmental and Architectural Planning," GREENING TO THE BLUE CONFERENCE, Yale University, 1996.

bration brings change in the geometric ordering of the material. Change the song, and it changes the dance. As change occurs – as chi ebbs and flows – the energy fields alter, and so do the patterns they evoke, resonate with, and support.

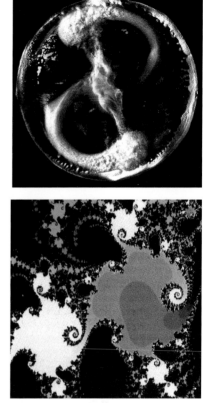

The magnetosphere of our planet pulsates at 10 cycles per second. Our brain waves are entrained with that rhythm. Human DNA vibrates at a rate of 52 to 78 gigahertz (billions of cycles per second).[3] Our sun vibrates like a bell, with 5-to-70-minute oscillations – a dozen octaves below the lowest note on a piano.[4] Such rhythmic systems interact, entrain, and resonate with each other, however, and frequencies many harmonics above or below a vibration may be entrained, fed by, and resonate with it.

Hans Jenny's beautiful *cymatic* studies of vibrating systems give a visual sense of the role of energy and vibration in the upbuilding of order.[5] In particular, his videos of two- or four-lobed yin-yang structures give a wonderful sense of the material and energetic flows within and between the lobes and the fluidic interaction of the polarities.[6]

Vibration is iteration – repetition. Repetition generates geometries and structures of its own. *Fractal* structures are records of systematic micro-divergence of geometries in repetitive systems. The geometries result from repetition and ordered change. Their beauty is valuable as a visualization of systematic and interactive evolution of underlying relationships over time.

Material organization arises, then, out of sound, vibration, and iteration through geometries that require the least energy to generate and sustain. The Aborigines are correct in their concept of *singing things into existence* on their Songlines! And all vibrating systems are interactive; they develop harmonics and sympathetic vibrations; move energy and information; and mutually transform as their energies interact. All this results from the emergence of yin and yang into the manifestation of our material world from chi, li, so, and chih chung.

Above: Two images of dynamic generation of form – Hans Jenny's sound-vibrated powder structures and fractals generated by rhythmic repetition and iteration of relationships. Below: Islamic geometric ornament. Floral "geometries" are the yin-yang balancing of the underlying linear geometries.

SO : *NUMBERS, RESONANCE AND INJUNCTIVE EXPERIENCE*

Numbers, in most traditional philosophies, are more than manipulative tools. They represent deep connectedness among things, and contain power well beyond that of calculating quantities.

In our own overzealous use of numbers for quantification in everyday life, we tend to forget that there are *qualitative*, and even magic, dimensions to numbers. That qualitative nature of mathematics was the

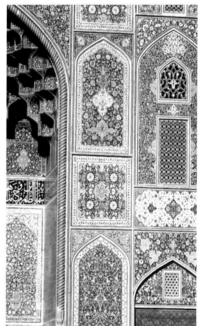

---

[3] Caroline Myss, ANATOMY OF THE SPIRIT, Harmony Books, 1996.

[4] Jonathan Wiener, PLANET EARTH, Bantam, 1986.

[5] Hans Jenny, CYMATICS, 1967; and CYMATICS, Vol. 2., 1974, Basilius Presse.

[6] Hans Jenny, "Cymatic Soundscapes," and "Cymatics" videos available from MACROmedia, P.O. Box 279, Epping, NH 03042 USA.

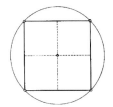

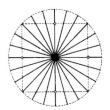

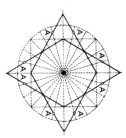

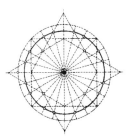

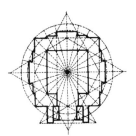

Development of the ground-plan of an Indian temple from a circle and square, with chronological/angular division of the circle corresponding the the energy of the deity involved (Volwahsen).

Right: Star-shaped plan and exterior of the KeshavaTemple at Somnathpur. The radial geometry is echoed at every level.

heart of its use in Greece, in Europe during the Middle Ages, in the world of Islam, as well as in China and India. As a representation of the nature of relatedness of things, it has a role in apprehending the sacred – and, by extension, in our surroundings via the rightful act of placement. Seyyed Nasr speaks of this power in the Islamic tradition:

> One might say that the aim of all the Islamic sciences . . . is to show the unity and interrelatedness of all that exists, so that in contemplating the unity of the cosmos, man may be led to the unity of the Divine Principle, of which the unity of Nature is the image.

> The Pythagorean number, which is the traditional conception of number, is the projection of Unity, an aspect of the Origin and Center which somehow never leaves its source. In its quantitative aspect, a number may divide and separate; in its qualitative and symbolic aspect, however, it integrates multiplicity back into Unity.

> It is also, by virtue of its close connection with geometric figures, a "personality." For example, three corresponds to the triangle, and symbolizes harmony, while four, which is connected with the square, symbolizes stability. Numbers, viewed from this perspective, are like so many concentric circles, echoing in so many different ways their mutual and immutable center. They do not "progress" outwardly, but remain united to their source by the ontological relation which they always preserve with Unity. . . . [7]

The enriched central plan geometry of many temples in India contains this kind of "centered" relationship, expressing in their abstract or sculptured complexity the multitudinous unfoldment in Nature from that central Unity.[8]

[7] Seyyed H. Nasr, SCIENCE AND CIVILIZATION IN ISLAM, Kazi Pubns. See also his "Sacred Art in Persian Culture," MIDDLE EAST FORUM, Spring, 1971.

[8] See, for example, Andreas Volwahsen's LIVING ARCHITECTURE: INDIAN, Grosset & Dunlap, 1969.

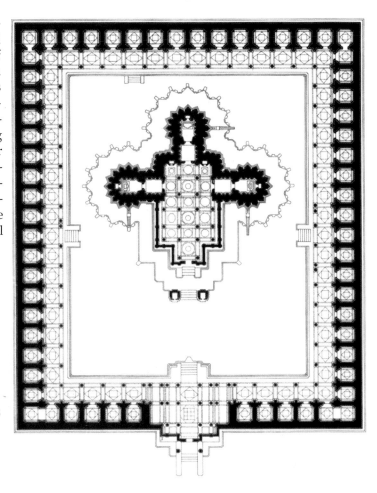

The mathematician, G. Spencer Brown, also notes that:

A universe comes into being when a space is severed or taken apart. The skin of a living organism cuts off an outside from an inside. So does the circumference of a circle in a plane. By tracing the way we represent such a severance, we can begin to reconstruct, with an accuracy and coverage that appear almost uncanny, the basic forms underlying linguistic, mathematical, physical, and biological science, and can see how the familiar laws of our own experience follow inexorably from the original act of severance.[9]

Buildings that appear similar can actually be qualitatively quite different because of different relational patterns in their geometry. You can't dance or move things around the same way, for example, in a room with a column in the middle as in a room without one. The column changes the room topologically from an egg to a torus, or donut. Warren Broday explains *kleinforms* - one type of topological geometry that is sort of like a donut eating itself:

Topology is a non-metric elastic geometry (more analogous to our perceptual geometries). It is concerned with transformation of shapes and relational properties such as nearness, containment, and inside and outside, which remain constant even when shapes are radically transformed.

The kleinform is a topological relationship in which the inside and outside are continuous. It is perhaps the simplest of topologies where context is an integral

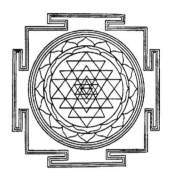

The Sri Yantra – one of the geometries that activate resonant energy systems in our bodies and psyches – used in Hindu temple and sculpture design as well as meditation.

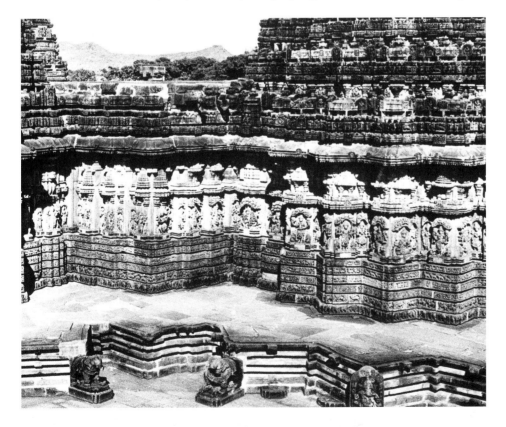

---

[9] G. Spencer Brown, LAWS OF FORM, George Allen and Unwin, Ltd., 1969.

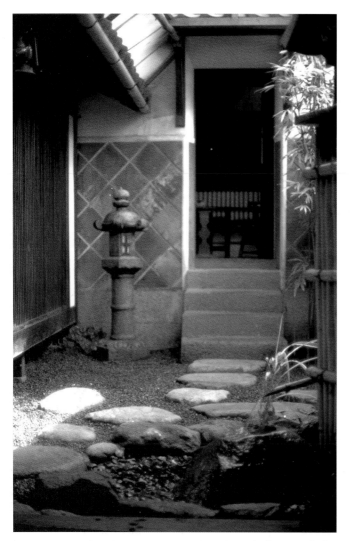

Above: An exterior-interior courtyard-hallway of the Kurashiki Inn.

Below: Inside and outside of a kleinform are a continuous surface.

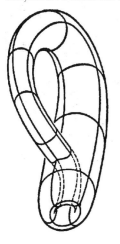

and essential aspect of all relationships . . . there is not just inside or outside, but infolding or intracontainment and a flow through each other through time and position.[10]

If we acknowledge, as Broday hints, that context is an integral and essential aspect of all relationships, then it is probably important to design our buildings to acknowledge that. Surprisingly, buildings actually do exist that embody such geometry, and which feel entirely different as a result. One of the most interesting is an old Japanese inn:

The Kurashiki Inn was not designed as a kleinform — in fact it was never designed. It was a collection of old plastered rice storehouses which was later adapted for use as an inn. But the way changes had been made, and what they did, were reflections of a cultural development which had never dissociated thought and action from context, and which had never lost its triadic logic where subject, object, and context are continually related. What resulted, in the renovation of the old storehouses was an environment with a richness of information and variability of context which changed with every movement and position.

The experience of the Inn is difficult to describe. The things that remain most strongly in my mind are feelings of my mental concepts being totally devastated—such as our common concept of Inside/Outside. At places in the building where we would think ourselves normally to be far and totally "inside" the building we would suddenly feel raindrops on our heads. Or we would discover ourselves in an alley outside; or we might step up onto the verandah from the garden, slide the door shut, and turn around to find the other side of the verandah opening into another outside garden, but this time without any door or other enclosure! Things which were originally "outside," between the storehouses, were now "inside" the Inn and its corridors, yet in some ways they had only partially become "inside".[11]

More traditional Euclidean geometry held an important role in sacred building traditions worldwide. Geometry has been prominent in the ornament and vaulting of Islamic buildings, in the cosmology of Chinese city layout, in the design of the Egyptian pyramids,[12] in use of the Golden Mean in Greek temple design, in the

---

[10] Warren Broday, "Biotopology 1972," in RADICAL SOFTWARE 4, Raindance, 1972.

[11] See my "Kurashiki Kleinform," ENVIRONMENTAL DESIGN PRIMER, Schocken Books, 1973.

[12] See, for example, Peter Tompkin's classic SECRETS OF THE GREAT PYRAMIDS, Harper & Row, 1971, for an exploration of numerological significance employed in construction of the pyramids and/or imputed in retrospect by later geometers.

astronomical significances in Stonehenge[13] and other Neolithic monuments in Europe, in Native American cosmology, and elsewhere.

The actual historical use of geometry as an energizing basis of sacred design is likely to turn out to be lip service in many cases, and much deeper than we comprehend today in others.

Numbers, simple ratios, and geometry are practical everyday tools inherent in virtually all construction. What is difficult in regard to sacred geometry is separating out what was actually *used* in construction vs. what is implied in retrospect; what was used for *sacred* vs. simple constructional purposes; and what was actually *achieved* through its use.

Geomancer Nigel Pennick notes that existence of some of these geometrical systems is not hypothetical:

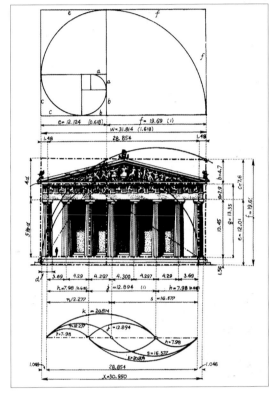

The geometrical systems underlying late Christian architecture are not the subject of speculation, but part of a well attested and continuous tradition. Several sets of working drawings still exist, showing the principles of geometry involved in the layout of churches in the medieval period. One well-known source of information is the so-called sketchbook of Villard de Honnecourt, an itinerant mason who noted down various systems of design, and also individual examples.

Less well-known are the surviving scale drawings of several German master masons. Among these are the original elevation for the west front of Strasbourg Cathedral, drawn in about 1385 by Michael Parler. There are also the designs for the steeple of Ulm Minster, made by Matthäus Böblinger between 1474 and 1492. When the plan was rediscovered in the last century, the spire was completed from it. . .[14]

The use of numerical and geometrical sacred numerical systems clearly had value in the minds and spiritual practices of their users. Their actual efficacy in the design of buildings from an energetic standpoint is more in question, as the points of measure frequently appear arbitrary, and usually there is little sense of resulting power.

QUALITATIVE CHANGE

In our example of the Chinese tradition, we find many other variations on the significance of numbers. In the Neo-Confucian cosmology of Creation we start with the Great Unknown, and from that emerges yin and yang. With yin and yang we have polarity, opposites, transformation. From them, we move outward into trigrams and hexagrams. These are an expansion of the yin/yang concept into the possible permutations of different combinations or transformation points between such polarities. Half yin/half yang; two yang over one yin; one yang between two yin.

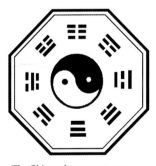

The Chinese hexagrams are a diagraming of the progressive balance points in a cycle of change between two complementary dualities.

---

[13] Gerald Hawkins, STONEHENGE DECODED, Doubleday, 1965.

[14] Nigel Pennick, THE ANCIENT SCIENCE OF GEOMANCY, Thames and Hudson and CRCS Publications, 1979.

What this ends up with is fine *numerical* distinctions of *qualitative* change – between building orientations that represent yin and yang, seasons that represent the same, or topographic patterns reflecting such polarity. Put into words and symbols, we have the I Ching. Put into our minds, we have *qualitative* characteristics of change. Put into physical, geometric terms, we have a framework for creating particular harmonies in landscapes, buildings, and gardens that embody subtle balancing of different polarities.

Moving again outward, we come to the Five Elements: *earth, air, fire, water,* and *metal*. Such names are perhaps misleading if we're used to thinking materialistically. It is possibly better to think of them also in terms of the *qualitative* differences that develop as a transformation or morphing occurs from yin to yang through all the intermediate stages (or hexagrams).

RESONANCE AND INTERFERENCE

Paying attention to the qualitative aspects of intermediate points in a transition helps us understand the interactions that inevitably occur between an intention and the heavenly and earthly circumstances it encounters in particular times, seasons, and conditions of place. The energy of certain times, places, or seasons will align with and give greater power to intentions with a similar energy. The energy of other times, places, or seasons may be in partial or full opposition to a particular intention. In such cases the intention becomes altered, diverted, weakened, or destroyed, depending on the qualitative nature and relative power of the intention versus the conditions it encounters.

On a conceptual level that makes sense. In paying attention to timing and examining conditions of proposed actions, it can give us a clearer perception of forces at play and their potential interaction. It is something we subconsciously pay attention to in timing many public and private actions and events. It underlies some of the astrological aspects of building placement and use. In terms of geomantic siting of buildings, it is not always of major significance compared to other forces at play such as site energy, active raising of energy, design intention, or personal energy and intention in a place.

The same Magic Squares are found in many cultures – with their hint of comprehendable underlying relationships between all of Creation

4	9	2
3	5	7
8	1	6

NEW PERSPECTIVES ON RELATIONSHIPS

We can only imagine how exciting it was for early mathematicians in China, India, Greece and other cultures to discover new dimensions of mathematics, such as the "magic squares" of numbers. They found that, for instance, if the numbers 1 through 9 are laid out in particular sequences in a grid of three numbers each direction, the numbers in any row or column – or even the diagonals – would always add up to 15. The immutability and wholeness of this complex and unexpected interrelationship gave it power in their eyes beyond that for which we may find reason today.[15]

The *Lo Shu* (magic square), in particular, was built upon by the Chinese into whole systems of application in their feng shui. The locations of the different numbers were corresponded with the Eight Trigrams from the I Ching classifica-

---

[15] Keith Critchlow, ISLAMIC PATTERNS: An Analytical and Cosmological Approach, Schocken Books, 1976, gives an excellent introduction to the fascinating patterns involved. For feng shui applications, see the work of William Spear – FENG SHUI MADE EASY, HarperSF, 1995, or THE FENG SHUI HOUS BOOK, with Gina Lazenby, Watson-Guptill Publications, 1998.

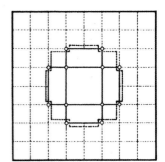

tion of the universe. The magic square was placed over the plan of a building or site, and the directions from which different kinds of energy corresponding impacted the site or building were examined.

The question remains as to what, if any, real power such a schematization and application of apparently unrelated observations of nature holds.

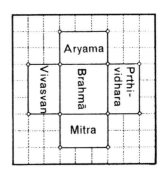

In such ways, visible use of mathematics plays an ever-shifting role in energy of place. At every stage in the history of mathematics (or culture), the newest insights hold a special power and excitement in our minds – compared to accepted ideas, they are *transformative*, opening new dimensions of understanding of the inner operation and relationships that structure our world. Each of these new discoveries was celebrated by incorporating it into the planning, layout, geometry, ornament, and relationships of buildings, gardens, and city design. Such affirmations bring our surroundings into conceptual congruence with our evolving sense of the universe we inhabit. From an energetic standpoint, this confirmation of our ability to find ever-deeper understanding of some aspects of our universe is possibly of more importance (or more variable) than the absolute and timeless relationships of mathematics.

We can see, in looking at historical buildings, when the power of small numbers was discovered, when constructive geometry and perspective drawing[16] were figured out, when algebra, calculus, topology, field theory, fractals, and chaos theory became known. This is culturally valuable, and gives power to place. However, each stage of this kind of application of numbers and mathematics loses its power as the newness of each discovery wears off and is taken for granted, and as new discoveries take their turn in the limelight. Consequently, while a particular form of mathematics may have influenced the energy of places a millennium ago in China or Greece, it is unlikely to hold the same power today.[17]

In Indian tradition, "mandala" is the name given to form, and the square vastu-purusha mandala (below) the form taken by existence when it has been set in order. The act of building is an act of bringing disordered existence into conformity with the fundamental laws that govern it. Home, temple (above) and city form (next page) evolve from division of the circle and the square according to the purpose of the construction.

RELIGIOUS RULES
We can also compare the theoretical numerical, "cosmic law" rules for city or temple design, for example, expounded in the *Shilpa-Prakasa*[18] or *Vastu-Shastra*[19] texts in India, to the actual plans of cities and temples. We see there that it was more common for the theoretical rules to be ignored than applied, even in the initial designs of the cities and temples. And it was even less common for subsequent generations to maintain such patterns.[20]

---

[16] The Italian Renaissance buildings of Palladio and Bernini come immediately to mind.

[17] See my "The Pantheon Revisited," Oct, 1990; or the "Geometry and Order" section of my THE HEART OF PLACE for a further discussion and critique of sacred geometry.

[18] A. Boner and S. Rath Sharma's RAMACANDRA KAULACARA - Silpa Prakasa, E.J. Brill, 1966, gives detailed evidence of one tantric temple design tradition from the Orissa area of India.

[19] D. N. Shukla, VASTU-SHASTRA, vol. 1, Bharatiya Vastu-Shastras series, Punjab University, 1960.

[20] See, for example Andreas Volwahsen, LIVING ARCHITECTURE: INDIAN, Grosset & Dunlap, 1969. This is also a more accessible and convincing introduction than the English translations of the Indian texts.

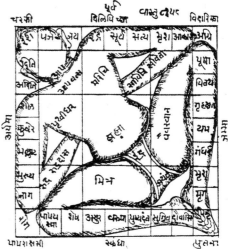

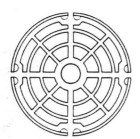

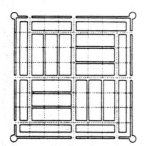

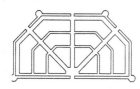

We can more realistically look at most of these geometrical/mathematical rules for building as "theory" books that give heavenly "conceptual" prototypes, rather than as exact patterns for earthly execution. Consequently, we can only surmise that the true power held by those theories for their users was relatively minimal – a mere intellectual underpinning or model, rather than a true experiential or operative key to the workings of the universe.[21]

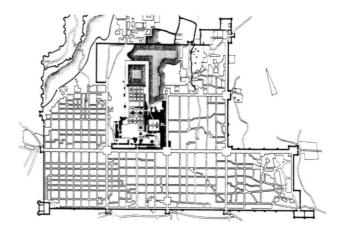

THE REAL POWER OF NUMBERS

The real, as opposed to symbolic, power of numbers exists where they lead us to new and more profound experience, insight, and understanding of the inner operation of Creation. Numbers have authority where they enable us to interact more deeply and wisely with our universe.

We are familiar with this occurring in engineering and science. We are far less familiar with it affecting our consciousness, our energy interactions with the world around us, or our emotional sense of meaning and our relationship with the rest of Creation.

Shape has significance when it grows directly from the structure or relationships inherent in a particular organism or situation. It is a circumstantial manifestation. Geometries or numerical systems imposed from a different system can only be symbolic, and contain far less power and meaning.

G. Spencer Brown notes, however, that:

The primary form of mathematical communication is not description, but **injunction***. In this respect it is comparable with practical art forms like*

---

[21]   We see a similar looseness of application in Chinese cities. See, for example, Andrew Boyd's CHINESE ARCHITECTURE AND TOWN PLANNING, University of Chicago Press, 1962; Yi Fu Tuan's "A Preface to Chinese Cities," in Beckinsale and Houston's URBANIZATION AND ITS PROBLEMS, 1968; and Sen Dou Chang's many examples of non-orthogonal planning in "Some Observations on the Morphology of Chinese Walled Cities," ANNALS, ASSOC. OF AMERICAN GEOGRAPHERS, Mar, 1970.

cookery, in which the taste of a cake, although literally indescribable, can be conveyed to a reader in the form of a set of injunctions called a recipe. Music is a similar art form. The composer does not even attempt to describe the set of sounds he has in mind, much less the set of feelings occasioned through them. He writes down a set of commands which, if they are obeyed by the reader, can result in a reproduction, to the reader, of the composer's original experience.[22]

This *injunctive* dimension of mathematics allows it to lead us to experiences far removed from numbers and calculation. It makes possible the communication of "indescribable" relationships and experiences. It also alerts us to the more-than-quantitative patterns inherent in mathematical relationships.

Energy and geometry are tightly interwoven in the evolution and "upbuilding" of life. There are "least-energy" geometrical patterns into which atoms, molecules, and biological systems inevitably fall, and which guide transformations as scale and complexity build.

Today, we are close to apprehending the real roles, relationships, and power of geometry and numbers in this interconnectedness of life. Again and again, certain irrational numbers – in particular *pi* (3.14159...), the ratio between diameter and circumference of a circle; and *phi* (1.618...), the fibonacci ratio of the growth spirals in sunflowers, pine cones, or tree branches, and of the Golden Mean ratio used in certain architectural traditions – appear in supposedly unrelated situations. The research of Anne Griswold Tyng, Buckminster Fuller, and Dan Winter corroborate the energetic and geometric interactions in layer after layer of energy, material, biology, and consciousness. Their work appears close to revealing the energy-ordering role of geometry and numbers. Tyng states:

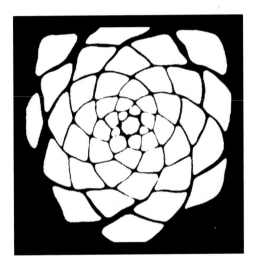

Dimensions of sequential elements in many plants, such as sunflowers and pine cones, follow the fibonacci growth ratio of 1:1.6.

> *These five Platonic Solids . . . are involved, not only in the spatial organization of forms at the level of nuclei of atoms and molecules, but also in cells, organs, plants, animals, the human embryo, the psychic structure of man, the works of man and in the astronomical forms of the universe which pre-existed man. Previously invisible ordering of the primordial atoms within us, revealed by the electron microscope, gives proof of internal geometry in natural forms, while recent psychological insights suggest instinctual images of the unconscious mind as the profound biological roots of man-made forms.*

> *. . . Not only does there appear to be progression in the life forms corresponding to the geometric progression toward complexity and increase in scale, but this progression can be seen as a repeating one with each new cycle building hierarchy upon hierarchy which indicate at each stage of development the record*

---

[22] G. Spencer Brown, LAWS OF FORM, George Allen and Unwin, Ltd., 1969.

of its earlier evolution, the hierarchies of form and the hierarchies of energy evolving from the interplay of polarity and rotation.

. . . Biological hierarchies built up out of the process of cyclic form intensification eventually lead to hierarchies of psychic structure. Psychic hierarchies evolved from cycles of energy-form tensions and synthesis lead to the principle of synchronicity. . . .[23]

In their dynamic form, these same cyclic hierarchies of geometric relationship occur in the research of Viktor Schauberger, Walter Russell, and others, as well as fractal geometry.[24]

Today's discoveries in mathematics are giving a deeper understanding of complex natural phenomena – like waves or wind – which confirm our experiential sense of deep and coherent interconnectedness of all things.

Such geometries and numerical and harmonic relationships occur in our own bodies. Certain repetitive points occur where resonance occurs simultaneously on multiple levels of our inner organization. Here the elements of chi and so, yin and yang, rhythm and cyclic change come together. Within that, important resonances can occur which reinforce particular relationships and large-quanta transfer of energy.

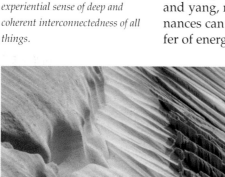

The potentials of this resonance to affect our personal energetics, psychic abilities, and consciousness are real, and are referred to in the writings of many spiritual traditions. The *Ramacandra Kaulacara*, in the Indian tantric tradition, calls for every space in a temple to have yantras, or specific geometric images, placed and consecrated in the structure below them to achieve this energetic linkage. It also calls for all images, including decorative motifs, to be composed on yantras and visualized by the sculptors according to their dhyanas.[25]

In this same tradition, the meditational wall sculptures in the teaching galleries at the Kailasanath at Ellora in India[26] have the ability to psychically imprint on the meditators minds and open their energy chakras, while in the process appearing to visually move off the wall into three dimensions. At temples in the Orissan area of India, however, sculpture and temples designed on the same tantric principles appear to lack this power.[27]

[23] Anne Griswold Tyng, "Geometric Extensions of Consciousness," ZODIAC 19, 1969. Or see a similar version as "Urban Space Systems as Living Form," in ARCHITECTURE CANADA, Nov, Dec, 1968 and Jan, 1969.

[24] For Schauberger's work, see Callum Coates, LIVING ENERGIES, Gateway Books, 1996. For an introduction to Walter Russell's work, see Tim Binder and Walter Russell's IN THE WAVE LIES THE SECRET OF CREATION, Univ. of Sci. & Philos., 1995.

[24] Boner and Rath Sharma, above.

[25] See Boner's outstanding PRINCIPLES OF COMPOSITION IN HINDU SCULPTURE, E.J. Brill, 1962.

[26] Some question exists, however, as to which Orissan temples were based on these principles.

✦

Quite different from their "quantitative" aspect, then, numbers hold a variety of roles and potential powers in the creation of place. This power, as noted above, is not always achieved, because of inappropriate use. Because of their relational nature, numbers have more value in a qualitative mindset than one that is merely quantitative; and may have significantly more power in ritual shamanic actions to connect us with non-material realms. Mathematics also can have very powerful injunctive or resonative action.

In their long evolution, many cultures have shown a flair for enumeration that became more sophisticated, yet arbitrary and further removed from experience, as time went on. Which of those many numerological systems will prove to have verifiable significance remains to be seen. With such broad and lengthy history, the amassing of chance positive anecdotal support for an*ything* is inescapable. Significant correlation of their effectiveness remains an open but important issue.

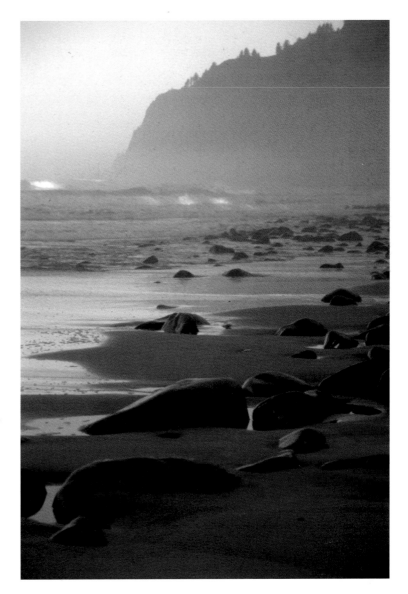

As we come to grasp the fullness of the relationships among things in the material world, we are also likely to confirm that their harmony runs deeper, that their nature extends into and emerges from the world of spirit, and that their energetic connections are as important as their physical and numerical ones.

Below: Different patterns of landforms "embracing" a site, with different effects on the chi energy of the site.

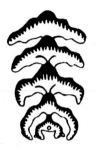

Growing Dragon

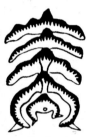

Strong Dragon

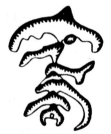

Sick Dragon

Right: Different landscapes, how their qualities fit into the cycles of energetic change, and how they consequently affect our spirits and the success of our activities.

HSING: OUTWARD FORMS OF NATURE

This aspect of the Chinese energetic cosmology works inward from the material and manifested world around us to find its internal energy and meaning. It involves examining the outward forms and patterns of nature. An attempt is made to apprehend within them – or to examine believed correspondences of their forms with – the underlying intention, energy, yin and yang, and numerical conditions. Then a determination can be made of potential harmony with proposed uses.

For example, traditional feng-shui practices classified shapes of mountains relative to the qualities of the five elements, or stages in cycles of change (see below). They looked at the structural arrangement of mountain chains to see if their organization was coherent, broken, or jumbled (left). They looked to see if faces or shapes of animals could be imagined in rock outcroppings or prominences. The topographic arrangement of landforms might look, for example, like a tortoise escaping a trap, or a happy dragon.

Some of these images work on our minds and our cultural beliefs. Others were believed to correspond with the qualities and strength of chi in the place. The inner geological complexity of a landform does not necessarily correspond with the outer shapes caused by circumstantial wind and water erosion, glaciers, or other geological processes. Considerable documentation would therefore appear neces-

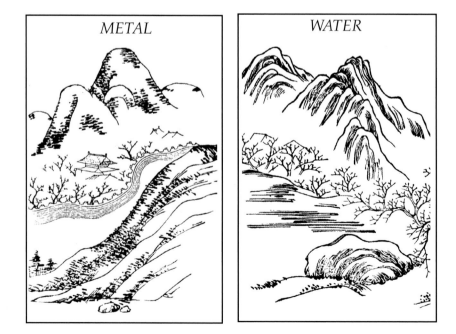

Simply put, hsing asks us to connect with our feelings towards a landscape or a place and how it affects our energy.

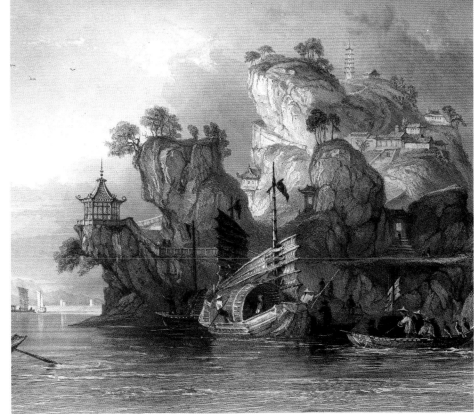

sary to demonstrate where and how actual energetic correspondence with landforms consistently exists.

There are, as usual, technical, intellectual, and intuitive means of apprehending inner energetic conditions of shapes of nature. Sitting *darshan*, an Indian term for being in the presence of something or someone in full attention and openness, is one technique. Meditation, trance, dowsing, or use of intuition are others. Aerial sensing of various energies may become viable.

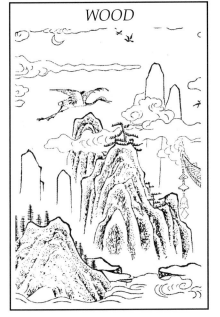

WOOD

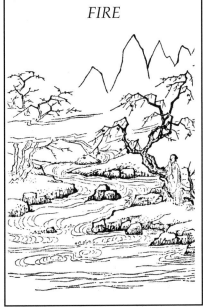

FIRE

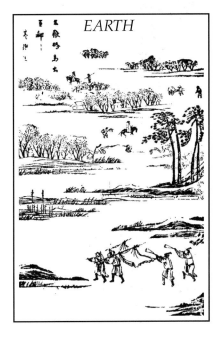

EARTH

From an intellectual perspective, categorization of known relationships – pointed mountains have fire type energy, interrupted mountain chains have bad chi, etc. – allow the less skilled practitioners to achieve some success. The correlation of forms of hills and watercourses with believed differences in energy, elements, and other astrological aspects have historically been widespread, as have rules for their uses.

A quick look at another cultural tradition suggests that more lies beneath the forms of nature than even the Chinese discuss. There is, obviously, the outer beauty of a place, and also the flows of earth energy or chi which the Chinese sought. In addition, however, it appears that connection with the primal forces of creation of the universe can be possible through association with specific natural places.

Australian Aboriginal cosmology suggests that great complexity, meaning, and importance lie in the connections possible with the energies, consciousness, and personalities that indwell in places. As commentators on Aboriginal cosmology and culture have noted:

> According to Aboriginal thought, every force, form, and substance, every creature and thing, is considered to have its own intelligence, its own spirit, and its own language. Whether animate or inanimate, perceivable or imperceivable, everything in the creation possesses, as do we humans, an interior invisible consciousness as well as an outer form.[28]

> Aborigines associate [these] ancestral powers with specific land formations and natural features, and they do not consider their inner psychic landscape to be fixed by generalized collective archetypes. . . . For the Aborigines, however, the knowledge and understanding gained and reiterated as metaphor derives from an intelligible energy actually emanating from the observed form – the seed, tree, or stone – to which subtle sensory centers in our body respond.

> . . . The Aborigines are inwardly transfigured by the vibrational energies intrinsic to the numerous sacred sites they travel to and from, and they manifest very different characters according to the role they play in the ceremony associated with a particular earthly place.[29]

> When one's familial or social relationships fail to reflect those of the metaphysical and natural world, the underlying ongoing powers of creation are prevented or blocked from sustaining humanity and nature, and a cycle of disharmony, disintegration, and destruction ensures.[30]

Like societies in Africa and other parts of the world, the Aborigines are able to make connections with the energy realms of our universe and their inhabitants. But they, possibly to a greater degree, access the wisdom available from those dimensions through the inherent nature of specific natural places and patterns. This clearly represents a source of value and meaning that is absent in our culture's past relationship with place.

[28] Johanna Lambert, ed., WISE WOMEN OF THE DREAMTIME, Inner Traditions International, 1993.

[29] Robert Lawlor, VOICES OF THE FIRST DAY: Awakening in the Aboriginal Dreamtime, Inner Traditions International, 1991.

[30] Johanna Lambert, ed., WISE WOMEN OF THE DREAMTIME, Inner Traditions International, 1993.

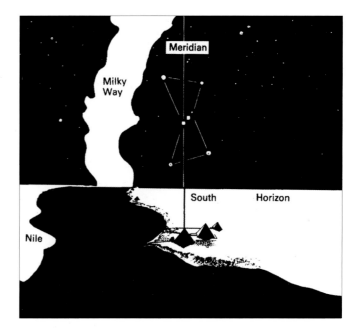

CHIH CHUNG:
RELATIONSHIPS AT A DISTANCE

One last concept from Chinese philosophy is important to mention here: that of *chih chung*. It loosely translates as "magnetism," but deals more fully with *invisible attractions between things at a distance*. It is an acknowledgment both of the invisible web of connectedness among all things, and the fact that specific significant relationships exist where we have little rational or visible reason to expect them.

There are many kinds of invisible attraction between things at a distance, such as gravity, light, magnetism, or plasmas, which even our sciences acknowledge but do not totally understand. A whole realm of psychic experiences still lie outside our scientific understanding and, therefore, our cultural acceptance. Instantaneous communications across vast spaces, cellular communications requiring only infinitesimal energy, and connection with non-material realms of existence similarly remain unexplained today, though they have occurred and been acknowledged in cultures worldwide.

We are no closer to clearly understanding such things today than the Chinese, 2000 years ago, who acknowledged the similarities between something like magnetism and many of these occurrences. For now, we can only acknowledge that there are yet many things in the universe which we can't clearly explain, but which do exist.

It is difficult to imagine that gravitation or other forces from as far away as the outer planets in our solar system can exert enough force to significantly affect our lives. Yet time and distance are turning out to be not as simple as we once thought, and our connections with the spirit world and other energetic dimensions of existence suggest we have much to learn in this area.

Astrology has had strong acceptance in virtually every culture in history. More people in this culture than will openly admit it find strong correspondences between a person's birth sign, their character, and their prospects. Astrological components have been important in feng shui and other energy-of-place traditions, dealing with influences from heavenly bodies immense distances away.

Reflections of the night sky in the Nile River or its seasonal floodwaters may have inspired the relative size and placement of the Giza Pyramids to reflect on earth the pattern of the stars in Orion's Belt. Those same stars appear again and again in the cosmological dimensions of the design of different cultures. The cooking hearths in Maya homes, for instance, were made of three rocks – symbolizing connection with those very stars.

Some aspects of astrology might be explained as providing a vehicle for non-rational reading by the practitioner of what is within a person. It's also possible that the heavens don't cause changes in chi on Earth, but that, by entrainment, they are in phase with such changes.

However, we've found already – perhaps to our own surprise – that phenomena far stranger than astrology, such as connection with the spirit world and communication from plants and rocks, *do* exist and have significant impact on energetics of place. *If*, as many energetic traditions assert, astrology does play a significant role in our lives, then there may well be other forces than minute gravitational tugs at play. It's probable, then, that we might find some other unsuspected and interesting forces operating in our universe.

To even begin conceiving of what such forces might be requires a major stretch of our minds. The work of writers such as Gregory Benford, Greg Bear, or David Brin are good mental exercise in this area. Similarly, very different work – such as that of Barbara Hand Clow[25]or William Tiller[26] – presents a mind-stretching but coherent framework for exploration and testing of dimensions in our universe which could account for influences involved in astrology and geomancy.

✧

Though described in terms of Chinese philosophy, the elements of energetics we've looked at thus far have been used in numerous cultures and in a great variety of forms. Taken together, they give a sense of the breadth and depth of energetics, and of its contributions to the well-being of people throughout time. The correspondence of these approaches, from culture to culture, and from ancient times to newly emerging concepts in contemporary physics and healing, is astounding. Their applicability to how we relate to our surroundings is of vast importance.

[31] Barbara Hand Clow, THE PLEIADIAN AGENDA, Bear & Co., 1995.

[32] William Tiller, SCIENCE AND HUMAN TRANSFORMATION: Subtle Energies, Intentionality And Consciousness, Pavior, 1997.

7 ENERGETIC DESIGN TOOLS

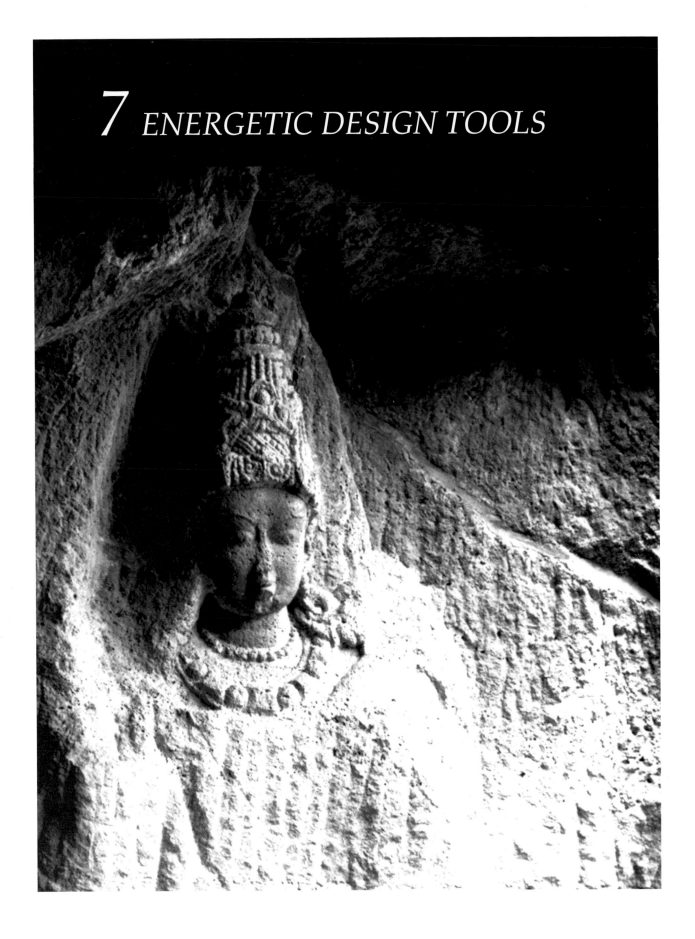

CLEAR GOALS

BECOMING NATIVE

Being born in a particular locale is not the same as being native to it. The latter requires that we be in harmony with that place – that we have shifted our beliefs, actions, and ways of being in the world into ones based on love for, celebration of, and participation in its natural community.

When a locale begins to speak to us and through us, and we through it, an indivisibility and oneness emerges which resonates through both us and the surroundings we have shaped. That resonance is a measure of success in connecting with the energetics of place, and a goal important to keep before us. Until we have become native, the surroundings we shape around us will always feel awkward and "out of place."

RESOURCES AND COMMUNITIES

Ensuring the health of all Creation requires major reduction in our resource consumption. Our built environment consumes two-thirds of all the energy used in our society – for heating and lighting of buildings, transportation caused by our land-use patterns, and the "embodied" energy that was used to process and place the materials in our buildings and infrastructure.

Eighty to ninety percent reduction from current levels of energy and resource use has already been demonstrated in test houses, offices, factories, and land-use patterns in a wide range of climates.[1] *Environmental Building News* suggests several simple actions that can move us toward those savings:

Within all things lie possibilities waiting to be released and brought to life. The vital ingredient is our own vision and clarity of goals.

---

[1] See Lovins and von Weizsäcker, FACTOR FOUR: Doubling Productivity, Halving Resource Use, Earthscan, 1997, and Lovins and Hawken's NATURAL CAPITALISM, 1999, for the context of these improvements. My "Living Lightly," 1973; "Hidden Costs of Housing," 1984; "Amazon Married Student Housing," 1994; "Bamberton," 1993; and "Transforming Tourism," 1993, show potentials in several specific sectors (available at <http://users.knsi.com/~tbender>) In regard to buildings, see also the many progress reports of the Rocky Mountain Institute, 1739 Snowmass Creek Rd., Snowmass, CO 81654; work of the Center for Maximum Potential Building Systems, 8604 F.M. 969, Austin, TX 78724; and John Todd's work with biological water purification at Center for the Restoration of Waters, One Locust Street, Falmouth, MA 02540.

* *Save Operating Energy:* Design and build energy-efficient buildings
* *Recycle Buildings:* Reutilize existing buildings and infrastructure instead of developing new areas.
* *Create Community:* Design communities to reduce dependence on the automobile and to foster a sense of community.
* *Reduce Material Use:* Optimize design to make use of smaller spaces and utilize materials efficiently.
* *Protect and Enhance the Site:* Preserve or restore local ecosystems and biodiversity.
* *Select Low-Impact Materials:* Specify low-environmental impact, resource-efficient materials.
* *Maximize Longevity:* Design for durability and adaptability.
* *Save Water:* Design buildings and landscapes that are water-efficient.
* *Make the Building Healthy:* Provide a safe and comfortable indoor environment.
* *Minimize Construction and Demolition Waste:* Return, reuse, and recycle job-site waste and practice environmentalism in your business.
* *Green Up Your Business:* Minimize the environmental impact of your own business practices, and spread the word.[2]

Maybe we could add: "Avoid the need for building," and find ways to meet our needs without the institutional and infrastructural costs that buildings entail.

Getting it right on the material level is an essential corequisite to effectiveness on deeper levels. Ecological building, natural building materials, simpler and smaller buildings, and using wisdom rather than technology all are helping bring into being building patterns and practices that *can* be used in ways that move our hearts.[3]

FREE NATURE
   With more than half of Earth's net photosynthesis now put to human use, the physical pressures on the rest of Creation are immense. The pressures that result from our ignoring the spirit and consciousness in all life are even greater. One of the biggest changes we need make is learning to say "No!" to ourselves. We need to set limits on our appetites and actions, and to leave enough to allow the rest of Nature to seek its own goals, live its own lives, and have its own relationships free from our pressures.

Years ago, protecting the sacred cows of India seemed an odd and peculiar practice. But there is a deep wisdom of restraint within it – one that needs expression on a far larger scale. It *is* as wrong to bend all of nature to our use as it is to allow our appetites unlimited rein.

What each of us will want or need to say "no" to will be different. For one, it may be a 1500 sq. ft. size limit on a place to live. For another, it may be living where there is need for fewer or no cars. For someone else, it may mean not travel-

---

[2] ENVIRONMENTAL BUILDING NEWS, Sept./Oct. 1995.

[3] For more conventional ways of improving the health impacts of our surroundings, see David Rousseau's HEALTHY BY DESIGN, Hartley & Marks, 1997 or Carol Venolia's HEALING ENVIRONMENTS, Celestial Arts, 1988.

ing on a vacation but staying home making their community a more beautiful and comfortable place to live.

Enoughness is a good word to learn.

AFFIRMING THE WORLD WE BELIEVE IN

It is exciting to watch what happens as new sets of beliefs coalesce, as a community becomes aware of its grounding in those beliefs, and as we develop the self-confidence to affirm those beliefs clearly and strongly.

Before that point is reached, actions taken are exploratory, limited by what can be achieved within the framework of prior beliefs. At this stage, practitioners of energetics of place tend to apply traditional actions from feng shui, geomancy, or other inherited traditions in a rote manner.

But once a certain point of clarity and understanding is reached, the whole arena of dialog shifts. Action becomes rooted in a coherent pattern of new beliefs and a clear acknowledgment of the underlying issues that conflict with those beliefs.

For example, only a couple of years ago, people proposed changes affecting energetics of a home, rearranging furniture – but with no acknowledgment of the role TV plays. But now people are willing to say:

The truth is, the TV must go.

TV is an electronic drug that tunes us in to disasters and wars we can do nothing about. We sit before it hour after hour, as it cultivates personal feelings of inadequacy, endlessly destroys self-esteem, and lets our physical bodies atrophy. Ads make us feel that we aren't okay – that we need more material possessions. Programs show us how much wealthier, more beautiful, and clever "everyone else" is. Professional music, sports, or dance programs show us how well something can be done and how lousy we are in comparison. Satellites now give us endless choices – overwhelmingly between the deeply ugly and the vapid.

TV damages our auras and undermines family, community, and individual self-respect. It destroys the physical, mental and spiritual health of all family members. No actions we can take have any significance beside the presence of this damaging force. No health can be achieved within its presence.

Similar changes are occurring in dealing with the energetics of work environments. Feng shui practitioners can now be heard to say what would have been unthinkable only a couple of years ago:

*Well, we **could** make some subtle adjustments in the furniture arrangement of this office, which would slightly improve the energetics. But that improvement would be insignificant compared to the negative impacts of the basic pattern of work involved.*

Large-scale organizations bring large office environments into existence. Such environments are dominated by secondary, paper-shuffling work, unfulfilling jobs, and organizational structures and business goals that are destructive to individual and community well-being. Work that doesn't use and develop skills or directly produce products and services of real value; that causes ecological harm; whose end result is unnecessary or harmful products, deceitful or degrading interactions, or the removal of energy and wealth from a community is harmful – period. Neither individual or institutional health can be achieved within those patterns. Their wrongness is so basic that no true success of any kind can be achieved through them.

✧

The energetic universe we are emerging into is one of wholeness. From within it, we can see clearly the destructive nature of patterns and beliefs we once embraced. With that vision, we can let go of them and restore health and wholeness to our lives.

WHAT DOES *GAIA* WANT?

Our culture is undergoing a transformation. We are acknowledging the energetic nature of our universe; embracing values of sustainability rather than growth; deepening our connection with other physical life and life beyond the physical plane; and globally interconnecting human life and society.

Teilhard de Chardin, James Lovelock, Lynn Margulis, and many others have pointed to this as the emergence of *planetary consciousness* – a single integrated awareness embracing all of Creation on the planet.

We can project many of the changes that this may involve: enough "psychomass" to establish a "planetary mind;" restoration and enhancement of the health of all Creation and its interactive ecosystems; an operative link between the physical and other realms of existence; help to all life to fulfill its unique potentials and combinations; reduction in the "noise" and negative energy generated by our extremely material-intensive human culture; acknowledgment and honoring of all Creation; deeper wisdom; the integration of human society into unique bioregional ecological "cells;" deeper sciences, richer and more moving arts, better biotechnology, communal experience, meaningful and rewarding lives, and a better world to live in.

Planetary consciousness, Gaia-mind, or whatever label we want to use represents a new and unprecedented level of organization and relationship. Out of this, however, we should expect a change in *kind* – not just a change of degree – in intelligence, compassion, knowledge, wisdom, awareness, and goals. This change in our nature is significant. It is staring us in the face, and needs to be perceived to be achieved. But what is it?

It is definitely more than just a cleaner, happier human culture, healthier ecological communities, or wiser and more capable caring for the health of planetary systems. Those are all internal maintenance issues from this new viewpoint. It must involve something fundamentally *different*, not just bigger and better (even if a *lot* better).

Individual life forms on our planet all operate in what is, to them, an external environment: the other organisms that surround their individual entities and communities; the greater "super-organisms" that envelope them; the seas, the air, the land, or the interfaces among these individual realms.

A planetary entity's external operative environment is stellar, not global, in nature. Its context is solar systems, galaxies, and energy fluxes on unimaginable scales, not just more surface area to occupy. Its environment undoubtedly encompasses levels of experience and existence of which we are unaware. We can conceive of peopling stellar systems, developing their "consciousness," evolving new nebulatic entities, but not yet the dimensions of existence and awareness that they might engender.

What could be the nature and value of the new capabilities we are emerging into? Can closer ties between potentials in the spirit world and their manifestation in a material world bring something quite new into existence? What could our new dreams, goals, and arenas of action become? Perhaps this is part of our malaise: the lack of a coalesced new awareness of what we really have become and are, and what new dreams and challenges are worthy of our new nature.

Machaelle Small Wright suggests that one outcome is the purposeful working together of human and nature consciousness as a team, creating new dynamic states of balance within the things that we manifest.[4] And, in his writing, Greg Bear muses that too much density of consciousness changes space-time. Perhaps, as he suggests, the universe has no fixed underpinnings:

> When a good hypothesis comes along, one that explains the prior events, the underpinnings shape themselves to accommodate and a powerful theory is born. Bad hypotheses, that don't fit what happens on our level, are rejected by the universe. Good ones, powerful ones, are incorporated. And the universe doesn't stay the same forever. A theory that works can determine reality for only so long, and then the universe must ring a few changes.[5]

As we mature and grow, our consciousness and identity reach out from family to embrace group, community, nation, all humanity, other life forms, and other forms of consciousness and existence. Our true growth comes by making "otherness" part *of* us. As we expand our sense of self to include others, we grow by helping those others grow. As one tribe, our greatness becomes their greatness, and theirs is ours – and together we create an even more wonderful greatness. Such unforseeable changes will constitute the deepest and most radical evolution imaginable, and we will benefit from being alert to their manifestations as they emerge.

What changes is *Gaia-mind* ringing?

---

[4] Machaelle Small Wright's CO-CREATIVE SCIENCE, Perelandra Ltd., 1997, gives wonderful examples of how we can work with nature intelligence to co-create the places we inhabit.

[5] Greg Bear, BLOOD MUSIC, Ace Books, 1986.

CO-CREATION CONFERENCE CALLS

When I started working with subtle energies, I discovered I was totally blind. Doing shamanic journeying or other processes with a group, everyone else came back with wonderful experiences; I just sat there with nothing coming through. I had learned too well, growing up in a totally left-brain part of our world, how to block "wrong" things out. I mentioned my frustration to Nicki Scully, a wonderful energy healer. To my surprise, she said she was the same way, but that she had learned to ask for feedback from the people she was working on, which gave her guidance. But when we're working alone, and wanting to contact the spirit world, and seem to be blind and deaf, what do we do? One answer was so obvious that I hit myself in the head when it finally sank in:

Use kinesiology. Hook up, ask for what you want to know, in yes/no questions. Muscle-test for confirmation. Slow, but it works!

I later found that Machaelle Small Wright uses that procedure extensively in the processes she has developed to work together with nature intelligences to co-create gardens (in her process, anything that humans touch is a garden). Here is how she suggests to set up a "coning" or conference call with nature intelligences. You can find more details in her *Garden Workbook, Second Edition*, which also shows the amazing results that this process can achieve:

Ground, center, enter sacred space, and open chakras.

State, "I wish to open a coning."

Link with each appropriate member of the coning individually: the specific deva(s) of the place and/or organization involved; Pan, representing nature spirits; the White Brotherhood, a group of highly evolved souls in the spirit world focused on assisting our evolutionary process; and your higher self, to ensure the work done is compatible with your own higher direction and purpose. (She explains each of these.) If you don't feel a connection occur, that's fine. Allow about ten seconds for the connection to occur, then verify your connection using kinesiology before going on to the next step.

Do the process, work, or ask the questions you desire.

When the work is completed, thank your team for its assistance and close down the coning. This is important. Simply focus on each member of the coning separately, thanking them, and asking to be disconnected. Then verify that disconnection by using kinesiology. Check and see that you are fully grounded again in this world.

MIND TOOLS

LOOKING AT THE WORLD WHOLE

There are major gaps in the mind and body tools we use to understand our universe. Our sensory organs and cultural patterns condition what we see. A North lander looking at the size and color of snow crystals sees temperature and weather conditions, the past and the future. Looking at the same snow, we may just see "cold."

A scientific or engineering approach tends to separate out and look at just one issue at a time. An ecological viewpoint recognizes the interrelation of things, and tries to look at the world as a whole. A spiritual viewpoint seeks deeper levels of wisdom, not just knowledge. A chi-based viewpoint adds the need to consider more than just the directly observable material conditions of our world.

Bucky Fuller used to talk about sunsets in his lectures:

Most of us are used to seeing the sun **set***, he would say, but few of us visualize what is really happening. The sun really isn't setting on anything, is it? What is really happening is that* **the horizon is rising!**

Seeing the horizon rising shifts in our minds the source of movement from the sun to the earth, and keeps that framework in our thoughts. Taking another step back, the horizon isn't even rising; we're just rotating back away from the sun's side of the earth so that the horizon comes between our position and that of the sun. Pretty soon we begin to carry in our minds a picture of ourselves standing on a spinning ball in space, circling a star in orbit around the center of a galaxy spinning around a . . .

Consider another Fullerism: "Winds suck, not blow." We've all felt a strong wind snatch a hat off our heads and blow it away. But is that hat *blown* off our heads or *sucked* off? Here again, Fuller has tuned in to a deeper perception. Air is a fluid. A "push" in any fluid ends up swirling off in all directions as vortices, and can't sustain a concerted direction. What we feel when the wind blows on us is air being pulled past us by the low-pressure area on our other side. (Some of the "wind" we experience may also be one of those localized vortices bumping into us.) Such expanded perspectives have major implications for water and aircraft design, but also for a more holistic knowing of our universe.

✦

This process of backing off and gaining a more comprehensive perspective on a situation is uniquely important to us today. Our cultural mindset of single-process "engineering" has resulted in our becoming stuck in all sorts of irreconcilable positions: whether abortion, growth, law and order, or endangered species. Expanded perspectives get us out of looking at things as "right or wrong," of seeing only mutually exclusive opposites. The sun *is* still setting, the horizon also *is* rising, and yes, we *are* rotating into the earth's shadow. Together, expanded perspectives give us a fuller, multi-faceted understanding of the situation. The problems we face today are intractable only because conventional techniques applicable to "physical" problems are the *wrong tools* for resolving such problems.

These problems are solvable. They require a process of *surmounting* or *transcending* the apparently mutually exclusive viewpoints that have arisen from each of our faceted fields of experience. That process of transcendence usually involves expanding our experience to include an overarching third element. Broadening our perspective allows us to see opposites as *complementary dualities* – essential polarizations of unity (as in the Chinese *yin/yang*) – which are encompassed and catalyzed into an essential whole.

According to E.F. Schumacher, every society needs both stability *and* change, tradition *and* innovation, public interest *and* private interest, planning *and* laissez-faire, order *and* freedom, growth *and* decay.[6] Every society's health depends on the simultaneous pursuit of apparently mutually opposed activities or aims. The tension between these pairs of opposites that permeate everything we do is a vital aspect of life, yet one that requires a transcendence – in which higher forces such as love, compassion, understanding, and empathy become available as regular and reliable resources to create a dynamic unity out of the opposed forces.

Even good design sometimes needs to have the tension and expression of the opposites – and sometimes their encompassing into wholeness.

Schumacher also observed that there are four different fields of experience that create our awareness of our world:

* Awareness of what is happening in our own inner world
* Awareness of what is happening in the inner world of others, or of other life
* Knowing how we appear to others
* Observing how others appear to us

Importantly, each of these fields is accessed by different means. We can directly access our invisible inner world and how others appear to us. Yet what we see can be very different from what others see. We frequently perceive and judge ourselves by our *intentions*, while others see and judge us more by our *actions*. There is often no way we can directly compare our experience of love, pain, or anger to that of others. And what we track and pay attention to in the world around us varies radically depending on our values, sensitivities, and inner knowledge.

The other two fields of knowing we cannot access directly at all. They involve putting ourselves in others' shoes and the difficult communication of inner knowledge through symbols. It is often difficult to convert inner experience into communicable symbols, and we can't foresee how those symbols will be experienced internally by others. They are resistant to any attempts at quantification and prediction, as they involve living, changing natures; predictability belongs only to the fixed nature of less complex levels of being.

As we move from the material world of minerals, physics, and chemistry to the plant, animal, and human world, there is an intensification of life, consciousness and self-awareness. Quickly, the dynamic nature of those aspects of life overshadow the fixed, predictable, and quantifiable aspects that are amenable to the "scientific" tools we have used. As that complexity increases, interactive experiential dialog, and probing into the levels of existence where these things arise and

---

[6] E.F. Schumacher, A GUIDE FOR THE PERPLEXED, Harper & Row, 1977.

interact, become essential to our awareness and action. In terms of design, it may mean admitting we can't always anticipate the needs of a building's users. It might be wise by starting by giving *them* controls for lights, windows, heat and cooling.

To experience the world whole requires a unity of knowing – the integration and balance of these four fields of knowledge gained through appropriate processes. That unity is destroyed if one or more fields are uncultivated or examined with instruments or methods applicable only to other fields. The method used must correspond to the field studied. Our "logical" sciences only apply to the fourth field: observing the appearances of how the world looks to us. Self-knowledge, essential both for knowing our inner world and for translating communications of other's inner worlds, must be balanced by the often different knowledge of how we appear to others. Social knowledge, vital for indirectly accessible knowledge, requires self-knowledge as a basis.

✦

All this, still, is words. All this is the churning of a singular language system in our conscious minds, and only a fragment of the reality accessible to us. English is a language of nouns – of labels or names for "things". It is not a language centered on verbs, not a language of the sacred, not a language of relationships or glyphic images.

Names are curious animals. On one level, they have power gained from drawing distinctions. There is power, also, in *giving voice or connection* to something, which names can enable. Names can act as links or ties, giving us the ability to call upon something. On another level, however, names are only a secondary reality, rarely able to encompass more than a fragment of the wholeness of the "things" named. Unfortunately, we often confuse names with the reality behind them.

Names foster an illusion of awareness, creating a power-over, an *apparent* knowing of something. But all that is known is a label, far removed from that thing's reality and farther yet removed from the webs in which it participates. Names can become prisons for our comprehension rather than tools with which we can unfold a consciousness of Creation. It is important, always, to focus on what lies behind and beneath a name, what it arises from and is connected to, and not just on knowing the name itself. There are much deeper levels of knowing, levels far removed from names, at once more intimate and more powerful in acting from fullness of knowing.

It is possible to let both literacy and its more ancient and vital antecedent of direct knowing occupy and coexist in our psyches. That deeper and wordless connection with the primary reality of things, relationships, and patterns, is available to us when we are able to put our active minds aside. When we let ourselves become an open conduit through which those patterns, relationships, and realities can emerge into our conscious world, we apprehend a far different universe. There are even places between the worlds, available through trance, which are places of becoming – places where the seeds of future events, future relationships and future realities are shaped and given form. Words cannot be used there, but we can, in those places, join in the dance of shaping those realities.

All this may seem far removed from helping decide how big a window you want to put in your bedroom. But the names of "bedroom" or "living room" may keep us from seeing that a different room, which we'd kept under a different label, may be a much more wonderful place to sleep (see Place Tools, below). And learning to connect with things on deeper "wordless" levels brings much greater power into all that we do and all decisions we make.

✧

There are, then, many tools which can help us experience more fully, more truly, and more deeply the world of which we are a part. Learning to speak from the heart, and to give others the safety allowing them to do the same, guides our mind tools and keeps them within the realm of personal and shared truths. Kinesthetic awareness (listening to our dynamic whole-body perception), storytelling, meditation, yoga, body work, trance channeling, and ritual are a few of the tools that can help us reach more completely into the wholeness of our world and bring convergence into our experience of it.

Seeing the world whole means trying to experience as much as we can the many invisible worlds that surround and permeate us. A subtle mud line on trees may tell us of occasional flash floods. Consistent asymmetrical patterns of tree branches may speak of frequent high winds absent on a fine sunny day. Vague feelings of discomfort with a place may be tracked down to subtle signals we're picking up unconsciously; even if we don't track them down, we need to pay attention to such intuitive responses. As Aristotle once said, "The least knowledge of important things is more valuable than certain knowledge of unimportant things."

We can expand our modes of perception to connect with our world. We can learn to use methods appropriate to the particular conditions we are examining. Doing so, we perceive more of the interactive patterns and rhythms and events which underlie and generate our world. This, in part, is how an energetics analysis of a location differs from a traditional engineering or architectural analysis. Most important, perhaps, is letting go of an assumption that the world is only what we have in the past perceived it to be.

In a nutshell, we must use every method we can find, use them carefully, and assume that we are still half-blind. Only then can we achieve the best out of our relation to our surroundings or any situation we face.

FOLLOWING THE THREADS

In a culture unaccustomed to looking at things whole, it is easy to think about an issue in isolation. The problem is, this often leads us to conclusions that are not appropriate when looked at from the perspective of the whole.

Cutting down ancient forests, for example, has led to the response that it is wrong to use old-growth timber in construction, and then to the conclusion that it is wrong to use *any* timber in construction. The timber industry now urges builders to use "wood-chip I-beams" instead of 2x12s.

As one who lives where some of the great forests grow, it is clear to me that *using* wood is not inherently wrong. What is most deeply wrong is letting our population and our appetites exceed what the forests can comfortably support. The Japanese culture has existed for thousands of years, building wonderful wood structures without overtaxing the forests the way we do. Moreover, that wood was used in amazingly effective ways to show the incredible power and beauty of the trees. Looking deeply at a problem, such as wood use, may end up showing us that the real problem – and the real solutions – lie elsewhere. In this case, dealing with excess population and appetites.

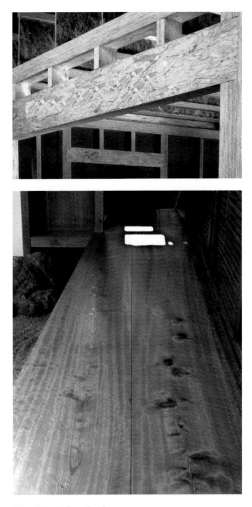

Most of the wood we use in construction is not old-growth timber. The forests also say that it's important that we *do* use wood. *Not* using wood removes it from our awareness. It is important, rather, that we use wood powerfully enough to keep it in our awareness, to deeply feel the beauty and magic of ancient trees, and to act to ensure that we continue to have trees. Not using wood, ignoring it, is akin to the harshest punishment used in many cultures: *shunning.* If a person is shunned, the community behaves as if that person does not exist. Even their family ignores them, no one speaks to them, no one ever lets their eyes meet, no one will do business with them. Shunned individuals quickly leave, go crazy, or die. This is not what should happen to our forests.

Choosing to honor and coexist wisely with our forests leads to reexamining our timber management practices. When we let trees grow for 240 years (much closer to old growth) rather than 60 years, it turns out that we *end up with twice the timber* (and better quality), *nine times the economic value from timber,* and *30 to 40 times the total economic value* from the forests.[7] Proposals to use "wood-chip I-beams" are merely a desperation act of companies that have cut down their forests for quick income, and are forced to resort to *any practice* that might bring in revenue quickly – however imprudent in the long run.

Top: Wood-chip glue beams are a response to overcutting forests, not optimum timber productivity.
Above: Floor boards cut through the heart of a tree expose its entire growth life.
Below: The beauty of a long life shared. Short forestry rotations lose a quarter of the growth period.

It is important, as in this example, to follow the threads outward from any issue of concern into the rest of the world. Those threads inevitably bring the insight and understanding that is crucial to wise action.

PLACE TOOLS

X-RAY VISION AND EMPTY MINDS

When we are examining an existing building, it is easy to slip into accepting what already is. "This" is a bathroom, "that" is a living room, "over there" is the front door. There are two important tools that can help us more fully visualize the possibilities of a place: *x-ray vision* and *erasing the labels.*

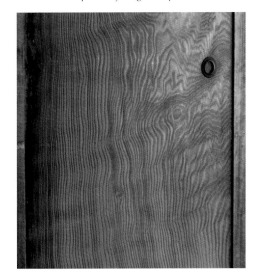

---

[7] See "Improving the Economic Value of Coastal Public Forest Lands," Tom Bender, IN CONTEXT, July 1996.

X-ray vision, for those of us who don't fly around in blue tights and a cape, can be achieved by a less esoteric skill: peeking around the corner. This gets us thinking about what is on the other side of a wall. Then we can start to ask what connections are possible by removing the wall, or cutting a door or window in it.

A small, old house we purchased a number of years ago was built close to a busy street on the north side. On the back side, however, it had a large yard, opening into a beautiful undeveloped city park with a creek running through it. You couldn't tell this from inside the house, however. There were almost no windows, and no doors on the back side! Peeking around the corners, or using x-ray vision, we figured out where decks could be built or where doors and windows could be cut into the walls, opening the house out into a wonderful private world of nature.

Using X-ray vision to see what is on the other side of a wall can turn a gloomy room into one connected with the world outside.

We added decks and openings to every room on the back of the house, and planted fir trees along the street in front. This totally reversed the orientation of the house, and opened it to sunshine, beautiful views, and private outdoor spaces.

So we need to constantly ask ourselves, "What is above that ceiling? Trusses, an attic, what roof configuration? Could the ceiling be removed to make the room higher? Could skylights be added to the roof to bring in light?"

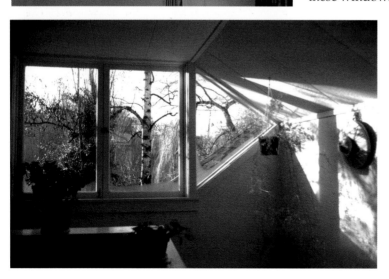

What is behind the wall you are looking at? Could it be taken out totally or be replaced by a beam, combining two spaces? Could a new door give access from this space rather than that one? Get on your x-ray goggles, peek around the end of the wall, or go outside and figure out where each room is. Do the same thing for upstairs and downstairs. What supports what? Where do walls fall? Chimneys? Stairs? Could the stairs be moved to a different location, rearranging the whole circulation?

The second tool becomes pretty obvious now. All it involves is to stop labeling the rooms we are looking at. Instead of "bedroom," say to yourself " a room about 12'x14' on the second floor, with south and east exposure, these windows, and that connection to circulation." Once the labels are off, we can quickly see how to do magic, like moving the entrance door to a different room to allow a former south-facing entry porch to become a sunny private verandah.

Learning these skills helps us see clearly what is really there and what changes can improve the livability and the energetics of a house. A delightful bedroom might be made out of a former breakfast nook with casement windows on three sides open to sunlight streaming through plantings outside. Asking yourself, with the labels removed, *where* you want to sleep, eat, and play can bring forth some wonderful changes.

MAINTENANCE AND CARING

Maintaining and caring for places needs to walk the narrow edge between love and obsession; between involvement and freedom. Like raising children, we can keep too tight a rein on the use of a place, ensuring that it never gets scratched, damaged, or dirty. But that can choke all the life out of a place. A clean and shining place can convey love and caring, or it can convey compulsive, emotionally empty drudgery.

What kind of maintenance is necessary to respect the resources, work, and love put into a place? What kind is necessary to allow the freedom needed for a particular activity? What kind of design and use of materials ensures caring, yet also ensures that the normal scratches, bumps, and scrapes of life can be absorbed without destroying the coherence of the place? A black or a white tile floor will show dust or mud instantly that would not be apparent on other colors and textures. A garden that needs to be manicured to feel right demands frequent maintenance unnecessary in a more freely designed garden.

Care needs to be given freely, not demanded – to be given out of thankfulness, not need. It needs to be offered as a gift to ensure that greater gifts become available to others.

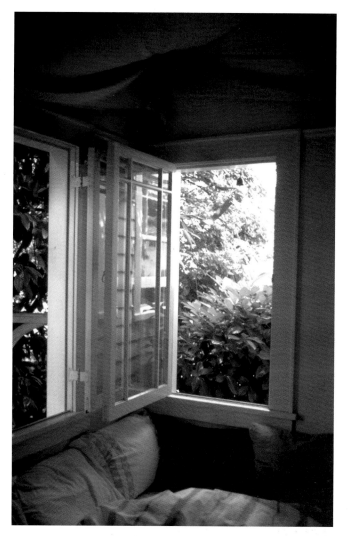

ENERGETIC TOOLS

SPIRITUAL CENTERING

Feng shui master Thomas Lin Yun teaches his students a wide variety of techniques and tools. Yet he counsels his students that those tools are not really important compared to their own spiritual training and development.

The situations we face are always unique; rules from the past or from another culture can at best be suggestions and guides to nudge our own intuition. That intuition gains power as we listen to and trust our connection to the world outside our skins. Cleansing ourselves of past issues, clearing our own energy, opening our chakras, acquiring meditation and trance tools, learning how to invoke sacred space, and discovering how to direct and channel energy are all means of connecting more deeply with our surroundings as well as furthering our own spiritual development.

A breakfast nook turned into a bedroom. Erase the labels in your mind of what rooms "should" be used for what purposes. Ask yourself where you would really love to sleep, eat, curl up and talk. Find ways to let those places happen. Eat breakfast in bed.

Most simply put, we cannot create anything different from what we are. As long as our root values are tied to greed, growth, and taking from others, the buildings, gardens, and communities we create will reflect those values. Our design work changes, grows, and deepens only as we do. Design starts with the designer.

TRANCE DESIGN

Energetic environmental design draws upon considerably broader, deeper process tools than the intellectual analysis/synthesis process of conventional design.

Many historical or mythological accounts of famous temples and sacred places describe them as "having lept into being in a single night." This is true of any project approached from an energetic perspective: once the heart-seed of a place is found, the design coalesces in one moment of trance or dreaming. In the world of unions and building permits, manifesting into physical form may take somewhat longer.

In design work the sensing, processing, synthesizing, and manifesting work involves every capability we have, not just our minds. It involves the rational, the subconscious, the deep memory in our tissues, the molecular communication of every cell in our bodies, the whole range of our psychic abilities, the assistance of guides, helpers, ancestors, and communal memory, and the interconnected capacities of all of life and Creation. Quite a committee to get together, but also a lot of free help.

This process itself often falls into several stages – most of them before even picking up a pencil. First, like any design, is identifying the boundaries, patterns and possibilities of the budget, program, site, codes, climate, and ecology.

Second comes a search for the real topology and relationships that can evoke the most powerful expression of what is to be accommodated in a place. At this stage, trance work comes into play, in sensing more deeply the topological and cultural patterns, the site, and the possible tools for accommodating and expressing them. What is its core spirit? What are the possibilities of expression in the site, culture, and time? What energetic relationship is established between the client, designers, and users?

What alternative tools are available? It is vital to look at each need and ask what different means can be used to accommodate it. Can it be taken care of solely through landscape means, or architecture, or interior design, or lighting, or institutional change, or by tweaking existing patterns, or some combination of these? Having a toolbox of alternatives available enhances the ability to obtain good, sensitive, powerfully coherent results.

The interactiveness of all these elements is so vital that it is difficult to design *anything* until *all* the relevant information is at hand and tossing around together in our hearts and heads. The process itself seems to refuse to start, saying "I don't know X or Y yet; it won't compute!" Starting to sketch or draw ideas too early often leads us to try to accommodate everything to those ideas. But if an idea keeps nagging or needs to be clarified, we may need to sketch it on paper to get it out of our heads and set aside.

The third stage is the crucial one - finding the heart-seed of the project – its spirit, its flavor, its smell, taste . . . its *soul*. Once that has taken form and permeated every cell of our bodies, it becomes an irrevocable touchstone which guides and aligns every element in the process of design, refinement, working drawings, and construction. To find it involves trance work. That involves moving into sacred space[8], and opening our full sensitivities to the spirit of the site, to its institutional heart-pattern, and to our own enhanced capabilities. It involves opening to assistance from all forces of Creation.

Trance work involves moving our rational processes aside and bringing into play the more deeply connective processes we inherit and share with all Creation. These are needed because only they can handle the complexity involved. Only they can bring into active dialog all the voices of all dimensions of Creation – past, present and future, materialized and immanent; from the most immediate and the farthest dimensions of existence which touch or are affected by this action. And only these processes can evoke the true power of creation into our work.

Trance design involves letting ourselves become one with each and all of these elements to the greatest degree possible, and then allowing them to dance and interact, to play and merge and coalesce on the dream level (or "between the worlds") into a coherent, resonant, powerful entity. This is the "building that leapt into being in one night." It contains the seed of all right answers for all the rest of the work involved.

Sometimes this happens merely from feeling the site. At other times it involves an agonizingly slow, step-by-step process of feeling through the program and physical needs. Sometimes it comes – pop! – instantly in a dream in the middle of the night. Sometimes it requires concentrated and lengthy working through of alternatives until their characteristics sort out and suddenly one pattern goes "click!" At times it may be an almost-visual image of a pattern of space and structure, materials and light. Other times it is more of a "taste" or "smell" of a particular timelessness and rightness. Usually, though, it doesn't come until we have as many of the pieces as possible in our bellies waiting to be digested. However it comes, we need to hang on to it, focus on it, and absorb it until we no longer need to worry about losing it.

The fourth stage is using that heart-seed as a *touchstone* to evolve the specific design. Now, using the exact site geometry, topography, vegetation, neighboring conditions, winds, natural light, and views, we can develop a preliminary topological (non-geometric) diagram of location, connection and barriers, and relationships. Here unanticipated opportunities often reveal themselves. What about that left-over corner of the site? What could it become or contribute? How do these two sequences of entrance and proximity compare? What does each have to offer? Here we can introduce second-order issues. "What can this situation give to the community?" "How can this contribute to the health of all Creation?" "How, in the particulars of this project and site, can we tie to our ancestors, to the past and to the future?"

After that, it may be useful to do a rough sketch to scale, getting the right approximate magnitude of spaces, thinking about possible structural systems, materials, or daylighting. This lets us know what has to be thrown out or juggled to fit. At each step in this stage, at every question or pattern focused on, we can reach back to the touchstone. If it doesn't resonate, we need to ask ourselves the

---

[8] Starhawk's THE SPIRAL DANCE, HarperSF, 1979, gives a good introduction to some elements of work in sacred space. Malidoma Some's OF WATER AND THE SPIRIT, Tarcher/Putnam, 1994, is an excellent resource on trance and the role of and connection with ancestors in a traditional African culture. Many spiritual traditions give specific training in trance and related work. It may be best to learn trance work with a person able to monitor your actual progress, give feedback, and act as a safety net.

questions that start to filter into our consciousness: "What if the wall between these two things were more open or more closed? Could this be darker, lower, or more open to the outside? Should this feel more unshakably rooted in the earth, or should it hover lightly above it?"

Each time, the touchstone will give a feel of rightness when the appropriate answer is evolved, and we can move on to the next unresolved issue, or just float through the holographically emerging design until a sense of dissonance brings attention to something that isn't yet working quite right.

From this point, the normal process of hard-lining, refining, and developing working drawings and specifications proceeds in a relatively normal fashion. Normal, that is, except that we have – deep inside us and humming warmly – that touchstone. It sits there quietly, guiding us more and more unerringly the more we trust it, to answers of power and rightness.

This touchstone works during construction also. Inevitably, we keep worrying about making the wrong decisions as each issue comes up. How wide should the deck be? Should this window be trimmed out this way or that? How should I construct this door? After a while, we finally learn the obvious: *We do get answers to these questions.* "Wow, this feels great!" "Yuck, this feels awful, guess I'd better tear it out and do it the other way." Or [. . . no reaction . . .] "Guess this isn't a significant issue and it doesn't matter which way we do it."

It may take a while, but we finally realize that we aren't working alone. The building itself, and the guides looking over our shoulders, talk back and forth, and both let us know if things are right or wrong. All through this process, the more fully we can drop into various levels of "trance" as needed to bring our complete faculties to bear on an issue, the better it works. This is not a mysterious process – just focusing, paying attention, and honing intention.

RITUAL

The role of ritual is a vitally important one in design, in sacred relationships, in shaping and using our surroundings, and in life itself. It is vital because it permits us to work on the subconscious as well as the conscious level, bringing together into harmony the various intentions that we hold on these different levels. As Denise Linn has so beautifully put it, *"Where our intention goes, energy flows"* – into our lives, our actions, and the places we inhabit.

Ritual is indispensable because it allows us to work in sacred space, and thereby to connect with and draw upon the wisdom, energy, and power of the entities which live in dimensions of existence other than our familiar physical ones. It is vital because it allows us to connect with the spirits of the earth, air, fire, water, and energy; to our ancestors, and to other life. It is valuable because it allows us to clarify and focus the energy of a group and use that energy to achieve our shared purposes. It allows us to align our intentions with the deepest forces of life, and gain power and rightness in our actions from that.

A ritual may be held in celebration, but it is not the same as a party. A ritual may be performed repeatedly, but unlike a habit, we need to keep its purpose conscious. It may or may not be ceremonious, but is not ceremony. It is focusing our conscious intention, using it to create sacred space, and invoking whatever can help us find a safe space to open ourselves to the creative forces of life. It is giving voice to our intentions and merging them with those of others, using that shared intention to draw energy into focus, intensity, and application to our deepest purposes.

Ritual is *taking action* on the energetic, communal, and spiritual planes.

Rituals need to be alive and born anew each time, coming from our hearts, or they have no power. Most rituals, however, have a sequence of some common elements:

* *Preparation:* becoming clear about our intentions; spiritual and physical preparation of our selves and our places; doing such things as cleaning, fasting, focusing, clearing out destructive patterns, and focusing on rightness.
* *Purification:* grounding, opening ourselves to energy flowing through our bodies, expanding our energy to flush and fill the place.
* *Opening:* establishing sacred space through calling in directions and guardians; connecting hara energy.
* *Invocation:* depending on the purpose of the ritual, this may include *invoking* (calling upon higher powers for assistance, support, or inspiration), *clearing* (assisting removal of unwanted energies), and/or *empowering* (creating an embodied energy linkage in a place or object).
* *Preservation:* taking actions to "set" the replacement of previous patterns with new ones, to remain clear about our intentions, and to keep our actions in line with those intentions.
* *Closing:* purposeful thanks and release of the spirits, guides, and guardians invoked.[9]

Ritual is tied with community. It may be a community of one person plus higher powers, or a large group of people and the spirit world that supports them. It produces energy, draws energy to us and through us into this realm, and allows that energy to support the community.

Malidoma Somé gives a partial list of the characteristics of true community, a self-definition by any group of people who gather with the intention of connecting to the power within:

* *Unity of spirit:* an indivisible sense of unity; the community needs the individual, and vice versa.
* *Trust:* everyone is moved to trust everyone else by principle.
* *Openness:* people are unreservedly open to each other; individual problems become community problems.
* *Love and caring:* what you have is for everyone; sharing.
* *Respect for the elders:* they are the pillars and collective memory of the community, holding the wisdom that keeps the community together, prescribing the rituals for various occasions, initiating the young, and monitoring the dynamics of the community.
* *Respect for Nature:* it is the source of wisdom, the locus of initiation, and

[9] See Denise Linn, SACRED SPACE, Ballantine Books, 1995; Starhawk, THE SPIRAL DANCE, Harper SF, 1979; and Malidoma Somé, RITUAL: POWER, HEALING, AND COMMUNITY, Swan, Raven & Co, 1993, for various discussions.

GROUP ENERGY IN RITUAL

When working in a group – using a place, planning changes to one, or gathered specifically to change energy in a place – paying attention to the energetics of group process can make a vital contribution to success. Two things stand out: linking individuals together energetically, and opening the process to bring in the wisdom and assistance of the spirit world. The later requires only entering sacred space and opening and asking for assistance from particular, or any, entities that can contribute positively to the goals of the group. Linking is a different process, called "using dropped and open attention" in the Reclaiming Wiccan tradition. A related description of the process can be found in Barbara Brennan's *Light Emerging*.

Ask the group to ground and center, and then for everyone to pull their attention inward with each in-breath. Pull attention in, first to the group space, then to your own body, then so it is just around your head, then just a grapefruit-sized ball inside your skull. Breathe with it and feel it there for a minute.

Then, when ready, let that ball of energy/attention float down the spine . . . slowly, easily. When it reaches the heart, hold it there for a moment, for a few breaths. Then let it float slowly on down, to the solar plexus, and then to the lower dan-tien or hara-point, a spot in the middle of your body a couple of inches beneath your belly button, that is your energy center.

Now let your attention expand from that point . . . out to your body, out to where it touches your neighbor's energy and then their bodies. Expand it on out, until the entire group is enfolded in your attention. You may see almost a disk or ring form, as the energy from each individual joins with that of the others. Focus your energy so it links from your hara point to a group hara-point in the center of the group. Feel unity of attention and intention emerge as that point comes into focus. That "group-mind" can then be linked to the spirit world, or to whatever is to be the attention of the group.

the source of medicine and nourishment of the community.

    * *Cult of the Ancestors:* they do not die; they live in the spirits in the community and are reborn into trees, mountains, stones and rivers to guide and inspire the community and the children.[10]

A community needs ritual, because it knows the virtual impossibility of existing without the wisdom and aid of the spirits, the ancestors, and the harmonized energy of the group.[11] In order for anything to happen in ritual, *it must be dominated by humility,* speaking from the heart, and open acknowledgment of what isn't as well as what is. Ritual must enable full acknowledgment, expression, and *release of emotions,* or it fails in its role of purification. Emotions open us, to power our linkage with others and the spirit world. A ritual must also *raise energy* if it is to be successful in nurturing the community involved. And it must direct that energy to the ritual's purposes, if its intention is to be achieved with power.

Ritual in the process of building keeps us in alignment with our purposes and opens us to allow the wisdom and energy of the spirit world to give vitality and power to our work.

RITUALS IN BUILDING

Ritual connected with the construction of buildings takes many forms, with various degrees of involvement of builders, owners, and the community, depending on the culture and use of the building. *In its highest form, ritual transforms the entire process of building into a spiritual practice.*

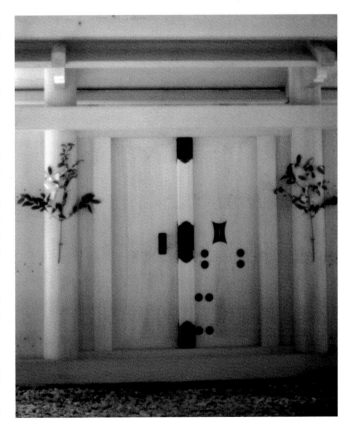

Teiji Itoh discusses more than twenty-two separate ceremonies that have been observed in rebuilding the structures of the Ise Shrines in Japan every twenty years for the last 1400 years.[12] These were used to bring the workers and the work in harmony with the spirits of the earth, mountains, wood, and various deities. They also demonstrate a Japanese process of making sacred space.

The first ceremony honors the deity of the mountain where the trees used for building the shrine grow, offering prayers for peace to the timber cut for the building. The second ceremony honors the deity of wood. It is performed by a child and a single Shinto priest. The child cuts a small tree with an ax, wraps it in a white cloth, covers it with a straw mat, and puts in into a sacred storage

---

[10] Malidoma Somé, RITUAL: POWER, HEALING, AND COMMUNITY, Swan, Raven & Co, 1993.

[11] Malidoma Somé's THE HEALING WISDOM OF AFRICA, Tarcher/Putnam , 1998, is an excellent exploration of ritual in traditional and modern culture. Starhawk & M. Macha NightMare's PAGAN BOOK OF LIVING AND DYING, HarperSF, 1997, gives a good introduction to rituals of grief.

[12] Teiji Itoh, JAPANESE ENVIRONMENTAL DESIGN, Vol. 2 - Architecture, draft, School of Architecture, University of Washington, 1965. See Kenzo Tange's ISE: Prototype of Japanese Architecture, MIT Press, 1965, for a visual sense of the product of this approach toward work as a spiritual practice. S. Azby Brown's THE GENIUS OF JAPANESE CARPENTRY, Kodansha International, 1989, gives an excellent sense of the depth of a temple carpenter's knowing of materials, process, and place in this way of working.

building until it is buried in the central part of the building site to house the spirit of the wood put into the shrine building.

Just before construction begins, a ceremony equivalent to laying a cornerstone occurs. A tree branch representing the earth deity is placed on an eight-legged table. The building area is defined by bamboo poles and a straw rope. The earth deity is invited in to occupy the space. To purify the land, a burial of ceremonial objects also occurs. Peaceful construction is prayed for.

This ceremony is followed by another to honor the tools, skills, and work of processing the materials. Generally a ridge beam or the most beautiful and largest timber to be put in the building is used as a focus for the ceremony. In the four parts of the ceremony, the representative timber is sawn, marked, hewn with an adze, and planed. Construction starts just after this ceremony.

Following the pre-cutting of the building framework, a ceremony occurs at the erection of the first pillar, followed by the assembly of the members of the framing. The most important ceremony occurs with the raising of the ridge beam, symbolizing completion of the framework. A festival area is prepared on the roof or the ground. A master carpenter inspects the measurements of all parts of the building. A post is set into the ground in front of the building and a rope stretched between it and the ridge beam, which an attendant pulls three times, symbolizing the setting-up of the framework. A bowstring is plucked, and mochi rice cakes and coins are scattered before tables at the northeast and southwest corners (direction of the spine of the islands and of chi flow in Japan). Gifts to the carpenters and a banquet complete the ceremony.

The date of the completion ceremony is set astrologically, and marks the occupancy of the new building. It is composed of separate ceremonies to purify the building, set the wood deity post into the ground, thank the deities for protection during construction, ornament the inside of the building, and welcome the soul of the goddess to occupy the building.

RITUALS OF RELATIONSHIP WITH PLACE

All change points in our relationships with places are important and appropriate times for rituals. In addition, cyclic points of renewal of relationships are valuable to sustain, enhance, and maintain the focus of these relationships:

> * *Founding*, or *commencing* any relationship with place is an important point for ritual - for grounding, for clarifying intention, for celebrating and blessing a new beginning.

> * *Site clearing or ground breaking* at the beginning of construction is the first active intervention, disturbance, and change of a place. It benefits from the blessing of the spirits affected and affirmation of the intention of the work. On a political rather than spiritual level, this has long been observed for public buildings in our culture.

> * *Construction* - This phase of a project has many opportunities, as Itoh suggests, for affirming relationships and thanksgiving for the gifts of materials, skills, work, and accomplishments. Traditional in almost every culture, from Scandinavia to Japan, is the *topping out* ceremony. This takes

place upon the completion of the roof framing, when the full construction of its support structure is completed and only enclosure and finish remain. Often a tree is decorated and hoisted to the ridge pole to honor and thank the trees whose lives have been given as the timber for the building.

* *Taking possession* of a completed building or project represents another milestone and transformation of relationship. Here the relationship changes from preparation to ongoing use and relationship with the place itself. In Christian churches, this is called *consecration*. In secular buildings its simplest form is a *ribbon cutting*. The phase of building is done, and the sacred phase of use can begin.

* *Cleaning, cleansing, and healing* are rituals that can be done and redone as needed when we wish to cleanse bad energy left by a former use from a place, clean up the residue our own actions, or move to a higher level of interaction with a place.

* *Exorcising* is a specific kind of ritual used to cleanse or clear a place from the presence of lingering spirits or harmful intention projected onto a place.

* *Sustaining* rituals are opportunities to reaffirm and reclarify ourselves, our actions and relationships, and our connection with place.

* *Connecting* rituals are often used when new people become involved, when significant changes occur in the nature and patterns of relationships.

* *Celebration or blessing* rituals are wonderful opportunities to raise the energy of a place, a community, and ourselves in response to an occurrence of importance to those relationships.

* *Concluding* rituals are helpful before saying farewell, moving out, or demolition. These are important times to reflect and honor the relationship that is ending. Bringing good closure to a relationship with places is as valuable as in a relationship with people. Acknowledging and thanking the place for gifts received during the relationship and some sort of giving in return are often involved.

These rituals affirm us, affirm our beliefs, focus our energy, show respect for gifts that have been given, and honor the place and what has been given into its making and alteration. All those actions raise and consolidate the energy of a group and help sustain it in its work.

WORKING WITH CHI

Systems such as feng shui or European geomancy strongly emphasize finding building locations with good chi in the land. Curiously, there seems to be less familiarity with traditions that focus on active direct work to sustain or enhance the chi of place.

The Wiccan tradition works with sacred space, raising group energy, and placing energy where it is wanted. Many energy-healing practitioners can read the energy aura of a place, much as they might read the aura of a person or a tree. Shamans and priests in Mayan, Egyptian, and other cultures work strongly with

CALLING AND MOVING PLACE ENERGY

Dowsers such as Joey Korn have shown that we are able to alter and enhance the energetics of a place using solely our intention, and that we can call on Nature to create a unique energy environment that is configured to support us in our efforts, wherever we choose. He suggests a simple prayer for use to focus and affirm our intention:

If it be Thy Will, may the Powers of Nature converge and work with any of the benevolent forces that are in accord with the Divine, to bring into balance any detrimental energies and to enhance and increase the beneficial energies in this entire house for all of the members of this household as to their needs, for all those who will visit, and for all of life, for now and into the future, for as long as is appropriate.

Reword this as needed or desired for your situation. Joey found that the more generally he stated this intention, and the less he called for a particular outcome, the better the results. As always, remember to ground, center, enter sacred space, and set up connection with the spirit world before making this request. Allow several of minutes for the work to be done, before uncoupling. See if you feel any changes. For more information, see Joey's book, *Dowsing: A Path to Enlightenment.*

energy of place. Many traditions work with clearing energy of place and putting good energy into a place as a healing practice. The Chinese worked with placement of pagodas and temples, draining, building dikes, altering of waterways, or planting trees to alter and improve the natural flows of chi in an area.

There is strong evidence from dowsing of English cathedrals that their energy over the centuries has been augmented and focused by the energy of pilgrims and worshipers.[13] The Black Tantric Sect of Chinese Buddhism stresses the impor-

[13] J. Havelock Fidler, LEY LINES: Their Nature and Properties, Turnstone Books, 1983, confirms my own experiences.

tance of the interaction of energy of people and place. In many Neolithic monuments such as New Grange in Ireland, quartz or granite rocks containing large quartz crystals were used in construction, possibly as accumulators for energy-related purposes.[14]

Energy work *with people* occurs in many cultures through the personal actions of priests, magicians, or shamans skilled in working with subtle energies. Ritual and community energy are strongly focused on by the Dagara and other African cultures, and that community energy acknowledged as vital for the well-being of the group. We know that such practices existed in the "esoteric" sects of all major religions. Tantra in Hinduism and Buddhism, Kundalini Yoga and similar practices in Taoism and Egyptian medicine, and faith healing and Pentecostalism in Christianity all involved active work with energy in our bodies, often in connection with *mantras* (sound), *yantras* (geometric diagrams), or *mudras* (hand-gestures). Good people and good community energy lead to good place energy; and many techniques are transferable.

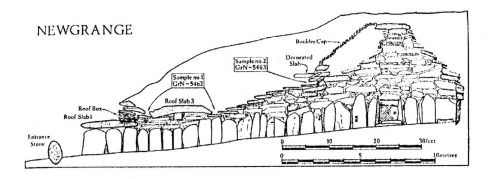

Ancient sacred places around the world show sophisticated actions taken to empower their ability to act as portals to the spirit world and to bring the benefits of those connections to their builders and users. At New Grange, a layer of quartz crystal was built into the mound to strengthen energetic connections.

The Chinese had their own word for shaman – *wu* – which appears tied with esoteric practices in other spiritual traditions. Important were dancing and the use of sound, which had particularly strong ritual significance in China. Women were prominent as practitioners. It appears that as Chinese society, and feng-shui in particular, later moved in a more intellectual and symbolic direction, the practice of working directly with energy receded into the background. Other than an occasional tangential mention of manipulation of earth chi, the practice of direct divination of chi through trance or actively directing energy and consciousness is rarely apparent in Chinese feng shui.[15]

The conscious creating and augmenting chi in a *place* and connecting it with sources of chi sustenance appears to be an important and undervalued aspect of working with the reciprocal energetics of place and people. Further exploration and development of it seems to be a fertile area of work.

---

[14] See progress reports on the Newgrange excavations in ANTIQUITY, 1964, 1968 and 1969 for location of the quartz layers.

[15] Feuchtwang (p142) quotes De Groot reporting on a geomancer standing at a spot on a slope where there is great accumulation of chi, then rushing down towards a proposed new grave site. This may appear all theatrics, but if the geomancer *had* made a linkup between his or her own chi and the power spot, it was one dramatic way to make a link-up to the grave site. Many other, less sensational ways exist, and presumably would have been discussed if energy work was an acknowledged part of the feng-shui repertoire.

CLEARING ENERGY IN A SPACE

The energetic detritus of our lives piles up in our living and working spaces. Both good and bad energy lingers, and anything that is not current or a loved remnant from the past needs to be periodically cleared from a space, just as periodic housecleaning is needed on the physical level. This is particularly true when moving into a new space, one previously occupied by others, or one where negative events have occurred.

Remember, a space that is energetically cleared is not the same as one that is compulsively cleaned to within an inch of its life! It is less important what you do, than your intention to cleanse and taking some action to achieve that state.

Cleaning is always a good, but not essential, way to clear or cleanse a space. With it, we physically touch most parts of the space enclosure, get the space to sparkle, and have ample opportunity to focus intention. Add a few drops of mint oil to the soap and water you're using . . . it will leave a light, fresh smell to the room that will acknowledge the cleansing. All sorts of techniques can be used for clearing – see Denise Linn's *Sacred Space* for excellent examples. Some useful elements are preparing ourselves by fasting, cleansing, focusing; cleaning the space physically; sorting out old belongings and "stuff"; greeting, honoring, and releasing any unwanted spirits in the place; opening doors and windows and encouraging old energy to leave, using fire, smudge, incense, music, bells, song, water, or a combination of devices. The main thing is our working in the space, while in sacred space ourselves, with the intention to release and clear the energy. It will happen. Here's an example using a drum:

Enter the space, and sit down against the wall. Begin drumming quietly, using a heart beat (two-beat). It's okay for several people to do this together. Close your eyes, breathe deeply, and focus totally on the sound of the drumbeat. Set the speed of the beat so that the second drumbeat quiets into stillness before the next one begins. In a few minutes, you will feel a difference, as your own sound, and that of other drummers, seems to come into focus. You've just grounded, centered, and joined the energy of the group and space, by a different technique! Focus and state your intentions to clear the energy of the space.

Now open the doors and windows, and move to the center of the space. Let the energy of the drumming take over. Every room has different energies, and will call out different drumming to resonate with that energy and release it. Listen to the sound of the drumming as it builds and fades. Let it build in intensity and volume as called for by the room. When that drumming feels it has come into clarity and focus, the main energy is cleared. Then walk slowly around the circumference of the room three times, counter-clockwise, quietly drumming along the walls. Stop at doors, windows, and wherever the drumming moves out of clarity, until it comes into focus again. Return to the center, and set the drum on the floor. Give thanks to the energies of life that have been in the room, and ask that they be welcomed to new places in the universe where their energy is needed and of value.

Then proceed to dedicating, consecrating, or setting new intention of the space.

SETTING INTENTION OF A SPACE

Once you have cleared a space, remember to refill it, with good, purposeful energy and intention. Denise Linn's *Sacred Space* gives an excellent introduction to the details of preparation, purification, invocation, and preservation involved in a ritual of setting intention of a space. She also gives a wonderfully detailed explanation of use of the four elements – earth, air, fire, and water – in cleansing and dedication of a space. See also the brief section on ritual in Chapter 7 of this book. An excerpt from instructions for a ritual, by Denise Linn, using colored candles to set intention of a space, can give a feeling for one way to do that:

Hold each unlit candle in your hands. Take a moment to center yourself and imagine yourself surrounded in radiant peace. Focus your intention on the results that you desire for the room. Bless the candles by holding them next to your heart chakra, or over your head asking for the blessings of Spirit. Before you light each candle, take three deep, full breaths, allowing a quietness to expand inside you. Visualize the results you intend for the room, let that fill you, and visualize the room filled with that feeling. When this feeling has reached a clear intensity, light the wick of the candle. In that moment the candle's flame acts as a magnifier and projects your thoughts and feelings into the room. Now simply gaze into the flame and allow your Intention to fill the room. Then just let go and relax. This is when true magic occurs.

She gives samples of prayers that can be used in lighting the different colored candles. Speak the prayers aloud:

Red: I dedicate this candle to courage, strength and passion. May the blazing life force of a red setting sun fill this room now! May all who enter this place be filled with strength, determination and zeal.
Yellow: I dedicate this yellow candle to the clarity of sunlight. May this room be filled with joy and clear focus. Bring wisdom, joyous communication and good luck to all who shall enter here.
Blue: I dedicate this candle to serenity and inner truth. May all who enter this room be touched by the gentle blue of the wide open sky, and may this room be filled with Spirit and peace.

And so on . . . . But use your own words, flowing directly from your heart in the moment. Other people's words, and even something you've put together and written down beforehand lack the power of even the simplest words that come from your heart in the inspiration of the moment. Once you put things in the hand of Spirit, the unexpected will always happen anyhow!

Opps! . . . did you remember to do all the energetic plugging-in and unplugging? Without that, all the rest is just fluff.

WORKING WITH INTENTION

Most of the exercises in this book are an introduction for working directly with chi energy in our surroundings. Some of them may sound pretty "woo-woo" or be frustrating at first if you are unable to consciously feel your chi energy being moved by your intention. If this is the case, concentrate first on working with intention, or li. It is the other leg to walk on in energetics of place; the instructions that call on chi and tell it what to do. Working with clear intention moves the chi by itself, without further mumbo-jumbo, and also works directly to accomplish things in the material world that feel good by themselves. So if the chi end of things makes you uncomfortable, just work with li to make places that feel good, and accept that there may be a "bonus" of things happening on an energetic level that you're not ready to deal with consciously yet.

Intention usually begins in our mind – a desire or wish to accomplish something. It is empowered from our third chakra – the one that deals with willpower or intention. It is enabled by our heart chakra – so the more of an empathetic or loving connection we can make with the people or place we are working with, the deeper will be the changes; the more powerful and beautiful what manifests on the material level. The clearer, more focused, and life-centered our intention, the more it moves into action by itself.

Ground and center. You can do this at work, on a job site, over a drafting-table. Search your mind for an intention concerning transforming a place or space you are dealing with. Envelop it with the energy from your "grounding cord" going deep into the earth. See if there is a deeper intention within it; an intention from the heart rather than the head. Focus on that, and see if the words, images, taste of it can come into clearer focus. Hold that intention.

Now move your attention slowly down from your mind to your heart chakra. Pause there for a few breaths to let the energy gather. Then ask the petals on your heart chakra to open and connect with your intention. Move your attention lower, to your solar plexus, where your willpower chakra is located. When the energy gathers, open that chakra also, and connect it with your intention.

Visualize the place or space you are working with, and connect your new intention to it. See what seeps into your conscious mind in word or pictures of changes that can embody that intention in this particular place. Let those changes take form, become clear and detailed. Then follow the normal paths available to you to implement those changes. Some new paths may emerge also, so keep open to "chance!"

This exercise is for *empowering* intention. If any parts of it are uncomfortable to you, leave them out and just work with the parts of it that you feel can help you become more clear on your intention or what you want to have happen. Later you can come back and add in the elements that help the process work deeper and more powerfully. For several dozen examples of changing intention and how it can transform how our surroundings feel, look at my *Silence, Song & Shadows*.

INTENTION AND CHI

There are indirect ways of working with chi energy which can be easier, more intuitive, and longer lasting than direct ones. I have elsewhere discussed several dozen basic changes in intention with which we can go about our everyday lives, while in the process creating significant changes on the energetic level of our lives and surroundings.[16] Honoring, giving, celebrating, changing community chi, connecting with our local communities of other life, and putting love into a place are but a few of the ways we can work from material actions into the realm of the spirit.

EARTH ENERGY

Locating sites for buildings, cities, tombs or other uses relative to existing patterns of energy in the earth occurs in many cultures. Most commonly, such earth energy or chi is located through the use of dowsing, though adept practitioners can use direct psychic attunement to evaluate it.

Dowsing with the use of forked sticks, pendulums, or other devices is an age-old practice used for locating underground water or energy lines. Simply put, dowsing is "whole body" perceiving of subtle signals from our surroundings, often using a device to visually amplify our body's responses.[17] Dowsing may be carried out on site, at a distance using maps, or merely by focusing attention on questions, depending on the problem and the skills of the dowser. Dowsers speak of such things as ley lines, energy leys, blind springs or energy domes, primary water, and yin energy flows.

With the growing resurgence of dowsing today, more communication with other fields of study is occurring. Repeated dowsing of specific sites by numbers of trained dowsers is beginning to develop consensus on what is experienced where. Better training techniques are being developed, and investigations of specific effects from different earth energy conditions are occurring.[18] Techniques for enhancing, diverting, and altering flows of earth energies using sound, earth acupuncture, or psychic action are being developed. Cyclic changes in different kinds of energy flows over time are beginning to be grasped, along with a deepening understanding of practices dating back to Neolithic times.

Comparison with Chinese feng shui work on various qualities of energy of place suggests that additional development work is possible in this area. And consideration of the Aboriginal access to primal wisdom through the energies of specific places discussed earlier suggests even further reaches of possibility for

Guy Underwood's dowsing studies of European churches show both placement on ancient power spots of earth energy (frequently already the site of previous shrines and temples) and also the accumulation of energy of pilgrimage over many generations of use.

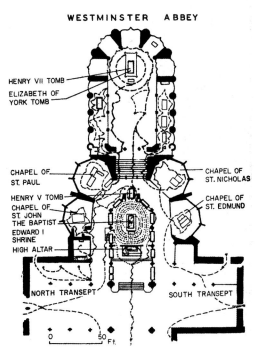

WESTMINSTER ABBEY

---

[16] Tom Bender, SILENCE, SONG & SHADOWS, Fire River Press, 2000.

[17] Eugene Gendlin's FOCUSING, Bantam, 1988, explains a step by step technique for gaining access to our body's awareness.

[18] Sig Lonegren's SPIRITUAL DOWSING, Gothic Image, 1986, gives a good introductory overview to dowsing and learning the techniques. Walter Woods' LETTER TO ROBIN: A Mini-Course in Pendulum Dowsing, 1990-96, downloadable from <www.dowsers.org>, gives an outstanding and simple process for self-training.

development of work with earth energies. As Johanna Lambert has indicated:

> *Aboriginal culture explains . . . this through its concept of "songlines," magnetic and vital force flows that emanate from the earth, crisscrossing the continent. Aborigines believe that they can project their psyche or inner consciousness along these songlines as a means of communicating songs, stories, and knowledge over great distances. It is said that songlines were once a sacred tradition that stretched across the entire earth, and, in this way, cultural knowledge was shared worldwide.*[19]

Learning dowsing or kinesiology, with their simple tools and procedures as aids, can be an important way to gain personal confidence in the existence of communication between people and place and our bodies' ability to hear those voices. But the real opportunities appear to depend on developing inner attunement to our body's overall perceptive organs and a clearer sense of what can be searched for and attained.

Parallel-held dowsing rods will swing towards each other and cross as they come to a positive alignment with the answer to what is being sought. Things like buried electric lines, with their own magnetic fields, will register those fields as well as the location of the wire itself. Remembering to open psychically and to connect with what you are seeking before you begin is essential to success.

---

[19] Johanna Lambert, WISEWOMEN OF THE DREAMTIME, Inner Traditions International, 1993.

DOWSING – SENSING SUBTLE PERCEPTION

Dowsing, like kinesiology, is a technique for making our whole-body responses to things more visible. Dowsers typically use hand-held rods or pendulums to exaggerate our imperceptible reactions so we can see them. My first real introduction to dowsing was when we built and walked a labyrinth on the beach a couple of years ago. Our friend who drew it said he had located the place by dowsing beforehand, but there was little energy in the spot. After we walked the labyrinth, he picked up his rods and walked from the outside of the labyrinth directly to the center, crossing all the lines. As he crossed each of them, the rods SNAPPED together and then apart. Our eyes bugged out of our heads. He then gave the rods to a couple of ten-year-old girls who had joined us, and let them walk to the center. For one, the rods responded strongly, for the other, more weakly. When we walked to the center, we could feel the energy palpably. To learn to use L-rods:

Take a fairly heavy-gauge metal coat-hanger. Cut it and straighten it out so you have two "L-shaped" pieces of wire, with shorter legs about 6" long, and the longer legs about 12", or whatever works with the coat-hanger size.

Hold one in front of you in each hand, loosely by the short end, like the Lone Ranger with a pair of six-guns. If working indoors, stretch a string or cord across the floor. Do the same out-of-doors, or use a garden hose, or a known location of a water line.

Ground and center. Open your chakras.

Take a couple of deep breaths, let go of tension and distractions, and focus your intention. Ask your body to teach itself to move the rods so they turn towards each other and cross as you move over a chosen object. Holding the rods level so they don't swing around of their own accord, approach the line on the floor. As you get near it, the rods should swing towards each other, and cross as you cross the line, returning to the original position as you move beyond the line. It may take several times before you develop a strong, consistent response. Repeat several times, until you become comfortable and confident with the response of the rods. If they don't respond at first, recenter yourself, speak your intention aloud in different words, in case what you said originally could have been confused, and try again. Don't tense up.

Then try to find some things of whose location you have a hint – buried electrical lines, phone lines, sewer pipes, septic tanks. State what you are looking for, and ask to ignore other distractions. Mark each time you cross something, then connect up the points and see of the line goes to the electric meter, sewer cleanout, etc. Ask someone who knows, whether you found the right spot. I found that I got a false reading on electric lines where I ran into the magnetic field around them, and had to average out the readings on both sides. Next time, when you cross what you are looking for, ask the rods which way to turn, and try to follow where the line goes.

With practice, you may be able to learn to dowse off of maps; to dowse for energy lines and power spots; to use the rods as a yes/no indicator of answers to questions you pose to the spirit world or your higher self.

For information on programming your body to pendulum dowse, download Walter Wood's *Letter to Robin* from the American Society of Dowser's website, or purchase it from their bookstore.

8 *GETTING TO KNOW A PLACE*

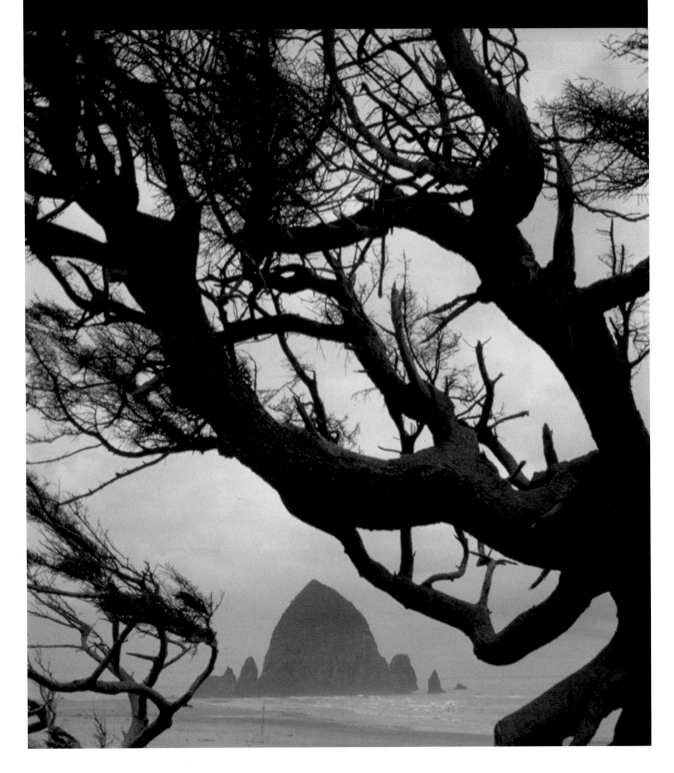

The goal of getting to know a place from an energetic viewpoint is to become aware of the physical and energetic patterns within it and of their interaction with the influences impinging on its site from its surroundings. We want to how the place is good or harmful for particular activities and people, and how it can be made more beneficial to the purpose of life, the communities, and the individuals involved. We can begin by communicating with the place, coming to know and love it in its complex, living wholeness.

This obviously involves both objective, physical information and intuitive awareness of energetic flows and patterns. It involves material and immaterial aspects of a place; psychic and spiritual aspects as well as physical; the dimensions of people and other life as well as architectural dimensions. The skills of apprehending all these things are rarely found in a single individual, and we may need to get help with what is outside our own skills and abilities.

On the other hand, don't underestimate your tummi. The most important thing is how comfortable you feel in a place. Someone else's sensitivities or concerns may have more to do with their own needs than yours. Trust your gut feelings. If you're working on someone else's places, get them, and their tummies involved, or try to include them in your "tummi testing". Regard this chapter as a checklist to remind you to "look both ways before crossing the street."

Opposite: Seeing what isn't there. Even on a quiet day, the shapes of trees speak of strong winds and wild winter storms.

Below: The hills in the background are the remnants of the ocean-canyon riverbed of the Columbia River. Lava floods from Central Oregon filled the canyon, and sediments on both sides eroded away as the land was raised by tectonic subduction activity.

SURROUNDINGS

No place exists by itself. Its neighbors, history, and impinging future, as well as our perceptions of those forces, all influence its present existence.

NATURAL FEATURES
It was recently discovered that the mountain we live on used to be a canyon – the offshore *riverbed* of the Columbia River millions of years ago, which filled with molten basalt from the cataclysmic rock floods in eastern Oregon. As the land rose, sedimentary rock on both sides eroded away, leaving a monolithic moun-

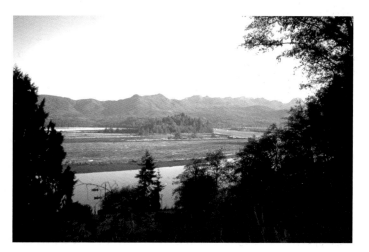

tain chain of volcanic rock where there once was a river channel draining the entire northwest section of the continent. We sit today on a river of fire from beneath the sea. What a shift in perspective on where we live!

Those long flows of history live in our minds and hearts, and color in subtle ways our current patterns of life. Look outward from the particular place you are concerned with, and try to see what larger patterns it is part of, both geographically and temporally. The surrounding land, geology, soils, water, topography, watersheds, and airsheds can teach much about the place itself. In hilly areas, cold air drains down and pools in valleys – cooling in the summer, but extra cold in winter. Fog and rain follow particular landform patterns, as do tornadoes.

The area where I grew up in Ohio was situated between two east-west glacial moraines. Old local legends said that tornadoes never strike between these "North and South Ridges." This was all interesting folklore until one day we saw a tornado funnel moving directly toward our house from the west. Suddenly, a couple of blocks away, it split into two funnels, one passing north of the North Ridge, the other passing south of the South Ridge! Enough for doubts about the importance of landforms.

Sometimes maps can help us see invisible forces affecting a site. Is there a swamp upwind that will share its mosquitos with you? Will the airstrip across the bay bring noise and unwanted visitors on the take-off path? Where will the city expand next? What about flooding potentials, or landslides?

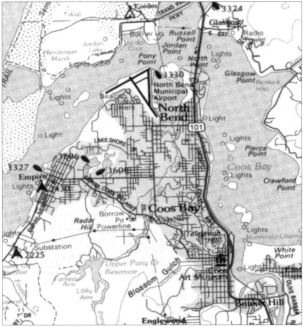

From maps, from high places, from the air, and by moving on the ground through the area, we can examine the patterns of *natural* features. In an urban area, these still exist underneath the buildings and roads. A friend built a house in Vancouver, B.C., only to have his basement flood while the neighbors' all stayed dry. He found out that his lot was crossed by a now-buried creek.

Look at the patterns of mountains, hills, prominences; the kinds of rock, steepness and stability of slopes, the geological history of the area. Follow the branchings of valleys and gullies; rivers, creeks, lakes, ponds, and waterfalls. Trace them in and out of their bondage in culverts.

Look at drainage, wet soils, marshes and swamps; isolated trees, forested areas, patterns of vegetation in general, and the kinds of wildlife. When a local builder moved a bulldozer onto one particular site to prepare for foundations, he found that the ground belched noxious gas every time the bulldozer went back and forth. It turned out that the site was a ravine filled with accumulated peat, over which a couple of feet of dirt had been spread before it was sold. Deep study of a site before buying it can save a lot of trouble later on.

Look at areas with no sun or no shade. Is the area subject to earthquakes, hurricanes, tornadoes, blizzards, ice storms, floods, or other intense natural events? Feel these things both in the wholeness of their patterns and in how the place you are considering is part of those patterns. New knowledge of local tsunami hazards in a community can cause property values in certain low-lying areas to plummet. Together, all these elements indicate the history of interaction of natural forces out of which the character of a region has evolved.

What is the temperament or spirit of the landscape, and the character of life that has matured in it – rugged, bountiful, languid, peaceful? What is and will be the related character of people who live as part of those patterns? Hill people, valley people; agricultural and hunting people; people of the deserts, of the snows, of the rain countries – all are and become different kinds of people.

HUMAN ELEMENTS

Look, then, at the *human* elements that have become part of the surroundings – at how they have responded to the natural features, changed them, and added to them. What are the meanings and implications of the agricultural and urban patterns? Look at the fields, hedges, drainage systems, and canals; the roads, bridges, airfields; phone and electric lines and microwave towers. What energy and spirit have tunnels, quarries, junkyards, industrial sites, and road cuts created? What is moving in over the horizon?

Look at how places change in short cycles. A peaceful campsite on the Oregon coast at noon on Friday can turn into bedlam by Saturday morning when the weekend dune buggy racers arrive. Many whole communities go through regular dramatic transformations due to tourism or other seasonal changes.

What would you do, if given the site visible below to build on, or the site from which the drawing was made? What changes would you make? What choices of building shape and placement, or decisions NOT to build, would enhance rather than destroy harmony with the forces in the landscape?

INVISIBLE FORCES

Try to become aware also of what *invisible* forces – both natural and human – are at work in the surroundings and what impacts they may have. The apartment is lovely, but what about the subway trains that shake the foundations eighteen hours a day? A house looks idyllic until you peek through the trees and realize that it is surrounded by TV broadcast towers beaming microwaves across the site. What are the energy flows and concentrations in the earth and air? What are the auras of the land and cities? What about its electromagnetic fields?

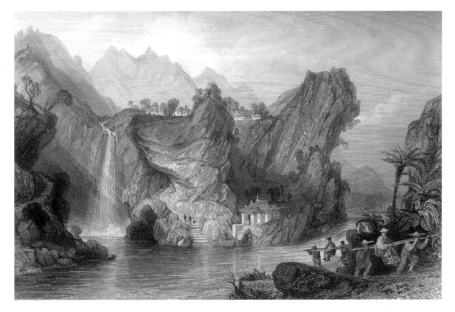

In a city, zoning regulations may not be visible at first glance, but a zoning decision made last week or next year could totally transform the area.

What population pressures might cause rezoning of the area from rural to urban, from residential to industrial? What transportation and political pressures might generate a new freeway artery that brings large numbers of people into the area? Where might the next airport be located, bringing planes overhead or development next door?

What is the health of the area? Does it feel nurturing or debilitating? How could it be changed for the better, or might it change for the worse? What are the colors of the area? Who are the plant, animal, and human neighbors? Can you see the stars at night, the rising and setting of the sun and moon? Can you feel the patterns of clouds moving overhead? What changes do the seasons bring? What

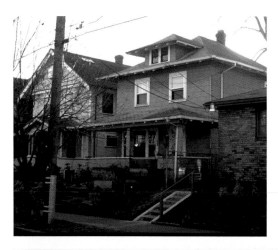

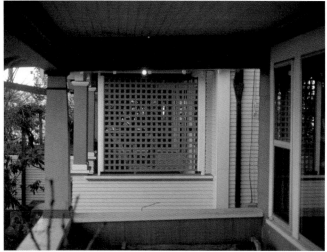

Top: Do close neighbors look in your windows? Could skylights bring sunlight and ventilation with privacy?
Above: A lattice screen on abutting porches gives a degree of visual privacy while still permitting ventilation.
Below: Industrial neighbors may be quiet or noisy, or problems at night. This one was for sale – and was replaced by expensive, multistory condos. What are the pluses and minuses and likelihood of such changes?

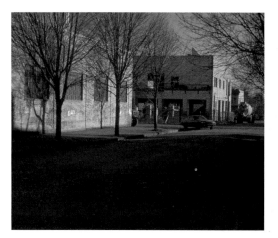

changes has the last century seen, and what might the next century bring?

Do the patterns at this place feel generative of life? Remember that life encompasses waterless deserts and windswept plains, not just farms and people. How do topographic elements – nearby mountains, rivers, valleys – feel from the site? Do they give a sense of protection, high energy, stultification, threat? Does your spirit rise or fall as you sense the patterns of life? How does this area feel as a place to be? And how easy is it to feel, and be part of, all these aspects of the flow of life around this site?

NEIGHBORHOOD

Particularly in urban areas, look at the human-created patterns immediately surrounding the place. What are the size and density of buildings? Are trees present? Again, what about phone lines, electrical wires, drains, and culverts? Are there electromagnetic fields from power lines or transformers? Will street lights shine onto the site? Are the houses so close as to feel claustrophobic? Are the neighboring townhouses fire- and structurally-separated?

What wealth, cultural, and social patterns are reflected in the surrounding residential area? Is there love in their making and use? Do people's houses look inviting and cared for? The neighborhood of manically manicured lawns might not be welcoming to your vision of an unmown wildflower meadow around your house. Is there welcome in the streets and the businesses? Is there space to walk and breathe? What are the intentions or values underlying what is there? Is the land-use pattern one for people, or is it automobile-based?

What about places to play, places to worship, schools, workplaces, or markets? What are the sounds of the neighborhood, and its energy – hostile, angry, loving? Are there institutions you would want to be near or ones you wouldn't want to have for neighbors? Is there singing, screaming, loud music, or laughter? Do you hear people, birds, and animals – or machines? Is there a feeling of community?

What about sources of negative energy? Are there graveyards, hospitals, old battlegrounds, police or military installations, industrial facilities, or similar places nearby? Being on the ambulance approach route to a nearby hospital might keep you awake at night, but also make you superconscious of death, illness, and accidents.

Are building materials and landscaping subject to conflagration? What is the proximity of other buildings, walls, and windows? What are the shapes of roofs, the direction of roads and driveways? Do the impacts of these things on the property feel protective or threatening? Are there ways to shield or alter them?

Look again for hidden things. Ask yourself, "What am I not seeing?" The beautiful trees surrounding a house I once lived in turned out to be screening a view into a railroad freight yard. All night, freight cars crashed together as the next day's trains were assembled. At another apartment I had in Virginia, there turned out to be a single railroad track tucked out of sight across a parking lot. What was invisible turned out to be quite audible, however. This was the precise point where the engineers would put all five of the train's engines to full throttle to get up the nearby mountains.

What impacts – positive and negative – would the use proposed for the site you are examining have on its neighborhood and surroundings? What could it give to the neighborhood?

THE SITE AND SITE BUILDINGS

TOPOLOGY AND TOPOGRAPHY
Now, focus on the site itself. Come to know it as intimately as possible, by day and at night; in rain and dryness, in all seasons. Does it receive adequate light and sun? Does it feel too exposed or too shaded? What is its orientation? Will it overheat from afternoon sun? Is it buffeted by wind or stifled by lack of air movement? Does it feel protected or threatened, energized or deadened by the people, places, and things around it? The north-slope site that is cool and shady in the summer might also turn out to be dank, chilly, and sunless for six months of the year.

Looking at the site, consider the same things as in its surroundings, but pay attention to their detail on this site and how it relates to those surroundings. Does entrance to the site or building feel exposed? Is the site located on the outside of a bend in a river which feels like the river could undermine it? Will the headlights from cars coming down a street shine directly in the windows? Are there steep banks above or below the site, and are they stable? Does anything neighboring loom over the site? What are the soils, drainage, views, vegetation, shading, or access to sunlight?

Do the site and buildings feel like they have good chi? Could it be enhanced? Does it feel like there is good chi nearby to connect with? Is there a feeling of bad energy on or impinging on the site? Could that be changed by drainage, planting, building, or energy-clearing on the site? That little asphalt "dam" across the driveway could alert you that the long sloping driveway drains water directly into the house every time it rains. Does it feel like exposure to good or bad energy is stronger in one direction or another? Could plantings, walls, storerooms, garages, or other seldom-used areas shield the main building from bad energy? Could important spaces be relocated to orient toward good energy?

Does "street energy" come directly into the site or the building through perpendicular walks, roads, or driveways? Are front and back door directly opposed, causing a feeling of public space through the building? Is there privacy on

SENSING CHI IN A PLACE

Some people, using dowsing, can make detailed maps of the subtle energies in a building or a building site. Others can see the energies visually, or sense them in other ways. Most of us, however, are left with only vague feelings of comfort or discomfort; depression or joy, in our tummies. Here's an exercise that may bring a little more clarity to such feelings:

When first visiting a site our building, sit for a moment, purposeless, just soaking up its energy. Don't try to make any sense or observations of it. Ground and center, open your chakras to tune in to the place, particularly your third eye. Call in the deva of the site, that of the organization potentially involved with it, and any spirits that inhabit the site. Honor them, and thank them for their attention to the place. Ask for assistance in sensing whether a good fit is possible between the organization and the place, and what energetic and material changes might benefit that fit.

Then, with your chakras open, wander around without purpose inside and outside any buildings, around the site, around its neighborhood. Just let your bodily energy-magnets pick up what is there, without judgment, without analysis. If you're with others, share impulsive comments that arise, and just hold those from others. Then find a comfortable place to sit.

Close your eyes and visualize the place before people had come to it. Was it forested, a prairie, a swamp, a creek draining a mountain valley? Feel that energy with your tummi. Then, with eyes still closed, visualize it today. Mentally take away the buildings, the parking lots, the signs, the utility lines, the trees. Let everything fall away until nothing is left but visible patterns of energy. How does that compare to the energy before people came? Compare the energy feeling of the site to that of the surrounding neighborhood – without buildings, streets, names, institutions. Is the site drained or fed energy from its surroundings? Does it feel that future changes, buildings, uses will harm or improve the energy? Now compare the energy of the site and the energy of the use that is anticipated for it. How do they fit, and nurture or drain each other?

Next, with that gut-feeling energy map of the site in your mind, walk the site again. This time, pay close attention to each part as you visit it. In the energy map in your mind, did your tummi feel uncomfortable in this area? Why? Can you pick up any more specifics? How about places which you have a vague sense of good-feeling? Can that come more into focus? Ask your spirit guides for feedback and direction. Are there parts of the site which should be left for the nature spirits, or specific things that might develop synergetic relationships with them? When your tummi feels as full and clear as possible, shut down, and proceed with a more conventional analysis of the site. Thank the spirits and disconnect before you leave.

Let everything soak and stew at least overnight. In the morning, as you wake, check what new perceptions have fallen into place overnight. Think back on the place you chose to sit. What is the energy of that place to which your body led you? What new clarity has formed about present energy, possibilities of change, and fit with potential use. Focus on that, and keep it as a touchstone as you proceed with explorations, discussions, and design.

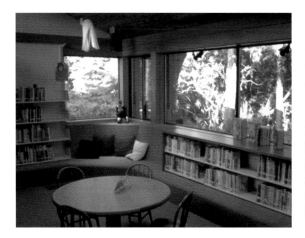

the site or in the building? Is connection maintained with the community world of the street? Is there anything about the site, building, or surroundings that would attract thieves? Or are there "friendly watchers" that prevent such encroachment?

Is there exposure to lightning, high winds, reflected light, noise, or anger? Are other forms of life present and bountiful on the site? What about other life attracted by poor maintenance and living practices – cockroaches, fleas, rats, or other less welcome neighbors? Is there any evidence of hazardous herbicides or pesticides having been used there?

Low windows in this library children's room create a connection with the trees, rain, and sunshine. A bird feeder brings other visitors.

PEOPLE – PAST, PRESENT, AND FUTURE

What about connection between people who use the place with other people and other forms of life? Are there outdoor spaces? Are they as carefully considered regarding their possible uses, access, and interconnection as spaces inside the building? What do those spaces connect you with? How do they feel? How would they feel in a different season? Are they easy to access and do they encourage use? Do the intention and design philosophy expressed in the buildings and gardens reflect a positive attitude toward life?

What is the people history of the place and its neighbors? Are neighbors happy? Is there a history of death, divorce, or unhappiness? Are personal, family, or business failures connected with the property or the neighborhood? Can causes be found and remedied, and energy cleared? What changes have historically happened to people who use the site or surroundings?

This house, now a Bed-and-Breakfast, has at least four doors visible as you approach it. Location of fences, walks, and landscaping can avoid confusion and make the right connections automatic.

There are two buildings on our local main street, where businesses have *never* lasted more than a year. The reasons are different for each building, but the situation has gone on so long that locals now assume that any new business in those buildings is going to fail, so they don't even patronize them!

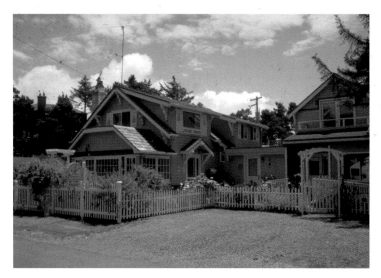

Look at how the human past, present, and future touch the site. What changes in it or its context have occurred or might occur?

CONNECTIONS AND BARRIERS

Look at connections and barriers: what are the sightlines in and out, what kinds of sound links exist? What about acoustical separation between neighbors on the other side of a wall, floor, or ceiling, or between close-by windows? How clearly are boundaries established between public and private space, and can they be clarified?

Is entrance to the building confusing or difficult to find? Are there multiple doors? Is access awkward: are there sticking doors, broken latches, storm doors, steps, railings, tree branches, snowdrifts, or anything else that makes it uncomfortable to go in and out of the building? Is there evidence of care and love in maintenance and upkeep? What does the place smell like?

What are the patterns of ownership, management, and care for the buildings and neighbors that may impact their condition? What values are reflected by the design and construction, building patterns, proximity, and connections?

Are there things in the layout of the building or site that give improper signals to people? A stair directly facing an entry door may make it appear that private upstairs rooms are really the main public spaces in the building. A bedroom with an outside door more visible to visitors than the entry door may receive unexpected guests. Unclear access paths to different apartments or businesses in a building may cause confusion and people going to the wrong doors.

Lack of clarity about whether a door opens into public or private space may result in tenants feeling invaded and visitors feeling embarrassed. I have known several apartments where closet doors looked just like the entry door. Departing guests would frequently walk into the closet rather than out into the hall, much to everyone's embarrassment. These and similar things also convey that the builders and owners have not been aware of their surroundings and their impacts on people, and may cause lingering concern about what other surprises lie in wait.

How does the place move your heart – or does it? Are there specific things or a general feeling that attracts you, moves your heart, and makes you want to stay? Are there things that make you want to leave? Or possibly worse, is there nothing present that moves you at all?

Places that have dramatic and abrupt features, like houses on the edge of a cliff, often have powerful energies. They are also generally not easy to live with, and at best require special and careful patterns of use in order not to be damaging.

The shapes and configurations of buildings, lots, and spaces should also be considered. Complex property shapes may be hard to utilize well. This can sometimes be overcome by utilizing the otherwise awkward configuration to create a series of connected outdoor "rooms" rather than a single oddly shaped space. Sloping properties can sometimes be used to create uses separated vertically instead of just horizontally. Here again, use the tummi-test. If you feel comfortable about being able to use it, okay. If it *feels* awkward to you, it is.

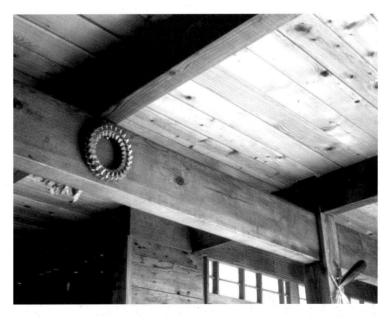

This floor/ceiling construction uses little more wood than one of plywood and chip-wood beams. It uses local products, and gives a floor and ceiling that grow more beautiful over time. Wise choices are not always ones proposed by those who would profit from them.

Buildings, like most creatures, come in all shapes and sizes. Some are put together poorly, others well. A giraffe is an unlikely but beautiful creature, well suited to its conditions. Similarly, a building can take an unexpected or unusual form to achieve something valuable. Another building with the same form, cre-

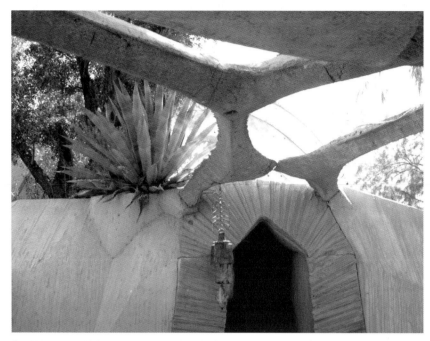

What is wise building design in one climate may be totally wrong in another. In the desert, buildings stick out like sore thumbs. Paolo Soleri found that building down into the earth makes them less intrusive, tempers the day/night temperature swings, and gets away from the sometimes unplesant winds. North and south-facing outside alcoves give shade or heat-traps for outdoor living year-round.

ated just to be different or out of poor design, feels wrong. Again, we feel the aptness when we sense its connection and purpose, or lack of it.

What is a strange-looking house to one individual or culture might be a wonderfully harmonious home to someone else, or in another culture. (Whether that person or culture is in harmony with the earth and the universe is, of course, a different question!) We have to be sensitive to context and meaning. And as Frank Lloyd Wright always warned, new things may not feel comfortable until we become familiar with them.

Coherence is probably the most important criterion. Is there a oneness of intention, purpose, and attainment – *and* congruence with the purposes and needs of the intended users?

Remember, also, that our little Earth-ball has extremely varied conditions within which long lasting cultures have existed filled with joy, wisdom, creativity, and beauty. What may appear to be a hostile or unlivable place to an Englishman may, to a Bushman, Inuit, or Khmer, be the receptacle of thousands of years of joyful existence. And vice versa.

To many, where I live might be a harsh and unfriendly world – 120 inches of rain a year, unstable ground, hundred-mile-per-hour winds. It is home, however, and I love it. In turn, I feel uncomfortable and smothered when I cross the Coast Range into the Willamette Valley, a tame and benign place where everything can and does grow. So what is good in terms of place is only what is good in terms of culture, history, connectedness and context. There is no universal answer. Get that old tummi out again, it is still the best measure of rightness.

INSIDE BUILDINGS

Inside a building, we need to pay particular attention to the needs of individual activities and the connections between them. A place where kids play should probably have close connection to where an adult is able to keep an eye or ear on them. In one family, this may be the kitchen; in another, a home office. We can easily get over-specific in this area, as our real needs are much less than our common cultural patterns, particularly in materially rich cultures.

Privacy doesn't require "separate rooms." It was achieved, for example, in a traditional Japanese family home merely by turning to face the wall. That was an accepted signal to others that a person wanted to be alone for a while. Similarly, people from cultures filled with "things" are often amazed at the wonderful meals that can come from the simplest "kitchen," or the enjoyable life possible in homes without dining rooms, TVs, separate bedrooms, computers, or garages.

In some cultures, people rarely bathe. In others, the bath is the most important space in the home. To some, the hearth is the core of "home." To others, it is the kitchen. Some cultures have separate rooms for different activities. Others have lightweight furniture and storage separate from the rooms, so that a room can be used for dining, living, sleeping, or other purposes at different times.

In looking at a house or a floor plan, try to throw out preconceptions. Just look at the individual spaces, their size, orientation, and connections, and try to figure out how best to use them. If room A isn't big enough for a home office, it won't work. If room B is the sunny and warm room, in many climates everyone will gravitate to it regardless of the intended use. And if we have to go through room C to get to room D, that interlinks the use of both.

A comfortable entrance, with separation from the interior space of the house, is important. Comfortable places to gather, eat, play, prepare meals and sleep are important. Connection with the outside worlds of nature and community is important. But the actual design which helps any of these places work well is dependent upon the specific circumstances.

What can give EVERY part of a home qualities that move our hearts?

In most buildings, detailed rules of what is good or bad for movement of chi in the place are probably far less important than two overriding considerations. The first is the chi generated from the happy and harmonious use of the place. And the second is the chi generated from the clarity of intention of the designer and builder and the harmony of that intention with the spirit of life in the place where the building is located.

The presence of *soul* in a building is necessary in order to attain either of these considerations. This involves, in part, absence of machine noises (TV, toilets flushing, washing machines, refrigerators, furnaces). It involves use of natural building materials and honoring their past lives. Elimination of excessive space, energy use, and TV are also necessary, along with honoring the heritage, the ecological community, and the spirit of all life.

One general principle of comfort and security in a place, which is buried deeply in our genes, is *freedom from surprise*. In geomantic rules, this translates into not having our back to the door of an office, and not having our bed facing away from the door of a bedroom. There is reason behind these rules, but they need not be followed to excess. There are usually a variety of clues and senses by which we become aware of someone approaching. In a quiet house, a squeaky floor can fulfill the same purpose, or at night, reflections in window glass. In our own house, we can see from our bed, through reflections in the windows, if the kids are sneaking into the cookie jar in the kitchen!

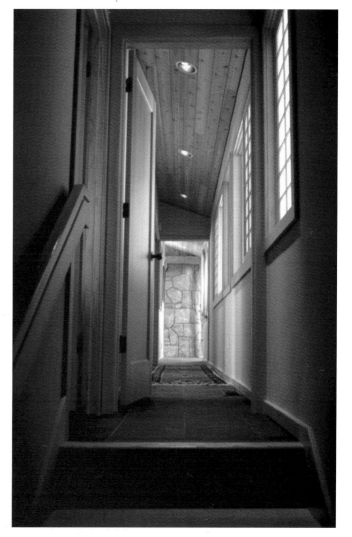

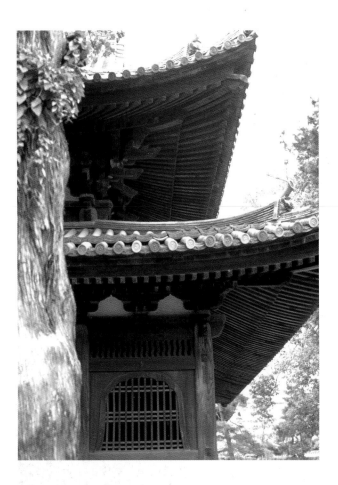

The "roof beams" visible in the photograph above are actually a false ceiling that cover up the massive roof beams (below) and give a sense of lightness and effortlessness to the structure.

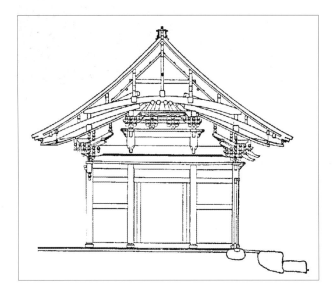

Another element of security is *faith in the adequacy of our shelter*. Fears of the roof blowing off in a storm or of a nearby tree falling on a house silently sap our energy. Worry about a sagging floor or beam, or a leaking roof, diffuses our attention, as does movement of a building in the wind. Even a well-designed building *can* feel uncomfortable if we are sitting or sleeping right under a large beam and becoming aware of the immense weight it must be holding up. (This effect doesn't seem to occur as much with repetitive rafters or floor joists, or beams with an arch or curvature to them.) As mentioned earlier, a typical geomantic response to this beam/weight situation in existing buildings is to hang a feather, or a flute, or something associated with lightness from the beam. Our minds intermix the two senses and escape worry about the weight overhead.

Several cultures have developed specific building practices to avoid this feeling of structural effort to support overhead loads. Certain temples in India use *corbelling* (further projecting out of successive courses of masonry from the wall) to span spaces without the feeling of heavily-stressed beams. Roof structures of Japanese temples employ a particularly clever sleight-of-hand. The builders wanted the feeling of shelter from wide overhangs of their massive tiled roofs. But they wanted to achieve that feeling of shelter with an *effortlessness* that wasn't really possible structurally. So they ended up building fake ceilings of small rafters to hide the big structural rafters, with upward curvature to the whole roof so that it feels almost weightless from underneath!

Some cultures have specific rules in their geomantic traditions for location of kitchens, toilet rooms, entrances, and other use areas. These and other rules are worth looking at and considering. Many of them appear to have emerged from commonsense considerations of health in cultures without electricity, running water, or sewers, rather than from geomantic considerations. Kitchens and living spaces were often placed as far up-wind as possible from pit privies. Mirrors were used to bring light into dark interior hallways or spaces, and high-status living spaces placed where they had best access to sunlight, breeze, or shade, as the particular climate demanded.

POSSESSIONS

This is probably the first time in history that accumulation of excessive personal possessions has become so widespread as to create a serious impediment to the energy among people and between people and place. Dealing with possessions is not built into our genes, so we have to develop new skills for clearing out excess possessions as easily as we accumulate them. I had a client once who wanted to build an addition to his house. He told me how lucky he was that someone had given him a pool table absolutely free. I scratched my head for a minute until I was sure he wasn't joking, then replied, "That wasn't a *free* pool table, it was a $50,000 pool table. That is what it will cost you to build this addition you're wanting to house it! It might be wiser, and certainly cheaper, to give it to the coffee house across the street!"

Some friends we were visiting a couple of years ago had a house filled with more belongings than any I'd ever seen. Their garage was so full of stuff that they had to park their cars on the street. Their basement, likewise, was filled. We'd go into one room after another, lined with shelves and bookcases full of stuff. Once those had filled up, they had set up a *second* row of shelves in front of the first, and now those were filled up.

They'd bought a television and a couple of comfortable chairs, and put them in the corner of a room. But pretty soon that corner was so full of stuff that it was unusable, so they bought another TV and a couple more chairs and set them up somewhere else. And again, and again! They were paralyzed in dealing with their belongings, and were even thinking of building a new house because their existing one didn't have enough room!

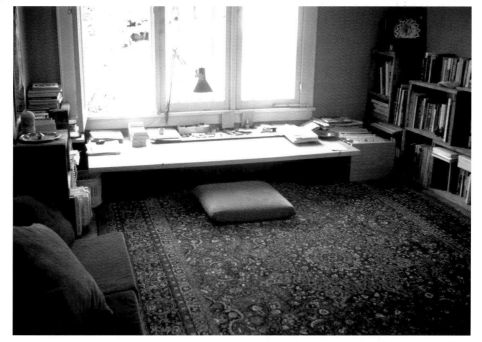

Rooms don't need to be filled with furniture to feel comfortable. Even a working office can feel spacious when different approaches are taken to what we put in the space.

Possessions can be a joy, but are unquestionably also a burden. They require care, use, maintenance, storage, access, and replacement. We're constantly having to lug stuff around, and move stuff to get to something behind it. Stuff is always diverting our energy and attention, yelling at us that we could be doing something else. We are constantly having to learn more consumerist hair-splitting to decide which stuff to choose. It is reaching the point where we're beginning to live in walk-in *closets* filled with *stuff*, not in rooms!

For most of us, it is time to learn to say *no*, to learn to pass on and get rid of stuff, to decide against getting more stuff because of the downstream effects of such actions. It's time to learn *enoughness*, to *live lightly*, and to let go of the past and gain the freedom of walking unencumbered through the world.

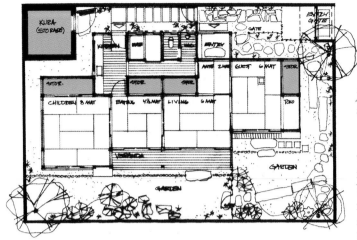

A separate storage building (kura), flexible "empty" rooms, and openness to an enclosed garden, can make even a small building site a delightful place to live.

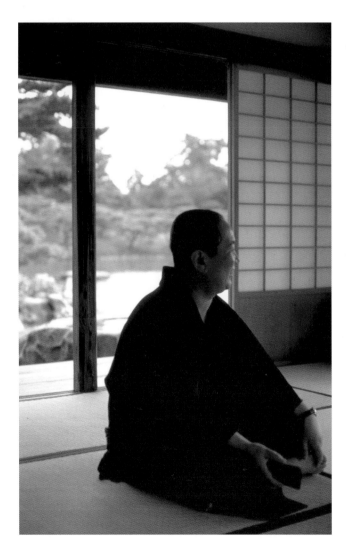

Sometimes it feels good to be surrounded by loved and meaningful things. But most of the things we have are neither. In the midst of a project, it is inevitable that we have a lot of stuff around, and that's okay. It's *inactive, overwhelming, excess, forgotten,* and *neglected* stuff that nags at our subconscious.

In part because of the fire hazards of their wood and paper houses, the Japanese developed an interesting way of dealing with possessions. They built a fireproof *kura*, or storeroom building, separate from the house itself, where they kept all valuable and out-of-season belongings, safe from fire. Each room was then an empty vessel, into which they brought just the one painting, flower arrangement, or carving they wanted to focus upon and enjoy, and the table, seats, or sleeping futons needed for immediate use.

Clearing out old "stuff" and dealing with clutter is like weeding a garden. It opens space and light for new things to grow in our lives and for us to focus on what is truly important. Things that needlessly divert our attention keep us from our true goals.

Possessions: cleared out, and out of mind. Place: focused on people, nature, relationships, and the moment.

✧

There is no perfect site, and there is no perfect building. After examining a place both objectively and intuitively, we need to summarize what changes we feel are needed and possible to accommodate it to its intended use – physically accommodating the new use, minimizing the effects of negative influences, and enhancing the effects of positive ones.

After seeing what we can receive through a place, we need also to ask what we can *give* to *others* through that place at the same time. Then it is time to sleep, dream, meditate, or otherwise let our intuitive processes integrate our overall impressions into recommendations and decisions. Then we will find creative ways to implement such actions.

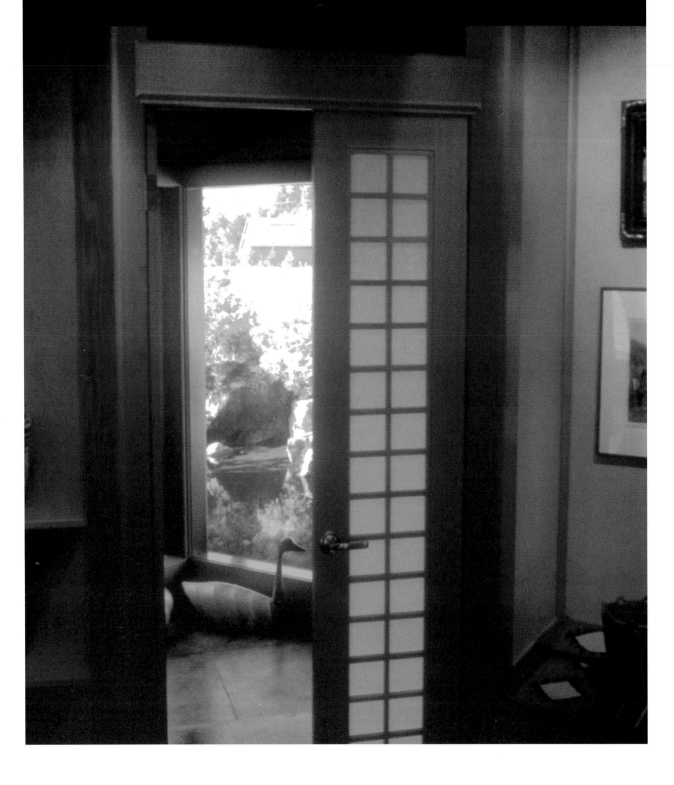

9 BUILDINGS WITH SOULS

T here *is* life in *all* Creation. There are wombs in space that give birth to galaxies and stars. The hearts of stars sing like bells. The rocks under our feet thrum with messages from within and around the world. Trees make love with a thousand others at one time. The microfauna in our cells create communities and transportation systems. All communities have life that transcends its individual members. A forest is a single organism. A planet has what can only be termed consciousness. And they all sing in harmonious celebration of life.

Even places have souls – small or great, gentle or fierce, nurturing or debilitating. Like all life, they have distinct and often strong personalities. They have auras and energy bodies. They are touched and altered by our regard or disregard for them, and they are able to move our hearts and alter our lives in turn. The soul of a place is, perhaps, the sum of the gifts it can give and the power and beauty with which it can make those gifts.

We have ignored this aspect of place in recent years. With rare exceptions, the places we have been making have not had souls of which we could be proud. But we are learning again to make places with souls that enrich and nurture us, empower and connect us.

Simply put, making places with souls is the most central thing we must attend to in making buildings to shelter our lives and nurture our hearts.

✧

A building with a soul has a number of characteristics:

FIT: A building with a soul fits its site and makes best use of it, making almost magical connections between location, relationships, and views. The arrangement and organization within it, outside it, and in connection with the life around it are apt. It fits its climate, its use and users, and the dreams that drive their society.

COMMUNITY: A building with a soul fits and belongs to the natural community of the local area. It uses local materials, local ways of building, and local traditions of design, while supporting local patterns of living. It chooses local wisdom for dealing with unique climatic conditions and ways of heating, cooling, ventilating and sheltering. It nestles into and celebrates, rather than standing apart

We like places, somehow, that are magic, that are more than our minds can comprehend, that bring us a richness that extends beyond the logical and rational. And we like places that beckon to us and say, "There's more magic around the corner, or through the next door." Places so rich that they can afford to reveal themselves to us slowly; places that we grow deeper into over the years.

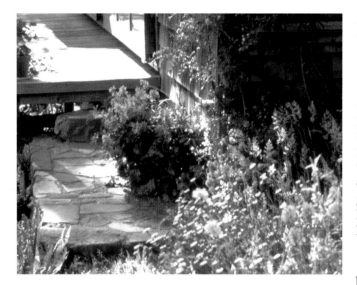

Sometimes fit comes by knowing when not to act – when to let nature take its course. Here a wonderful wildflower meadow grew itself into being while we were trying to figure out how to landscape the area. The obvious answers are often in front of us, if we just learn to see them.

from, its unique ecological community which has evolved through the ongoing test of centuries. It touches the spirit of where it is.

SIMPLICITY: A building with a soul takes a straight-forward modest route, rather than a complicated one, to fulfilling our needs. It lets nature do the work rather than machines. It finds simple responses to needs (with complex reasons why they work so well), rather than complicated high-tech ones. It knows that excess is as harmful as meagerness, and discriminates between things that harm and those that enhance our abilities, our relationships, and our lives.

INVISIBILITY: Like a good servant, a building with a soul is invisible – a presence known only through the smooth and faultless orchestration of energy, communication, and flow of experience. When our places act as good servants, they draw back into shadow, revealing themselves only slowly, giving us quiet surprises from time to time. They let the light and attention rest on their inhabitants and their partners in Creation. They place but small demands on us for attention, operation, and maintenance.

They evoke deep and moving experiences. Their making and use pay attention to important inner qualities rather than superficial outer ones. They surround us only with meaningful things, and convey love and clarity of intention. They make us subtly aware of important things in life, so that we can come to feel at home everywhere.

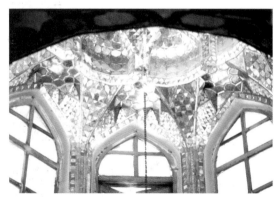

Using natural systems that work, rather than manufactured answers, is often more effective and beautiful as well. Here an air conditioning system that lets hot air out through the cupola of a dome, drawing in cool air from the garden below.

They are filled with the *emptiness* of Lao Tsu's teacup, and reverberate with the peace of *silence*. They are free of unnecessary possessions and mechanical noises, and open to the joyful sounds of birdsong, laughter, and the sound of the wind. They have learned restraint and simplicity, and the ability to say, *"No."*

CONNECTION: A building with a soul is enriched and given meaning through its connection with other things. It brings us into closer touch with each other, the rest of the world, and the rhythms of nature. It connects us to the daily and seasonal cycles of the sun, the moon, and the stars, and to the visible and invisible universe. It adapts readily to changes in use and additions to its structure.

GENEROSITY: The relationships of a building with a soul are based on "giving" rather than "paying." Its retaining walls give more than needed – a place to sit as well as holding back the earth. Its roofs shelter birds and other creatures, as well as passers-by on the street. It may well accomplish that generosity in surprising ways, like a Japanese room which is generous in space because of its emptiness, not because of its size. Its generosity is created out of the love and energy put into its making. It gives the *unexpected*.

RESPECT: A building with a soul honors its surroundings and the lives of materials which were given up to make its existence possible. It honors the skill, competence, and sacredness of the work that went into its making. It honors its users, like the Japanese who seat a guest to be seen by others next to a flower arrangement in a *tokonoma* alcove, giving the guest a sense that they and their activities are of value. A building created in harmony with tradition honors the insights and wisdom gained from the past. Surrounded by newly-planted trees, it honors a hope for a future. It celebrates age, and newness, creativity, death, and its neighbors. It honors all life, and the power that begets it.

COHERENCE: A building with a soul is consistent; it arises out of a single, whole, and clear vision of the needs it can fill and the possibilities it can unfold. It reflects a lucid and unencumbered *intention* of its owner, designer, and builder. It has sought and found the heart of the institution it is sheltering, and found ways to honor and unfold that heart in its making. The issues it has addressed are fundamental and not frivolous, and the solutions it has created are sound.

ENDURANCE: A building with a soul is built to endure beyond the needs of its makers – to become a gift to future generations. A building that lasts 200 years costs 1/10 as much as one that lasts only 20 years. A building with a soul would be as comfortable a thousand years in the past or future as it is today. It is comfortable with the changes of time, neglect, and love, mellowing and becoming enriched rather than tarnished and tattered.

The savings from the durability of this church could feed an entire village.

NOURISHMENT: A building with a soul enfolds, shelters, and gives peace and rest to all who enter it. It uplifts our spirits, nourishes our souls, and brings us into harmony with its own soul. It gives refuge and sanctuary. It welcomes us with water in the desert, fire in the cold, shelter in the rain, food and friendship everywhere.

A building with soul fills primal psychic needs for protection, for warmth, for companionship, for meaning. It moves our hearts and enhances our *chi*. It helps us marshal our inner resources, and stimulates us to use those resources for growth. It affirms *sacredness* and meaning in our lives and surroundings, and creates places for our hearts and minds as well as our bodies. A building with a soul draws on and connects its users to power that extends beyond just the material world.

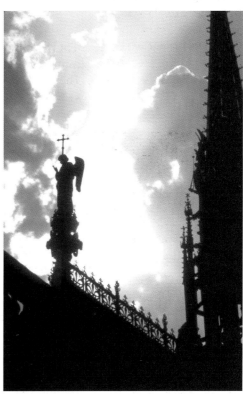

Together, these qualities combine to create a place that gives us deep welcome and refuge – a place that connects us with the beauty of a unique locale, and draws us more closely together with the rest of Creation.[1] Entering it, we are drawn into an inner calm, peace, and joy.

---

[1] My THE HEART OF PLACE, 1993, and ENVIRONMENTAL DESIGN PRIMER, Schocken Books, 1973, go into more detail on building with a heart and related issues such as geometry and order, giving life to existing places, economics of a sacred world, the inner and outer product of work, and other aspects of sustainable building.

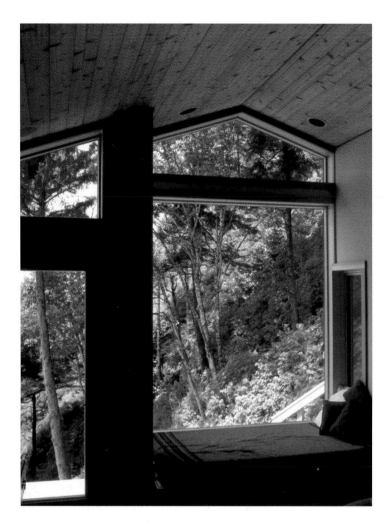

✧

As we acknowledge the energy basis of Creation, we ask buildings to fulfill new roles. There is a shift in the kinds of activities that we undertake and need to house in buildings, and in the image of our society and our universe that is reflected in those buildings. We might create restorative justice centers rather than prisons, healing centers rather than hospitals, learning centers rather than schools. Our buildings become more honest. No fake-brick, no pseudo-Georgian manors, no hyped-up shopping malls.

Energy fields in the earth are acknowledged in choosing locations for buildings that support psychic, healing, or spiritual uses. We can avoid places with bad natural energy, and locate and design of buildings to balance and augment the chi of the landscape. We can choose to *not* build in landscapes that have powerful energy.

The emotional and spiritual well-being of a building's users are considered in its design, so that the energy they impart to the building is good. Fulfilled users leave positive feelings behind, just as pilgrims leave good energy in temples, churches, and shrines. We take care with electromagnetic fields in our

Wholeness comes from connection, and feeds our spirits as well as our bodies.

buildings, with materials and design, and with the connections to the outside. We design to shield from bad chi and to connect with good energy.

Chi affects the interconnection of buildings and gardens. It leads us to have skylights to connect with the night as well as the daytime sky; to the northern lights or to the stars. We may reduce exterior night lighting so that we can experience the night, the darkness, and the stars. It brings our buildings to reflect clarity of intention, and at times to focus energy in yantric fashion, where specific geometry of design of space or sculpture affects the chi of building users.

Wholeness causes us to seek wholeness from our actions, and to build and use places in ways that continually enrich them, ourselves, and the world around us.

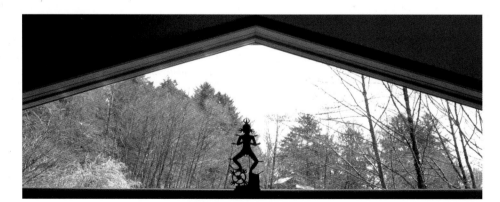

FILLING A PLACE WITH SOUL

Pick a space you want to work with or change. Empty it out – physically if possible, mentally otherwise. Open a window. Sit down in the empty room. Empty yourself as well, and do the usual grounding, centering, and opening of your chakras. Form a ball of golden energy in your heart chakra, and breathing into it, let it expand to encompass your whole body, and then the whole space you are in. Now open your eyes. Sitting there on the bare floor, with just bare walls around you, ask it and yourself if that is enough to bring peace, joy, and success to the use proposed for the space. Let go of any images in your mind of how magazines say rooms should look. Let go of wanting to show the finished space to someone, and of wanting to feel proud of what you accomplished. Let go of expectations.

Focus on the energy of the space. The space probably provides more materially than all but royalty have had throughout history . . . but if it doesn't feel good, what is pulling down the energy? Is it dirty – will giving it a scrub make it good? Is it dark, or dank, or smelly, or noisy? Or does it just feel energetically dead – a place nobody has ever put any love into?

Now begin testing. Light a candle, and ask yourself if the life it brings into the room changes it. Enough – just you, the candle, and the space? Or, how would it feel if the old carpet was ripped up – what is the flooring underneath, how would it change the feeling? What if that branch outside the window was pruned, so more light could get into the room? Or what if a window was put in that blank outside wall, connecting with sun and moonrise? Your empty room is never empty. It is always full of something, but what can fill it with life? Stuffing it with furniture and gee-gaws isn't the answer – it's what's done to mask energetic emptiness. Like watching soaps on TV instead of dealing with our healing in community.

Bring something else into the space with you and your candle – a flower, or some object that has had love put into its making. What does that change, or not change? What is still nagging? Try something else. Project your mind outside. What connections with other spaces and activities inside the building would bring life with it? What connections out-of-doors, whose absence causes deadness inside? How can you bring them, in some magic way, into the space? A skylight? A mirror? What will bring the smell or life of the forest? How can you connect with life in the street? After you've found what is lacking, figure out possibilities of how to restore life to the space.

And soul? There is an alchemy between the natural qualities of a place, its human history, who is using a space, and anyone involved in design and changing a space. Put all of these in your mind together; ask for magic, power, and beauty. Soak in the feeling that arises, and let it guide you in each if the decisions in choosing what goes into the space.

Then, and only then, consider what is needed functionally for use of the space – a bed? a desk? equipment? chairs? storage? How simply and with how much love can each of these needs be filled, harmoniously, without in turn drawing down the life of the space?

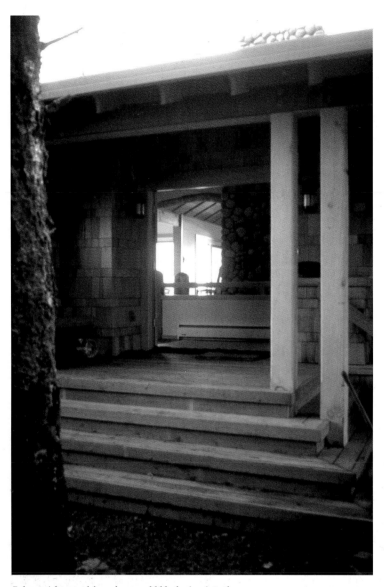

What beckons you into a place, and gives your heart a sigh of relief and pleasure?

ENTRIES

If we look in more detail at one element of a building – its entry – we can get more of a sense of how different aspects of a building come together to create a "soul". Entries to buildings, particularly homes, hold an importance in this process far beyond their actual size. Getting a sense of the multiple and important roles they play is vital to successful placement, design, remodeling, or accommodating their function, even in an apartment.

A typical North American residential pattern shows us almost everything *not* to do with the entrance to a home. A large living room window open to the street across an open front yard ensures lack of privacy for the occupants, exposing them constantly to the view of passers-by. Anyone approaching the front door has to walk directly in front of that window, seeing everything going on inside the living room. Once at the front door, the visitor stands in the rain getting soaked, with no place to put down packages or rest. When the owner answers the door, the visitor comes directly into the living room, interrupting whatever is going on there, and becoming the immediate focus of everyone in the room. How would your tummy feel as either visitor or resident in this pattern?

Chinese feng shui pays a lot of attention to which room an entry door should open into. The real answer, perhaps, is that entry requires a separate place inside the house, apart from *all* interior activities. Entry deals with strangers as well as family, and needs to accommodate their business without impinging on the occupants of a house. This doesn't need a lot of space. It *does* require separation. At minimum, it needs a bookcase, or portable screen, or even a curtain, that can visually partition the entry area from the rest of the interior.

Below: A louvered fence here could block view into the house and permit an entry garden that residents and visitors could both enjoy.

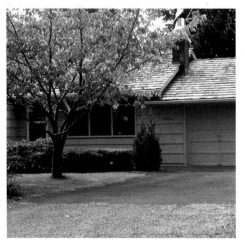

An entry has to address many needs: weather protection, creating a thermal "airlock," and people putting on and taking off outdoor gear. It has to deal with privacy, safety, protection; providing places to sit, to put bags and gear, and to discuss business or life. In snow country, roofs need to be designed not to dump snow or icicles on visitor's heads when the door is slammed.

Entries are also the settings for important rituals in our lives: passionate goodnights after a date, farewells, waiting for family or friends to return, setting off to school or work, return to comfort and rest at the end of a day. They are places of celebration, grief, joy, reticent departures and emotional returns. They are entwined with love, beautiful mornings, sadness, loneliness, excitement. They sometimes denote entry into and departure from sacred space. They become containers for ritual energy, adding to the power of those rituals. They can show connection and how our lives are nestled into the native community of life of the place. Most of these events require at least an eddy out of the way of traffic in and out of an entry door. Some require much more.

Entries can also be a place of *giving*, offering shade, coolness and water in the desert, warmth and shelter in the cold. They can be a place of giving to the street – of beauty, of caring, of connection and conversation, of guardians and a watchful eye, of mingling the emotions and energies of family and community. They can be places of *honoring* visitors and guests, honoring the neighborhood, nature, the materials whose lives were given up in the making of the place. They can be a place for expression of *caring*.

Welcome tells you that you have arrived – at a place you will want to be – and that your needs and nurture will be given to out of the fullness of the place.

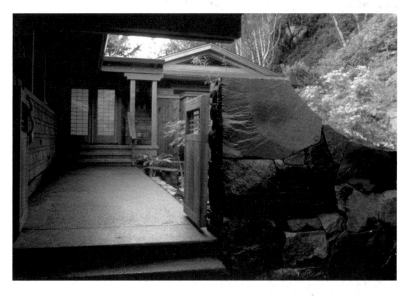

All this takes more than just the 1-3/4"-thick door we usually give to entry! Designing, modifying, and adding elements to an entry area to accomplish these things creates conditions of harmony between us and others, and between us and our surroundings.

The ambiguity of the suburban living room with its picture window facing the street is an important one. It speaks of absence of even the most minimal awareness, skills, or traditions to provide privacy to the occupants of the home. But it also speaks of the need for connection, of loneliness, of wanting to know what's going on out on the street and desire to connect with it. While the suburban "front lawn" is a particularly odd and wasteful pattern, connection with the human world outside is an important need. As well as providing for privacy, making positive connection with the outside world is an important element of entry.

If you are designing from scratch, placing the house closer to the street or adding a front porch can create a useful in-between space. Even with a row house in the city, if we place a couple of potted plants beside the front door, we can create a "front stoop" area where it is comfortable to "hang out," talk, or just enjoy the street scene.

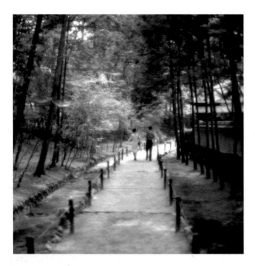

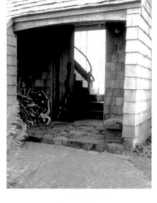

Top: The entry walk to Saihoji – space to leave the city behind.
Above: Shelter from rain, a place to sit, knowledge you will stay warm, something more beckoning.
Below: Wide eaves shelter entry steps along the edge of the forest from the rain.

Using topology, or "rubber geometry," we can often accomplish more than one thing at a time, and more than one thing can occupy the same space. By stretching an entry walk toward one of the sides of a front yard, the rest can be fenced or walled in for private outdoor space for the residents, while still giving access to the entry. In a small elementary school, rubber geometry can stretch the inside "entry" space to make it large enough for a "Commons" – a non-classroom place for parents to wait for kids or to meet with each other – a place for kids to have lunch, do individual work out of class, or hold small group meetings.

At the Saihoji Zen garden in Kyoto, the entry walk is rubber-stretched to extend *around two whole sides* of the garden, to give the city-world time to drain out of visitors' heads, and to bring them to where the garden could be viewed with full attention and with the vegetation backlit by the sun. A front entry can be stretched around to the side of a building, if needed, for better weather and surroundings, or to link better with the interior arrangement of activities.

An entry can respond to our anticipation of and need for comfort. The approach to this house gives a glimpse of warm light pouring out of the kitchen, with reserves of food visibly at hand on the shelves. A sheltered porch, smoke from the chimney, and a full woodpile easily at hand give immediate assurance of warmth, shelter, food, and companionship regardless of power interruptions, road closures, or the worst of weather.

Inside, a soil-cement floor keeps the entry as part of the ground; steps up to the house floor provide a seat for removing or putting on shoes; a shoji screen provides visual and thermal separation from the living space while bringing light into the entry; a stairs provides access to upstairs offices; and a pantry provides storage for bulk-food purchases.

Where site conditions dictate living space on the upper level, rubber geometry can stretch the connections entry needs to make, to a second floor level . Placing the entry on the downwind side of the house, and by extending the roof overhang to shelter the entry stairs from rain, an outside approach to the entry door can occur, open to a lovely wooded area. At the front porch, a bench and shelf give a place to set packages, rest, or take off muddy boots, then a right-angled turn brings visitors to the entry door.

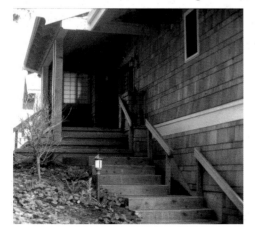

Interestingly, that right angle turn works differently when leaving the house. Opening the entry door, the porch gives direct connection out into the wooded part of the lot, *then* you remember the stairs going down on the left! This pattern makes it possible also, by opening both entry doors, for the house to connect directly to the woods on nice days.

Design of the garden side of the same house involved careful organization of levels of outdoor terraces and walls to provide seating without view obstruction or railings. At the same time, it used a rubber geometry to stretch the ground level to the upper floor, although the house floor is almost a full story above grade. By locating circulation paths so that people are drawn to a corner of the site, a distinctive view of the ocean and the end of the mountain gives a special sense of connection with the forces of nature. An entry from or to a garden may be as important as the main entry to a house.

The wonderful Dutch architect Aldo Van Eyck used to talk about doors and windows as a special category of "in-between spaces" such as entries. He talked about the specialness of walking along the edge of the last landward movement of water on a beach – that in-between realm where water, earth and sky meet – and how such places have characteristics of their neighboring realms and additional unique ones themselves.

Doors and windows do lie on that kind of edge between the inside and out. Enlarging that edge into a realm of its own, containing porches, verandahs, and entries, can recognize its specialness and capture its unique potential for making us comfortable in our complex world. Areas between inside and out can give us a place to sit when we are unsure whether we want to be out or in. They let us be part of what is going on both outside and inside. A window seat can allow us to linger in that in-between world, able to be securely inside our home, yet able to call out to a neighbor or friend, start a conversation, or just enjoy the passing world outside.

Houses in the Queensland area of Australia developed a unique pattern of front porches enclosed with a wood lattice, allowing breezes to pass through, giving visual privacy, yet allowing view out to the street. "French windows" in European villages give connection between upper story rooms and friends in the street below. "Spirit walls" outside entries in Japan and China allow entry without loss of visual privacy.

Some geomantic traditions such as feng shui emphasize a compact house design, ideally one that will fit easily onto a square "geomantic chart" diagram. Such "bagua" diagrams are used to see if different activities in a house or room are located in positions that are supposed to have energy benefiting specific activities.

Strict geomantic analysis of this kind would not result in an "L"shaped house, but this house works beautifully. In this case, numerous factors resulted in a strongly L-shaped design – or even an arrow-shaped design. One crucial element of making this shape work was the design of a garden as part of the entry. Interest-

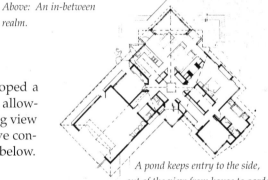

Above: An in-between realm.

A pond keeps entry to the side, out of the view from house to garden.

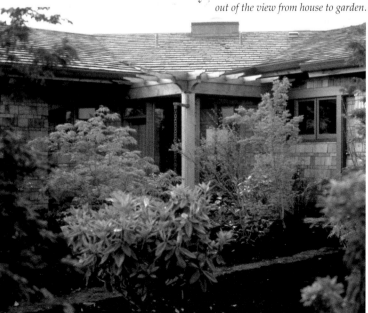

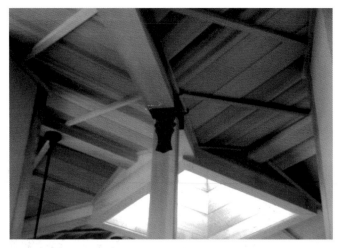

In-between spaces can connect to the sky as well as the ground around a building.

ingly, this brought the entry into the center space of the house, not one of the perimeter spaces. It gave "protection" from the north, while enhancing the view. And by carefully locating the entry walk, visitors are brought to the front door along the edge of the garden under a wide roof overhang, while the pond keeps them outside the sight lines from the entry windows. This simultaneously maintained a view out to the garden, visual privacy of the interior from approaching guests, and rain shelter for the approaching visitor.

A good design usually has indoor, outdoor, and in-between places. It may have sunspaces, outdoor rooms, carports or garages. Fitting a chart onto such complexity is clearly problematic. Paying careful attention to how things fit together may be more important for our well-being than an exact fit into some theoretical model.

✦

Then, of course, there is the story of the Japanese Zen master. As the story goes, a famous Japanese tea master was given a piece of land with an outstanding view of the Inland Sea. When his teahouse was finished, his first guests arrived, curious to see how he had sited it to take best advantage of the magnificent view. They were shocked to find that he had planted a hedge that totally blocked the dramatic view of the sea.

Then, as they bent to drink the traditional dipperful of water before entering the tea house, a hidden opening in the hedge exposed a view of the waves breaking on the rocks below, just as the water in the dipper touched their lips.

Later, when the master had finished the tea ceremony inside, he quietly slid aside the shoji screens and brought the sense of water that lingered on their lips and in their hearts together with the powerful vista of the sea below.

The design of an entry can do many things!

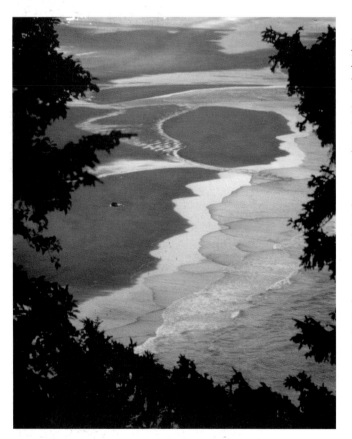

Every connection our places make between the worlds inside and outside of our skins – if done well – is unique, and adds a new richness and meaning to our lives.

BUILDING FROM INSIDE

Homes are personal places. Our living patterns, cultural traditions, and individual comfort levels vary tremendously. The energetics of personal space are dominated by our hearts and minds. Glare, noise, and smells affect each of us differently. What represents comfort and security to each of us is also vastly different, and it is those personal perceptions that need to be dealt with. Listening to our tummies as to what feels good or bad to us is vital.

Every part of the daily patterns in our homes contains opportunity for embodying the sacred in our lives, for honoring others, finding meaning in our lives, and for deepening our rootedness with the rest of our cosmos:

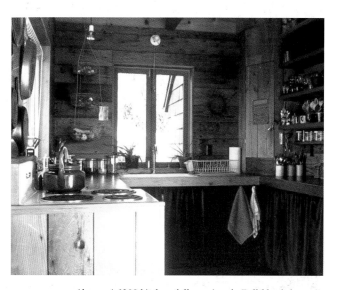

Above: A $200 kitchen, fully equipped. Full-blooded dishwasher, cool-box, used appliances, good food.
Below: One twisted branch brings nature into a toilet room.

   * A good kitchen does not need fancy appliances, or cabinets filled with equipment and packaged foods. It needs to be a place capable of honoring and enabling those who feed and care for others. It needs to cradle the social rituals of making meals. It needs to honor the foods, allow them to embody the energy given through them by the cook, and enhance their ability to nurture our energy as well as our bodies.

   * A bath can be the heart of a home – a place to honor and restore our bodies and our spirits, to wash off the fatigue and tensions of the day, and find wholeness out of its experiences. Our bodies, too, are sacred and wonderful. Even our wastes are food for other life, and nutrients that need to return to the fields.

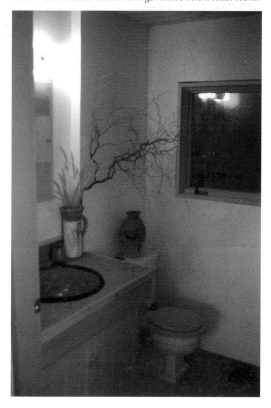

   * Where and how we sleep is not important. Where and how we dream, whose hands we put ourselves into when we sleep, what we wake to and say goodnight to *are* important. The place between sleep and awake is a place where the veils to the spirit world are thin and where our dreams can be brought to life.

   * "Living-room" is a seed of family and community. It is a place for enabling and evoking our relationships, honoring others, those relationships, and ourselves. It

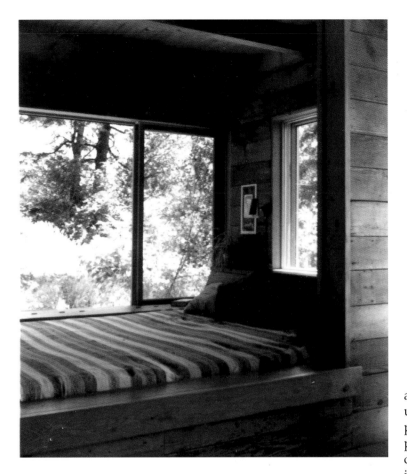

A bed alcove off of a living room gives a soft space for a family to curl up together in the evening.

is a place of opportunity to care for others, to give gifts of spirit, hope, love, and support.

* Where and how we find a place of peace and nurture within our buildings – a sacred place where we can touch the forces in the universe and bring them into our buildings – varies with each of us. It matters *whether*, not *how* we do so.

* The life, rhythms, and energy of the sun, the stars, moon and seasons and the forms of life that make the community of which both we and our buildings are part can be brought into our buildings in may ways. Again, it matter *that* we do so, not how.

There are many things we can do to align our buildings with our selves and our universe. We can change our lives – our perceptions, beliefs, actions. We can make physical changes to our surroundings – choosing or not choosing a site, modifying it; determining or changing the characteristics of what is built on it. Or we can work directly on the energetic level to alter or augment the forces at play and how we relate to them. Beneath all the rules, the goal remains achieving a sense of "rightness." That rightness comes in providing the nurture and love needed for us to feel comfortable within our surroundings and part of relationships and patterns that give meaning and power to our lives.

A friend commented with surprise that with thirty-five years of design and building behind me, the chapter of this book dealing specifically with structures is the shortest and least specific. In part, that is because I write about what is

Morning sun on an outside "drying-off" area off of a bathroom.

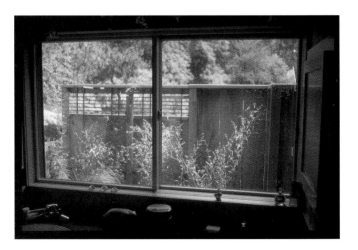

"in process" for me – what is coming into focus and hasn't yet been fully assimilated and become an inseparable part of me. In another sense, though, it is because I do know these areas more deeply, and know that specific "how-to" suggestions are not the real answer to making our selves and our places whole once more.

Those kinds of answers are sought by our heads. The real questions – and answers – lie in our hearts. How-to answers are wrong at least half of the time. And I've seen even the best distorted again and again into unrecognizability and twisted to serve the wrong ends after being filtered through values that we hold in our hearts that are incompatible with them.

Books like Helen Berliner's *Enlightened by Design* can help you feel your way around the boundaries between inner and outer design/questions/answers. But the answers that work for you will be very different than those found in that book, this one, or any other.

Buildings only reflect their makers and users. The real tools for good design are head tools and heart tools that change our values and goals, and teach us to work with our hearts open. They bring forth the right answers effortlessly, seamlessly, and automatically. You are your own best tool and source of answers.

Hone that tool.

10 GARDENS OF THE SPIRIT

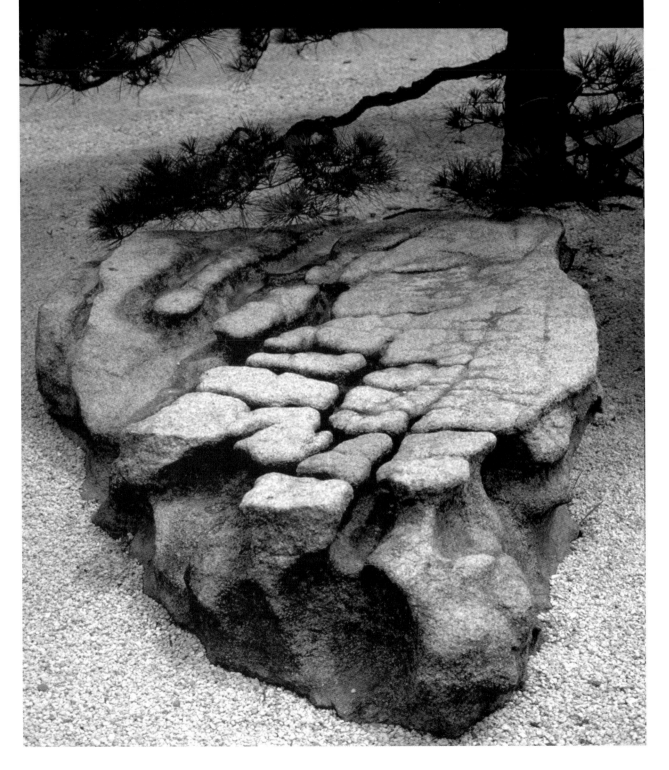

Gardens of the Spirit are places that change our lives. They connect us to our inner energy and power, our intentions, and our purposes in this life. They bring us to wholeness, so that we come to all our actions connected to and supported by the entire web of Creation. They take us between the worlds and touch us with the deeper flows of energy in the universes outside of our material realm. They connect us in deep and wordless ways to time and the flows of creation, and the infinite joy and love that feeds all that exists.

As opposed to buildings which must keep people dry, warm, and safe, the ability of a garden to focus solely on the needs of our spirits, gives them a particular ability to embody the principles of energetic design. In powerful meditation gardens, they can assist us in connecting directly with the energetic basis of all Creation. Gardens can be designed to create and enhance energy fields in the Earth's crust and give us an opportunity to connect with them. They can raise our spirits and enhance our chi. They can help our buildings nestle into the native ecosystem, provide room and food for other life, temper our climates, and generate native landscaping to bring us in tune with intention that has evolved over millennia.

They can produce food – more intensively than farming[1] – while feeding our spirits. They can bring us in touch with time and duration beyond our own scope; with death and rebirth, with our ancestors and descendants, and with the cosmologies we evolve. They can become a pure vehicle for expressing sacredness, for honoring and celebrating the multitudinous dimensions of Creation.

But most vitally, they can bring our hearts directly and wordlessly in contact with the power of Creation.

Opposite: A garden can speak silently of many things – whether rock or water is harder, the value of persistence, the role of time. And it can speak those things in ways that move our hearts, not just our minds.

HOMES FOR OUR SPIRITS

When we ignore our spirits, we suffer. Like our bodies, our spirits require nurture and health. Unlike our bodies, they don't need roofs to keep dry, walls to protect, clothing to keep warm. In a world where material things for our bodily wants are intensely marketed, it is easy to forget the needs of our spirits.

[1] See, for example, Farallones Institute, THE INTEGRAL URBAN HOUSE, Sierra Club, 1979; Rosalind Creasy, THE COMPLETE BOOK OF EDIBLE LANDSCAPING, Sierra Club Books, 1982.

Yet our spirits are vital. Our ancestors, with few of the material resources we have today, relied for millennia on the strengths of their spirits to connect with, and to find meaning and strength in, the world around them. Their spirits performed a powerful and essential role in marshaling their inner resources for both survival and celebration. Through the strength of spiritual resources, joyful and sophisticated cultures have been developed and sustained for thousands of years even in regions of the Earth's deserts and Arctic tundra where we would consider survival alone to be impossible.

Even today, our spiritual resources are more vital than our material ones. Emotional, mental, and spiritual relationships evolved over tens of thousands of years into vital processes for our survival and health cannot be ignored. They do not vanish even in a world suddenly awash in material satisfactions.

We need to create homes for our spirits – homes that don't need walls or roofs, but which, like a garden, can provide nurture. Buildings themselves can become this kind of garden, but they have more constraints of material and functional needs that outside places don't. Outside places, our traditional places of garden-making, can also more easily nurture the rest of nature and our connections with it, and have more freedom in expressing our values.

Winter gardens mean celebrating winter. That can lead to amazing things – like enjoying winter instead of griping about it. Then what about mud gardens, dust gardens, and gardens for every other kind of climate?

Making places where our spirits can grow and flourish has a long tradition in the history of gardens.[2] It is an aspect of landscaping often neglected today, and one with potential and resources far beyond today's conventional garden-making. Learning to create gardens of the spirit can teach us much of the power and needs of our spirits and help us make the changes in our lives to heal and restore the spirits of our bodies, homes and communities.

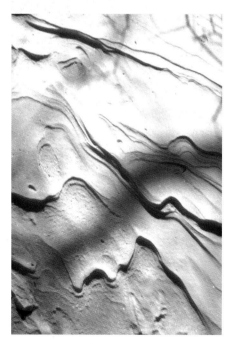

SPIRIT-OF-PLACE GARDENS

Each place has developed a unique nature over time. Its particular combination of location, geology, topography, climate, and neighbors has resulted in a special configuration of conditions. Over millennia, a singular community of plants, animals, and fungus; of creatures of the air, the waters, and the earth, has developed. That community has stood the test of time and survival, and shown itself singularly fitted to the conditions of that particular place. It has its own beauty with an unsurpassable sense of rightness.

When we come to newly inhabit a place, we bring with us our own sense of the rightness of the place from which we have come. For example, European settlers tried to recreate Europe in America. We may try to recreate lush temperate-zone lawns in the sun-seared desert. We ignore the joys of winter in northern climes, and sit huddled indoors impatiently awaiting the coming of spring. While the spirit of former homes may contribute wonderful elements to a hybrid spirit of place in the new one, much needs to be discarded or transformed, and a deep awareness of the spirit of the new place developed before we can be part of it.

---

[2] For a pleasant introduction to a traditional feng shui approach to gardens, see, Gill Hale's THE FENG SHUI GARDEN, Story Books, 1998.

It takes time and perception, involvement and love, to become part of a place and to draw sustenance from being an integral part of its specialness. Gardens which acknowledge and connect us with the special spirit of each place can assist that adaptation within us.

WINTER GARDENS

If we live in winter country, for example, how do we deal with the spirit of winter in a garden? What is a winter garden?

In snow country, gardening is a summer concept. Come fall, plants are dug up and brought inside; remaining ones are mulched, braced, buried, and otherwise prepared to bear the onslaught of cold. Garden tools are put away, snow shovels brought out; thoughts turn indoors, and gardens are banished from our minds until spring.

Perhaps the simplest winter garden we can create – a tiny playground for winter to touch our spirits – used to be a commonplace occurrence before the advent of modern window technology. Frosted window panes are delicate ever-changing scenes of sparkling feathers, interlocking crystalline shapes, and imaginary pictures. Melted off by sunlight in the daytime, they are regrown before our eyes in the cold of night. We can scratch drawings into them with our fingernails, or melt peepholes with our noses or a warm penny.

Modern windows don't let enough heat out to frost up, but that doesn't mean we can't save *one* window in our homes - perhaps just a small one in the bathroom - to give us an ever-changing ice garden at our fingertips. A garden can come indoors with us in the winter!

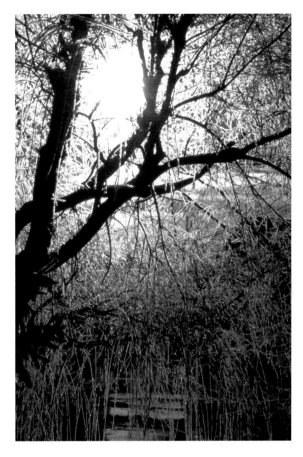

We're used to deciduous trees standing bare-limbed through the winter. But who hasn't awakened the morning after an unseasonable winter rain to see the sparkling magic of glistening ice-coated shrubs and trees? Too much ice can cause massive damage. But what happens if we install a tiny "fog generator" in a garden – a freeze-protected water source that emits tiny droplets of fog to waft through the garden at night and settle as a sparkling snowy or icy patina on the leaves and branches of garden plants, walls, and other objects?

The magic of a winter ice garden can remind us that every climate has its own magic, and its own unique ways to be celebrated at all times of the year through the gardens we create.

Similarly, we all love the wonderland we discover the morning after a heavy snow – a world transformed into strange, hooded shapes. It is a silent world, and one given more to thoughts of play than the struggle to force our way to work. A windless snow gives one kind of world: suddenly visible branches and clothes-lines precariously balancing an inch of snow, garden lights turned into bulky white mushrooms. A windy storm brings us into a different world: strangely sculpted forms that respond to normally invisible flowlines and eddies in space.

Fences and plantings and garden objects can be planned in anticipation of winter and of this ever-changing wonderland of sculpted snow that they can shape and transform. And when the sun reappears, the dark silhouettes of trees and the

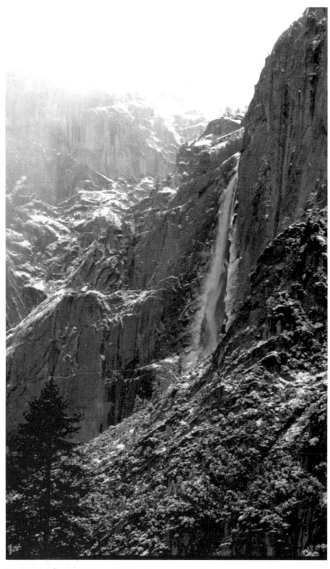

*How do we capture the majesty of
nature in our gardens and hearts?*

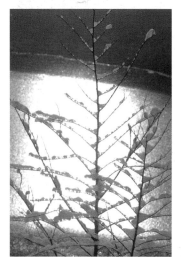

shifting shadows of their branches against these sculpted mounds of snow create a palette any garden painter would love to own.

The Inuit have as many words describing snow as we have words describing traffic jams. When snow or ice is brought close to our attention, we see its daily changes, personality, and beauty. One morning it may become a cloud of puffy giant flakes, another a coating of white hail-like ball bearings, a carpet of rainbow-reflecting crystal, or perhaps a glistening icy crust with strange and gaping caverns below. We can make gardens to bring us *close* to these tiny magic worlds.

On really cold days, when the thermometers are falling into double-digit minus numbers, the air itself becomes transformed. Ice particles in the air create glowing rainbow-tinged sundogs spanning the sky outward from the sun. Breath, car exhausts, and chimneys emit clouds and streamers of frozen smoke that create beards of crystal hoarfrost on surfaces they contact. A winter cloud garden! What a wonderful tool to create a garden floating free in the winter air.

In-between places, on the edge between different worlds, hold a special beauty of their own. I remember sitting one day at the edge of a mountain stream that was half buried in snow, with shells of ice encrusting the boulders. I sat there watching air and water bubbles migrate slowly about through the interstices between the rocks and their icy shells, seeming to defy the common sense rules of gravity. What beauty, this, in a garden! Some gardens are found, some made, others co-created with the forces of wind, rain, and sunlight. Bringing ourselves and others to where we can discover them is as vital as finding or making them.

A shallow pond, located where it can thaw and then refreeze, can create another ever-changing scene of tiny icebergs, dark water against snowy banks, or glistening smooth surfaces against its fluffy white surroundings. Waterfalls in winter create another ever-changing spectacle of icy beards, frozen mist, and dark crashing water. And what could be done to bring into our gardens the magic spaces under a melting glacier or snow bank – the silvery faceted vaulting overhead, glowing blue with transmitted light, the sound of tiny waterfalls, and the screens of icicles in front of openings?

These, then, are some tools for changing gardens into winter gardens. But what about ourselves and changing ourselves into winter *people*? The Japanese, instead of heating their homes and walling themselves off from their gardens, used to wrap themselves with quilts and sit with shoji open, listening to the snow falling silently around them.

WIND, WATER, AND STAR GARDENS

What then also of grassland gardens, celebrating the oceans of grass waving in the wind? Or underwater gardens, or rain gardens? What of gardens of the desert, open to the scent of faraway places on the wind, to the silence of emptiness, to the sea of stars, to the welcome of shade and water?

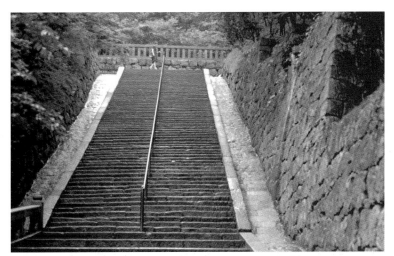

There is a stairway in Japan, at the Kiyomizu Temple in Kyoto, that is an amazing waterfall garden. On a rainy day, it gives one an unforgettable experience of walking down a mountain stream. Stone walls reflect and reverberate the sound of water rushing down stone gutters at both sides of the steps, while closing our vision off from all except the motion of that water. Vertigo, waterfalls, water gushing and leaping downward – you reach the bottom feeling like a drop of water having leapt down a mighty cascade.

A stairway built on top of a waterfall? Or a stairway that becomes, and helps us become, a waterfall?

GARDENS OF THE SPIRIT

COMPUTER ZEN GARDENS

Zen meditation gardens are extraordinary historical artifacts, but have little application in everyday lives in today's world . . . or have they?

A three-foot square garden can contain the universe, and can stimulate our minds with primal patterns and interactions.

Our high-tech world has dramatically increased the information load our minds have to process. Computers manage rational processing of information, but as yet do little to assist the vital subconscious connecting and implication-finding that we do at night or in quiet times. Every new thing requires its "mirror duality" to restore balance – by making some things easier and better, other things suffer in comparison. What computers have generated is a new need for times and places that encourage us to create wholeness out of our fragmented world.

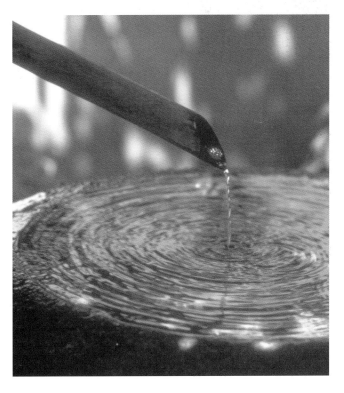

Here, of course, meditation gardens come into play. Some of the most effective meditation environments contain patterns and processes that parallel "thought forms" which stimulate our mental processes:

> * In a pool of water beneath a waterfall, trapped water bubbles float up to the surface and into the sunlight – a visual analog to thoughts and ideas floating to the surface of our consciousness, which stimulates our subconscious processing to do the same.

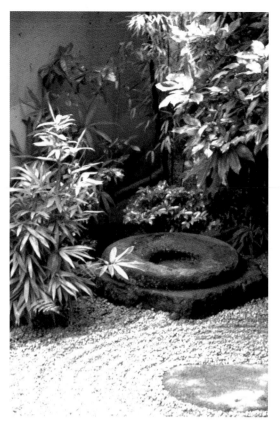

Old mill-stones can speak of many things in a garden.

* A single drop of water falls into a water basin, sending out concentric ripples that permeate the entire basin – an analog to ideas falling into place and affecting arrangements of whole thought structures.

* Two rocks – one concave, one convex – emerge from the shadows of a garden. The shadows give relief from new inputs and the peace to sort things out, while the quiet tension between the two rocks forms a visual mantra: "connect, connect, connect."

The Zen garden, or an adaptation of it, becomes a vital antidote to the data-overload of computer addiction. It generates a crucial and balancing process to the kind of mental calculation the computer imposes upon us. Together, they give us a far more powerful means of transmuting information into wisdom and bring the need for meditation gardens out of the esoterica of spiritual practice and into the heartland of everyday scientific research and corporate practice. Strange bedfellows, perhaps, but stranger marriages have succeeded before!

Computers allow us to work closeted away by ourselves. But we still need the non-structured, face-to-face get-together, brainstorming, and unanticipated synergizing of different fields, questions, and personalities. So the need for yet another, but more conventional, kind of "computer garden" also emerges: for a public eatery/garden where the computer "heavies" can get away, let their throbbing eyeballs rest, watch or join with others, bump into dancers, journalists, janitors, and secretaries, and let their worlds touch and spark with those of others.

GARDENS OF DEATH

It is easy to think of gardens as a celebration of life. It is harder, perhaps, to think of them as a celebration of death. Some gardeners go to great length to avoid providing the experience of anything but the full bloom of life. Blossoms are cut and removed the moment they pass the peak of bloom. Fallen petals and leaves are vacuumed up and quickly hidden from sight. Flowers are continually transplanted to keep only currently blooming ones visible. Dead or dying trees are relentlessly pruned and removed to avoid any hint of death.

Yet to anyone with their hands in the dirt of gardening, death is a familiar and integral part of the cycle of life. Death becomes the compost from which new life grows. It is a giver of fertility and potential – something to be celebrated rather than denied.

Some gardens do celebrate death. The cherry tree and its untimely fall of petals is a central theme of Japanese gardens and philosophy. The New England autumn, with vibrantly colored leaves falling to the ground and floating on ponds and streams, the image of red sumac or golden aspen with their leaves brilliant against the fresh snow, are familiar images. So are the beautiful skeletal forms of bare trees silhouetted in the snow in northern winters. Yet we avoid coming face to face and truly celebrating death in our own experiences and in our gardens.

The exceptions are some of the gardens created as part of modern crematorium chapels in Scandinavia. They seem more able than even the highly praised architecture of the region to express a deep and powerful connection with nature – particularly unique in that they deal with death rather than life.

One of the most powerful chapels and gardens is the Resurrection Chapel in Turku, Finland, designed by Erik Bryggman in 1940. The seating in the chapel is placed to one side, and the other side is a glass expanse opening into a garden of moss-covered rock and aged trees. The altar, and an open area for the coffin or urn and memorials are on the side of the chapel toward the garden, forming a balance point between the congregation and nature. The pews are set at an angle in the space – curiously, it seems at first, until you become aware that your attention is being called not only to the symbols and rituals within the space, but also through the open side of the room to the signs and rhythms of nature outside.

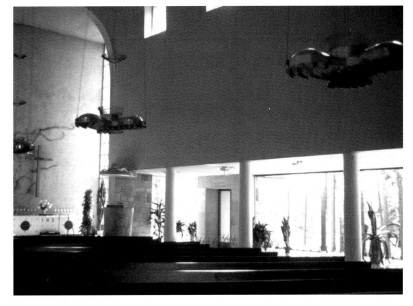

The glass wall in the Resurrection Chapel opens out into the forest, where ashes are scattered after a memorial service.

In this chapel, the changing seasons, the birth, death, and rebirth of the plants, the glorious burst of beauty of the flowers climaxing the long cycle of renewal, the falling leaf, the passing bird all become part of your experience. The duality of the setting becomes powerfully united at the close of the ceremony, when the dead are carried by the living through a ceremonial door in the open wall, out into the forest, into reunion with the cycles of nature and life itself.

A nurse-log garden demonstrates viscerally that new life emerges from the compost of old.

✧

The Scandinavian crematory gardens remind us of something else: to think of gardens not just as things in themselves, but to think of them along with our buildings and how we use them, and in relation to the rituals of our lives. They can be an important way to reconnect our activities with the broader context in which they take place.

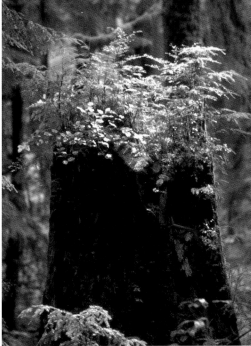

Celebrating the cycles of birth and death in gardens can be accomplished in many ways. One is combining both types of ritual in the same gardens. In many societies a ritual associated with birth is the burial of the afterbirth, often accompanied by planting a tree.

Such ideas can be incorporated into the design of a garden itself. A garden can focus on death and rebirth using rocks as a medium: igneous rocks, such as basalt or granite, breaking down into sand, reformed into sandstone, sedimentary, or metamorphic rocks. The concept of death as contributing to the compost of life can be a theme of a garden. A garden of death can focus on fungi, which live on and reprocess dead or decaying organic matter. A fungus garden, composed of various kinds of mushrooms, puff balls, and shelf fungi glowing luminously at night or unfolding after a rain, can be an absorbing kind of garden celebrating the processes of life feeding life.

A walk through almost any forest in the Northwest will bring you upon the cut end of a log four to six feet in diameter, which in itself forms a wonderful garden of death, being host to an abundance of raindrop-covered mosses, lichen, fungus, and seedlings of new plants taking root.

A garden celebrating death and rebirth can, in those rain forests, be formed from a fallen log or rotting stump which has become a nurse log out of which sprouts of new trees take root. A century later, we can sometimes see in the forest a row of giant dancing trees, standing tiptoe on their roots, with a hollow space uniting them; their common nurse log has long ago rotted into compost to quicken their growth.

A garden might focus on the indomitable life-force in something like the redwoods, which seem to generate new life out of old in ever more inconceivable ways. Regrown from stumps, downed logs, roots – any remnant of life exposed to the power of water, sun and soil – their perseverance and will to live are amazingly empowering.

A GARDEN OF TIME

Even something as abstract as time can be brought close to our hearts in a garden.

Think of a tiny garden, only a few feet across. Within it are but two rocks, some gravel, a bit of moss. It is separated from its surroundings by shadows. Yet the garden is not enclosed; what lies within is merely kept intently in focus before our eyes.

One rock lies half submerged in the grains of broken gravel which surround it like a sea lapping and wearing at an island. Enduring and patient it lies, as it has lain for more than 400 million years, since the formation of the earth itself.

From the depths of the shadows, its neighbor reaches out across the surface of the gravel to within inches of the first rock. This rock's surface is wrinkled and stretched, a lava river whose edges froze and hardened while the flow within pulled on and on. Looking closer, its dark surface turns here and there into rainbows, where the glacial taffy pull within has stretched the skin into fragile and delicate golden angel hairs of stone, which catch and reflect a shimmering light.

A newborn infant, this rock! Squeezed from the core of the earth and frozen in the release of pressure and heat, it is seeing its first circling of the stars overhead.

Mere inches separate the two rocks. But within those inches lies time – vast reaches and dizzying expanses of time. Sunrises and sunsets, day and night. Years, centuries, eons piling one upon another like waves upon the shore. The entire history of a planet, the wheelings of its galaxy, the birth, death, and successions of its surface, its ages and its forms of life.

Across this gulf, the rocks are yet the same. Part enduring, part reborn of themselves from the debris and wear of time, re-fused and re-formed again and again in our planet's inner fires, and brought again to the light of day and night and the stars which gave us birth. Both are formed, as our planet, our sun, ourselves, and the stars over our heads, of the ashes of the same stars now long dead.

Across the gaps of space and time we see, and know them – our brothers, our sisters, ourselves.

GARDENS OF CELEBRATION

Another important role of gardens can be to celebrate or honor, in a much more immediate and experiential way than with a bronze plaque saying "Joe Smith Memorial." Gardens can celebrate natural phenomena: earth, air, fire, water, or spirit. They can honor people by creating a place where we have time, space, and attention to experience each other's many facets. They can celebrate dreams we have of our destiny, our future, or values we hold.

Natural phenomena such as water, wind or rocks can obviously be used as tools in a garden to create experiences. *Celebrating* them in a garden is a quite different thing. Water can be used in a garden without calling attention to itself. But when a garden *calls attention* to water, which focuses our minds on its importance to life or its myriad wonderful qualities, it *celebrates* water. There are many ways to praise water without using it as a vehicle for that celebration. Water, for example has been honored wonderfully in Japanese gardens containing no water – only rocks and gravel.

In creating a garden to honor something, we are in a sense reciprocating – giving something back to recognize what it has given us. In a garden that honors something, we give ourselves an opportunity to become more fully aware of it and to appreciate the value, intrinsic beauty, and specialness of it. At the same time, we are making a statement that we honor things beyond our immediate material needs.

In honoring something, we make a vital change in our lives and in the world around us. We move from a secular world of "I want" to a world where we hold sacred ourselves, our neighbors, and the world around us. In giving honor to something, we act out of love, not out of calculated self-interest, for love is the pure act of unstinted giving. And we enter a different world.

Let's think for a minute how we could honor *air* with a garden . . . . .

CLOUD GARDENS

Look up for a moment at the clouds floating along all together, and remember how gossamer they are when we pass through one in an airplane or as fog. Now look closely at one cloud. Watch its delicate shape as it slowly moves across the sky. Look more closely. See the transformations taking place in its gauzy filaments as they emerge into view and disappear again in the unfolding and transforming circulatory patterns within the cloud. Watch the cloud drift through the air. But it *can't* be moving *through* the air! Anything that delicate, and with such complex internal movements, would be ripped apart as it pushed into the air ahead.

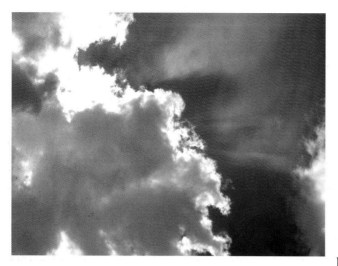

Cloud gardens, continually changing and transforming. Waiting only for a "picture frame" or other means of focussing our attention on them.

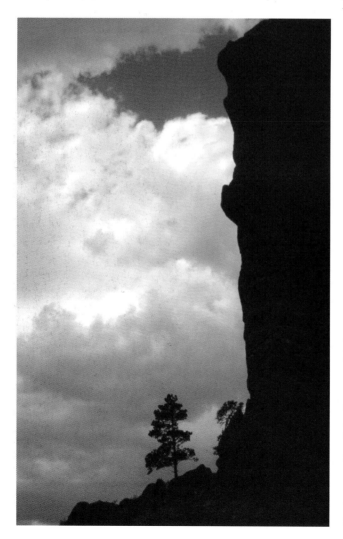

Focus your eyes wider. Look at two or three or four clouds at the same time. They probably seem to be moving in concert, maintaining the same spacing as they move across the sky. The clouds aren't moving through the air. They're riding *within* a river or stream of air, which itself is being *pulled* along from place to place by differences in pressure, temperature, and density of the surrounding air. From space, sometimes these giant streams of air can be seen rotating in great gyres of air and clouds. Even the streams of cloud and fog pouring over a mountaintop or down a river valley are being borne along within rivers of air which enfold them.

In a sense, clouds are not objects themselves, but only visible interfaces within the rivers of air which have become discernible through water condensation. At certain conditions of pressure, temperature, and contained water, conditions form by which the water vapor in the air condenses into water droplets or ice particles and forms clouds. As conditions change, the water or ice may again vaporize. Often a bank of fog will appear to be moving rapidly, yet the end of it may never move, as the cold air is warmed and the fog evaporates.

So look again at the clouds. We can begin to feel the location and movement of these invisible rivers of air whose inner structure they make visible. Sometimes we can see the edges of the river in the movement of birds or adjacent cloud masses. How wonderful is the delicate unfolding and transforming structure of clouds within these great rivers flowing endlessly within our ocean of air.

We are dwellers at the bottom of an ocean of air. It is a giver of life and of beauty. Its transparency to our eyes means that we depend on other means to make its beauty visible to us. Clouds, fog, soaring birds, wind chimes, scents wafted from far away places, and the movement of breezes through prairie grasses or leaves of trees all bring glimpses of the beauty of that ocean.

Even if we have no ground, no trees, no water – nothing but the roof over our heads – we still can have an incredible garden that touches these beautiful, often overlooked, yet awesome aspects of nature.

Both the French architect LeCorbusier and the Mexican landscape architect Luis Barragan pioneered wonderful rooftop gardens that don't try to carry the ground up on top of buildings but which look to the sky and its beauty. Barragan's cloud garden is a starkly walled rooftop, excluding the view of everything except the sky, the sun, the dramatic, ever-changing cloudscape, and at night the wheeling of the moon and the stars.

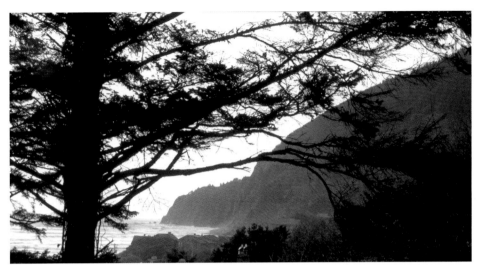

Yes, a cloud garden may be the entire rooftop of a building, with a panoramic view of the sky or a carefully framed view of sunset, moonrise, or a mountain top where fog or lee clouds form and disperse. But clouds can be equally powerful viewed from a carefully placed skylight over a bed, or a window attentively framing a view with the branches of a tree. Cloud gardens need little water or fertilizer, and are generally easy to maintain. Care, however, must often be taken in their design to "shadow out" the presence of other things people expect to see, and to focus dramatically on the clouds themselves.

Waves crashing against the end of the mountain are only a small part of the view. But the removal of a single branch from the tree focuses attention on that one dramatic point.

Below: A wind garden, rippling in the breeze.

Even more enchanting is a cloud garden at night, with the clouds softly luminous from the moonlight behind them, shifting shape as they pass in front of the moon, with soft-colored auroras forming and transforming around the moon itself.

These cloud gardens remind us how narrow our viewpoint on the rest of the universe is – in time, scale, frequency and meaning. They show us how often our "proven" views radically change when we come to see things from a new perspective. Even one little window from our optic nerve into a garden of a single cloud can change our sense of our universe and ourselves, and costs but a moment of time.

. . . Or what about, perhaps, a WIND GARDEN?

What of something as invisible as the wind? How could we celebrate such an ephemeral yet powerful force of nature without using the wind itself?

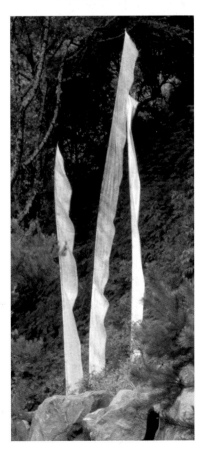

Wind is perhaps invisible, but its effects are often extraordinarily visible and powerful. There is a bowl carved into the rock in Mauritania – the Richat Hole – which is twenty miles across and two thousand feet deep, carved solely by the scouring forces of wind.[3] In Utah, you can find sandstone boulders with strange striations on their surface – once sand dunes hundreds of feet deep, piled up by the wind, compressed into rock, eroded to the surface, and scoured again by the wind into strange and curious shapes. The surfaces of sedimentary rock, scoured by the wind to expose contrasting colored layers, as at the Dasht-I-Kiver in Iran, can present ethereal patterns more akin to interpenetrating fluids than to rock.[3]

---

[3] Kevin Kelley, THE HOME PLANET, Addison-Wesley, 1988.

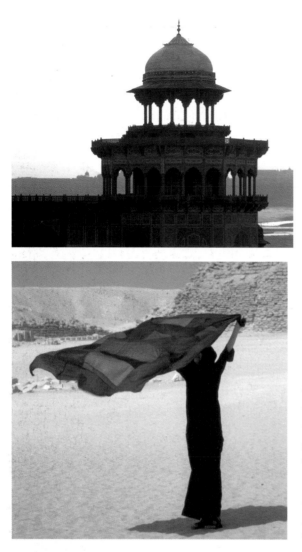

Snow drifts or sand dunes, in their ephemeral living forms or frozen by temperature or geologic processes, can present with startling beauty the effects of the passage of winds. Seen from a satellite, these make exquisite patterns. Seen from inches away, the erosional patterns on the downwind edge of a sand dune can rival the greatest sculpture. The ripples of sand in a lake bed, frozen into rock, can be uncovered in certain strata, and become the focus of a garden.

Cloud gardens, or a garden of birds or butterflies hang-gliding on thermal updrafts, can be other ways of touching the presence of invisible winds. Or the fog blowing through trees. Or a view of fog rhythmically condensing and evaporating in the lee of a mountain peak.

The windswept shapes of coastal trees form indelible images of the power of wind. Inland, the waves of prairie grass, the sounds of leaves rustling in the wind, the turning of maple leaves before a storm, or the sighing of a pine forest in the wind can all become part of a garden.

Wind harps, wind flutes, or wind chimes bring sounds linked with the wind into even an urban garden. Light silk canopies or hangings that float in the lightest breeze can offer a special effect. The gauzy window curtains of years ago billowed out from the window at the slightest air movement, bringing a wonderful anticipation of relief on hot summer evenings.

The great Mogul and Persian gardens didn't bother with such effects. They built elevated pavilions atop the walls of their gardens and the roofs of their buildings to bring them into a garden which was just the wind – a slight desert wind bringing relief from the heat, the subtle scents

Top: Another kind of wind garden – just a place where you can enjoy to wonderful relief of the slightest breeze.

Above: Yet another kind of wind garden! The Moghuls created wonderful outdoor garden spaces using only lightweight fabric canopies that shaded, while making the breeze itself visible through their undulations.

from afar, indistinct signs on the ground or the river of an approaching zephyr. Their hearts traveled with the wind, and the wind became the heart of some of their most subtle gardens.

✦

The uses and potentials of gardens in an energetic universe are far different, and hold far more possibilities for the nurture of our hearts and spirits, than gardens of a materialistic universe.

When we think of our senses as gateways to the universe, perhaps *they* should be celebrated. Gardens of light, or shade, or shadows, or moonlight. Gardens of sound, of silence. Gardens of warmth, of coolness, of fragrance. Gardens of taste, of touch.

And then, of course, what of our inner senses? Some of the most wonderful gardens are gardens of immensely powerful *emptiness*, gardens that bring us into touch with the incipient moment of *becoming*, the seed from which all emerges.

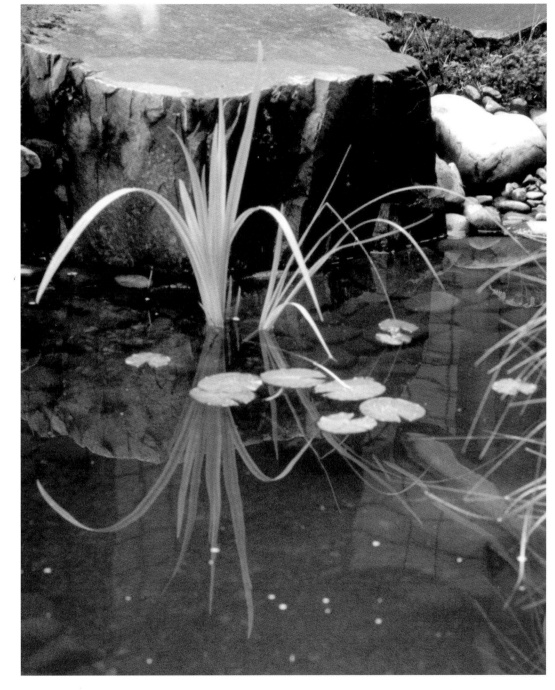

*Austerity, in a
garden, takes away
the clutter that
blinds our vision.*

11 CITIES OF PASSION

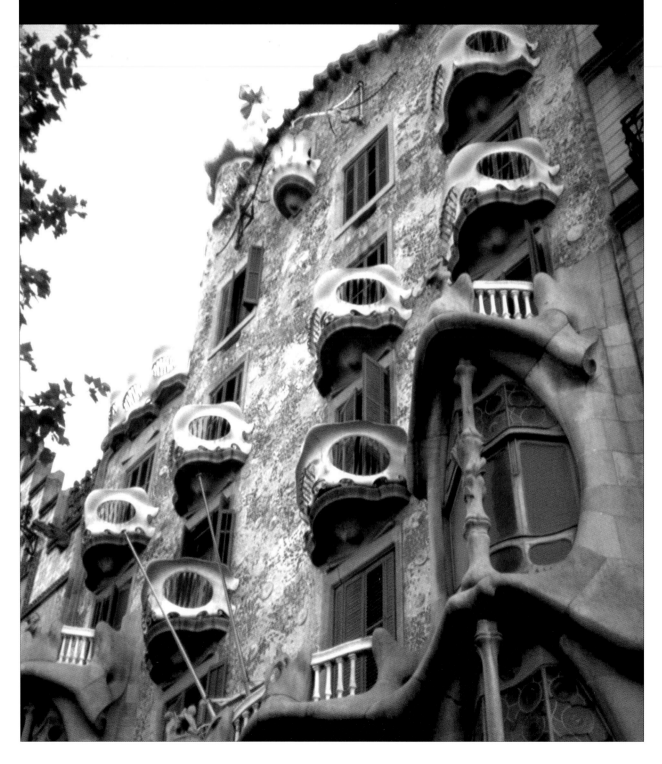

WHAT MAKES A CITY LOVABLE?

It is our shared dreams and passions, our distinctive communal cultures and ways of life that give shape to our cities and give them the power to move our hearts and affect our lives. Cities, like buildings, have personalities and reflect the way of life of their makers. Efforts to improve the sustainability of our urban and cultural patterns have so far ignored this vital human component of enduring patterns.

Not unexpectedly, the cities that stand out in our memories are those tied to *passions* – our own or someone else's. *Passions* build and focus energy, even more so for a group than for an individual. A place we value is often one that has developed distinctive and unlikely character out of the quirks, enthusiasms, ardor, or zeal of some individual or group which shaped its nature and its destiny.

What distinguishes a community from a city is <u>intimacy</u>. A community arises when we share bonds of friendship, history, hardship, or caring. It arises when we open our hearts to share our longings, fears, and stories. It arises when we create places of safety where we can speak from the heart, develop compassion about other people's needs, and experience the joys of giving. It emerges when we join *together* our energies with common intention for good.

Privacy, for example, is a powerful value in today's cities, but a two-edged sword. We seek it as escape from the irritation of strangers. Yet inside, our hearts yearn for the sound and connection of family and friends. When it is *our* children making noise, we're content – tuning but half an ear to track their energy and their comings and goings. Yet the same sounds from strangers create irritation. When we allow neighbors to be friends or family to us, their noises become lines in a play in which we, too, are players, awaiting our cues, swept along by the interweaving webs of plot and passion. Village life may be too close, constraining an individual's need to change and grow. Today's urban life, on the other hand, gives little heed to the individual or to community.

The wonderful sacred and organic designs of Antonio Gaudi – parks, apartment houses, cathedrals, homes and public buildings – have given a special flavor to the entire city of Barcelona.

CHI OF PLACE

Our modern cities *have* reflected our passions, but unfortunately those have been mostly passion for greed, mobility, and freedom from responsibility. Our newly emerging energetic view of our cosmos gives rise to different passions, new visions of community, and new form for our cities.

A deepening awareness of the energy basis of Creation, the interconnectedness of all life, and interconnectedness between material life and other dimensions of existence can only have a profound effect on our communities. It represents a change in the *intention* of our lives and communities. It underlies a change from cities for production and consumption of material goods toward communities based on satisfaction from interaction with other people and other life. It embodies change from "growth" to evolution; from human-centered to all-life-centered realization of individual and interactive potentialities. It represents a central refocusing of our dreams and understanding.

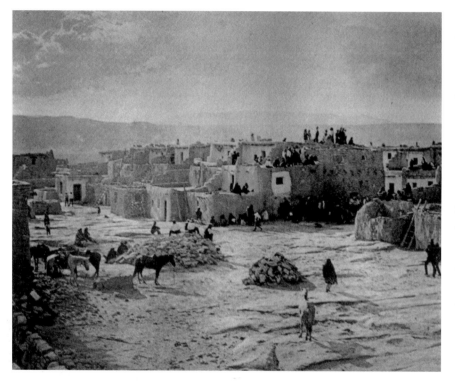

Attention to energy fields in the earth has been part of the energetics of community in almost every culture. Energetic awareness was commonly used in China, Japan, and elsewhere in choosing sites for establishing new cities. Anomalies in earth energy do occur, or can be called into existence, on the scale of a community. It is an aspect to consider in founding a new city, or expanding or relocating an existing one.

African, Aboriginal, and Native American traditions suggest a richer, finer-grained, and more complex connection with the energy of place in their communities. Joseph Rael, a Southern Ute and Picuris Pueblo Indian, talks of this connection:

Preparations for a dance at Acoma Pueblo.

As children we were taught that we existed as pressure point activators for the sacred sites within the village. Every twenty feet or so were consecrated points on the ground which carried special blessings. These shrines were buried in the ground and were only visible to the inner eye. As we walked through the village, we pushed them into aliveness with our bodies' pressure on them. . . . The holy shrines were placed there because the vibrational essence of those holy sites would enhance the psyche of community and of each individual within the community.

. . . The energy was always shifting, was always different. The resonating vibrations in the sacred sites were always changing so that the people in the village were always alive with energy. These sacred spaces, generating life sustaining powers, maintained our integrity as a group, orienting each individual toward the community's highest ideals.[1]

[1] Rael, Joseph, BEING AND VIBRATION, Council Oak Books, 1993.

Modification in the existing energy of a community's setting, however, can more frequently be an opportunity to affect the resultant chi. Washington, D.C. and Rome, Italy, were both originally unhealthy sites chosen for reasons of commerce, access, and politics. The draining, filling, and moving of the earth and waters, along with siting important facilities on the tops of hills rather than in the low-lying areas, was vital to improving their energy and their health.

In other cities affected by dry *föhn* winds, the planting of trees and development of fountains, waterfalls, and other water features have been used to restore the negative-ion content of the air and lessen the psychological impacts of those wind conditions. Cities in Germany have examined the entire airshed of their cities. They have zoned building height and location and planted or cleared urban forests in order to gain or escape cool air drainage channels, modify climatic effects, or reduce temperature variation.

Tree planting for shading and cooling a city is widely done. With the scale of earth-moving possible today, even creating gaps in landforms that block air movement and cause inversion layers can potentially be accomplished. "Tuning" subtle energies of place by digging ponds or lakes, placing large rocks, or changing threatening landforms can also be done.

Korea once had a national "chi patrol," which traveled the country looking for good and bad patterns of energy, good places to site new cities and activities, and things which could be changed to benefit the overall chi energy of the country.[2] As noted in Chapter Three, the first Han emperor of China, Qin Shihuang, went to extraordinary measures to create positive chi for the country far into the future.

The Chinese are known for their long history of selecting locations for cities, tombs, and temples to connect them with the strongest chi energy in the ground and to enhance the overall harmony of their communities and their landscape.

Modification of waterways – by damming or undamming rivers, modifying and restoring channels, or creating lakes and ponds – can change the effects of the water flow patterns on the lives of residents. Location and design of bridges across water or ravines, can change energy patterns in a community. Any large-scale actions like these should be done with caution, however, as their unanticipated impacts can be considerable.

The location of temples, churches, shrines, or other key elements of a city on "power spots," such as the Kiyomizu Shrine, many of the English cathedrals,

[2] Yoon, Hong-Key, GEOMANTIC RELATIONSHIPS BETWEEN CULTURE AND NATURE IN KOREA, Orient Culture Service, 1976.

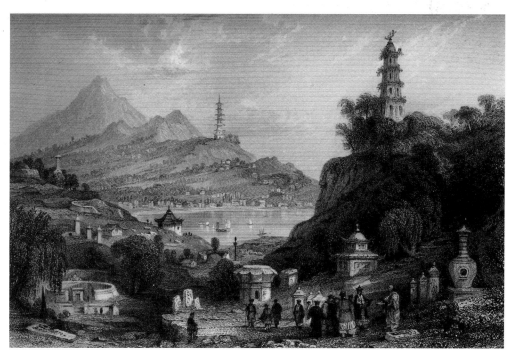

or Hawaiian healing and birthing places, can bring the benefits of that energy to all residents. A look at Chinese modification of landscape in and around cities can be instructive today. Careful location and construction of pagodas, bridges, and large buildings has been used to improve the balance of natural features such as hills, rivers, lakes, or waterfalls. Creating a harmony between a city and its setting can improve the self-image of the community and empower the lives of all its members.

Conversely, understanding the impacts of energy fields in the earth can lead to tempering invasive actions used today for other purposes, which unintentionally change environmental energy fields. Quarries, mines, or highway cuts can alter nearby energy flows. Irrigation, or pumping of groundwater, can alter or deplete water movement in the earth, affecting surface energy conditions as well as the growth of trees and other vegetation.

Acknowledgment of the energy fields in the earth necessitates changed attitudes toward the microwave towers, TV and power stations, electric rail lines, and the entire amped-up pace of life in our cities. Alternatives to these elements are available, frequently with the additional benefit of dramatically lowering our energy and resource consumption.

Perhaps most importantly, awareness of environmental energy fields can lead to modification of the increasingly intensive energy pollution of our communities. Our cities and our bodies are saturated with radio and TV broadcasting waves, microwaves, and infra-red emissions. Electromagnetic fields generated from electrical systems, transformers, trains, and other equipment are overwhelming.[3] Even the frantic pace of life in our communities may change as we rediscover the value of resonance and attunement.

These are physical or "material" approaches to dealing with the chi of community. We need to remember that the greatest impact on the energy of places where large numbers of people congregate is the energy of those very people, individually and in concert.

The institutional web of a community is magnitudes more complex and interactive than that of a single home or business, and the attention we need to pay to the chi of interaction is similarly greater. The presence of common dreams or pursuits of the community plays a powerful role in marshaling that chi of community. What leads to physical, emotional, and spiritual well-being of each and all leads to more positive energy, which leads to enhanced well-being of each and all.

COMMUNITY INTENTIONS

Aligning our community intentions with that of all life brings the power of rightness and the love, support, power, and knowledge of all Creation to our actions. It maintains individuality and individual purpose while remaining connected to the larger communities of which we are part. It brings synchronicity to our actions, and keeps our actions in alignment with our individual and community life purposes.

---

[3] A working group of experts assembled by the National Institute of Environmental Health Sciences in June, 1998, recommended, after reviewing hundreds of studies, that these fields should now be regarded as a "possible human carcinogen."

Changing our intentions from maximum personal wealth and power to that of equity of wealth and opportunity within a community creates profound change in that community. Merely changing legal minimum wages to $12/hr would eliminate the need for most government assistance programs, and with them the stigmas and self-worth-destroying effects of public housing, the bureaucratic morasses of welfare and public assistance, and much of the resultant drug use and crime.

Equity in wealth means a change in the symbols of success – to actions that benefit the community. The traditional status of a person in India was not based on what they owned, but what they have been able to *give* to others. Removing the incentives of personal gain lessens the appeal of taking wealth from others and from nature. With more equity of opportunity, there is more incentive for students to be in schools, transforming their nature. The role of potlatch, or giveaway, as a means of healing and balancing community energy in Pacific Northwest Native American communities is an interesting precedent to consider. The conventional elements of eco-cities – reducing need for transportation, using renewable energy sources, natural building methods, increasing durability, and reducing environmental impacts and pollution – are all elements of attaining sustainability on the material level.

Not every climate needs buildings to create magic places to live. Shah Abbas laid out the Royal Quarter of Isfahan as a series of gardens and garden pavilions.

A third element in securing the health of all Creation is our coming to enjoy and celebrate the *specialness and differences of places and the life that composes them.* Arni Fullerton's Winter Cities project in Canada a few years ago found that in all the tourism brochures produced in Canada there was only one picture of winter! So he got people together from winter cities around the world. Together, they found they constituted a real market for winter cars, winter clothes, and other products for winter living.

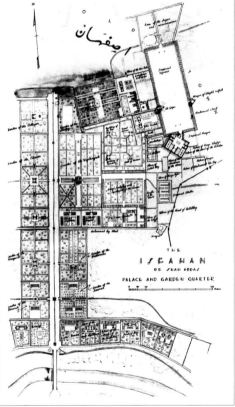

But more importantly, they figured out how to *celebrate* winter with ice skating, ice sculpture festivals, skiing, snowmobiling, and sled dog races reflecting a learning of what life in the winter means. Beginning to *live* in winter, they have begun to see what constitutes life in their region, to develop concern for it, and to discover what constitutes its health. It wasn't long before people in those communities changed into *winter* people, enjoying and looking forward to winter instead of just waiting impatiently for summer.

Distinctive qualities of places touch our hearts: climate, geology, history, and community of inhabitants. These qualities make a place different from others and give root to a special personality and spirit in its inhabitants. A culture arising in harmony with those conditions becomes uniquely robust and potent.

Isfahan, the 15th century capital of Persia (now Iran), brought an unforgettable pattern of desert life into being by combining unusual elements of its traditions and conditions. Bringing ice-cold snowmelt water across the desert from the mountains through hand-dug underground channels, they were able to make gardens bloom in the desert. Their nomadic desert culture had little interest in or need for buildings, so the royal city became a collection of wonderful walled and protected gardens.

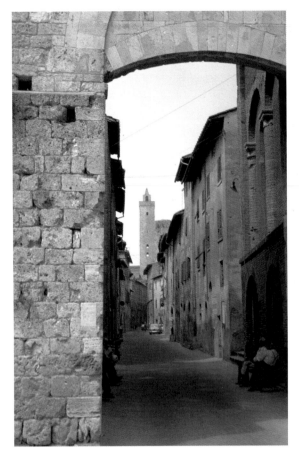

Trees and flowers are not the same thing as Nature. A city with neither can be as integral and beautiful a part of nature as one filled with greenery. And adding greenery to a city does not, in itself, heal our separation with the rest of Creation.

Water chutes and irrigated trees brought coolness to the air. Water features brought a wonderful sense of welcome and respite from thirst. Tents and pavilions in the gardens gave the only shelter needed. Vaulted streets, markets, and bridges, and irrigated tree-lined promenades, brought shade and coolness to commercial activities and community gathering places. The "Paradise Gardens" of Isfahan, by adding in a limited area the missing qualities of the desert without overpowering or denying its special nature, leave an unforgettable impression of the beauty and power of desert life.

Nurture of place gives the special power and beauty accreted from layer after layer of everyday acts of caring for other life with which we live. Amish villages and farm country show an indelible mark of their nurture of place. Irrigated paddy agriculture in Southeast Asia brings into existence an essential community of caring and responsibility, without which the entire agricultural system falls into ruin. That sense of caring quickly expands into the entire ecosystem and gives a special flavor to an entire region.

WILDNESS

Wildness in the city can go far beyond conventional attempts to "bring greenness into the city." This is the connectedness we miss when we go "into the wilderness" with our freeze-dried meals, aluminum canoes, and high-tech camping gear. Existence of trees or "green spaces" does not represent a deeper relationship with the rest of nature. A community entirely without trees or greenery, like an adobe pueblo or stone Italian hill town, can be deeply connected with and as much a part of nature as a bees' nest or a termite mound.

What we truly seek and need from "nature" is not greenery, or even wilderness, but wildness. We think of wildness in terms of danger, but wildness does not mean either danger or lack of danger; it means *unbrokenness*. "Unbroken," in turn, means seamlessness or unity, and unity means oneness – with *all*. Wildness means to open, to let the generative power of our love flow, to manifest without hesitation our seamless intuitive interaction in the events of our world.

That wildness can be found only *within* us – by abandoning ways that separate us, break us, and keep us apart. Letting wildness flow within us, infusing it into our lives and our places, we come again into the unity with our world that we seek in vain in wilderness. Without that unity, there is little hope of our sensitivity to the health of other life.

Wildness means being real.

ROOTS OF COMMUNITY PASSIONS

Our minds, hearts, dreams, and emotions are vital to our cities. We often think of cities in terms of their technical and material elements, such as streets and highways, hospitals, water, sewer, electrical and communication systems, building functions, and institutions. Yet how they stir our love and passion, affect our minds, give form to our dreams, and evoke our emotions are vital elements in their power.

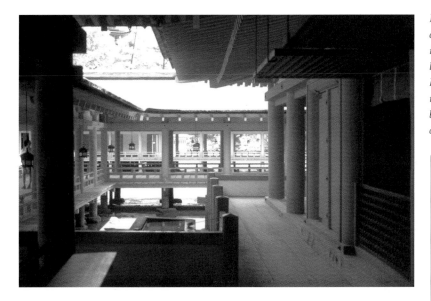

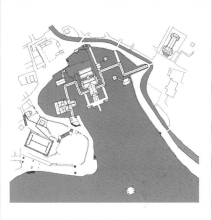

Pavilions floating above the waters of the bay, their crimson color irridescent and shimmering in the light reflected off the water. Itsukushima Shrine is an unforgettable setting for the blessing of a fishing fleet, and image of the Sacred Land of Paradise.

One element of that power is our ability to bring into being powerful and unprecedented patterns and images through grasping new potentials of a setting. The Itsukushima Shrine in Japan, instead of being built on land, was constructed on pilings in a bay. Its red-orange buildings float on their reflections in the tidal water, as the festooned fishing boats arrive thorough the giant *torii* gateway framing the entrance of the bay for the annual blessing of the fishing fleet.

Or think of San Francisco and the images of its bridges appearing and disappearing magically in the fog. Or Shrinigar in Kashmir, where the royalty of India created a fabulous summer retreat of gardens encircling the lake. Gardens cascade down the hillsides and float on reed mats on the lake. Communities of houseboats are connected by causeways, arched bridges, and boats floating on the mirrored surface of the lake.

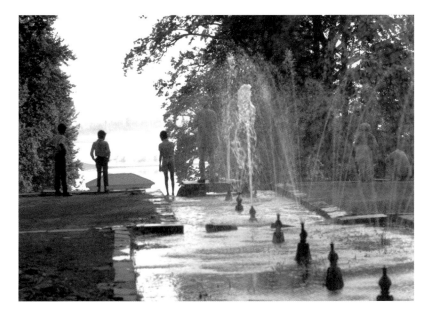

Built as a pleasure retreat for the royalty of India to escape the summer heat, Dal Lake in Shrinigar manifests a magical vision of a community living in cool, fragrant gardens on terraced slopes around the lake, joined together by boat.

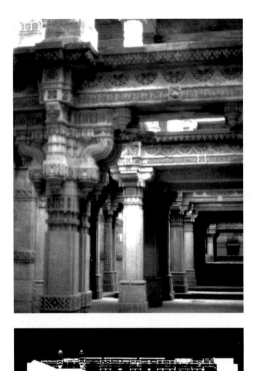

Above: Adalej Village stepwell. A solution to dry-season access to water also created a wonderful place for community, away from the heat and sun.

Right: The long avenues planted with towering cedars create an unforgettable setting for the Shogun shrines at Nikko.

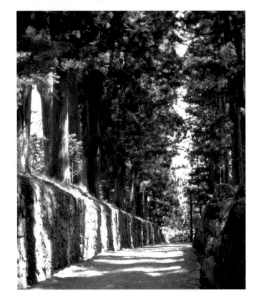

In the Gujerat area of northwestern India, the groundwater subsides dozens of feet into the ground in the months before the yearly monsoons. The local villages there developed a pattern of building "step-wells" – flights of steps giving individuals access to the water far below the surface. In bracing the walls of these stone stairways, the villages evolved a wonderful pattern of cool, shaded, carved-stone platforms and alcoves which became the village's gathering place in the hot, dry months.

The passions and driving force of single *individuals* like Baron Haussman in Paris, or Pierre L'Enfant in Washington, D.C., have shaped the dominant nature of some wonderful cities. The architect Antonio Gaudi gave Barcelona a unique flavor and sense of sacredness, mathematics, geometry, and color through his parks, apartment buildings, homes, and churches.

In Nikko, Japan, the funerary shrines of several of Japan's great shoguns, or military rulers, are intricately carved and gaudily lacquered, built through the coerced "contributions" of the shoguns' underlords. But what is most striking and memorable about the shrines is their surroundings. They are approached through long graveled avenues set between stone walls in a deep forest of towering Japanese cedars, which contribute great power and contrast to the buildings themselves. The trees, however, were not there originally, but were planted by one of the lesser lords, who conceived of their planting either through a stroke of genius or as a clever way to avoid paying a burdensome monetary "contribution."

What would Agra, India, be without the individual love and passions of Shah Jahan: the Taj Mahal built in memory of his wife, his own planned tomb on the other side of the river, and his palace structures in the Fort?

Yet individuals do not have to be rich or famous for their passions to give shape to a community. Simon Rodia's wonderful whimsical Watts Towers in Los Angeles, made from broken pottery and used rebar, have given identity to a whole neighborhood. Balladeer Forestiere's underground gardens in Fresno, California have become a local wonder.[4] The three-foot-thick stone walls of the Tassajara Zen Center's kitchen in California give silent testimony to the gentle persistence of faith against the unreasonableness of local building codes that demanded such overbuilding. A 40-mile loop walking trail

---

[4] See Jan Wampler, "People and the Places They Build," ARCHITECTURE PLUS, July/Aug '74.

around Portland, Oregon, exists because of the vision and faith of a few individuals.

The citizens of the Czech capital of Prague had such a *love of their community* that they bribed the Germans not to destroy it in the Second World War. Prague had its share of beautiful monuments and historical structures, but the specialness of the city was in how its entire fabric had, over the years, become an expression of love for community. Through dozens of generations, the exterior of virtually every building in the city had been ornamented and enriched with sculpture, painting, and architectural decorative work – for the enjoyment of the entire community, not just the building's owners. A hodge-podge of styles, techniques, and treatments amassed over time, which sounds like a recipe for chaos. Together, however, their individuality is subsumed into an overall richness with wonderful and unexpected details anywhere we look.

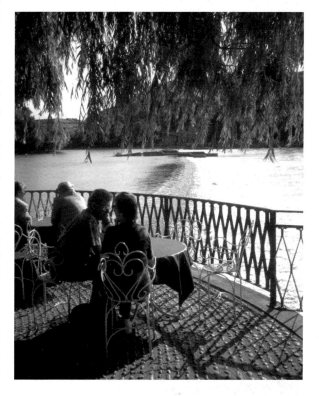

Institutions can be the source and vehicle for expression of a community's passions. To most visitors, the governmental buildings of Washington, D.C., are secondary to the extraordinary collection of private and public museums that have congregated around the city's center. University towns like Oxford or Cambridge in England, Amherst or Cambridge in Massachusetts, have imbued their communities with a sense of passion for academic learning. Other cities, like Jerusalem, are so prolific with institutions of various religions that the air is filled with prayers in many tongues.

A riverside cafe terrace in Prague provides one of innumerable places for the residents to enjoy the beauty of their city.

It is hard to think of Spain without thinking of the rituals and passions of the bullfight and the archetypal patterns renewed in us by those celebrations. Similarly, who can think of Indianapolis without car racing; of Milan without opera; or of Rio or New Orleans without Mardi Gras? Whenever we come together in celebration – sacred or secular – we bring into focus a vortex of energy that renews both us and the place. If well focused, it can bring healing and power to our endeavors.

An all-too-infrequent passion is the simple pleasure of a *community enjoying life* and itself. Getting off a train one night in a crowded station in Sendai, Japan, I was suddenly surrounded by the sounds of laughter, singing, and merriment instead of the sounds of frantic travelers normal to such places. I knew immediately that this was a community worth getting to know.

Many towns and villages in Spain and South America have an evening tradition of the "passerada," in which people gather in outdoor cafes and in the squares to enjoy the spectacle of the young and old eyeing each other, making overtures, beginning and renewing friendships. Paris has its sidewalk cafes, the Champs Elysees, and similar promenades in other districts. Italian and Greek neighborhoods are filled with a continual banter of give and take among their residents. Venice at night echoes with the sound of operatic arias from passing gondola.

Copenhagen, in Denmark, has created the famous Tivoli Gardens, filled with delight, music, song, and the sounds and smells of feasting, dancing, and merrymaking. The bar districts of Osaka, with their light reflecting in tiny canals, the riverside geisha district in Kyoto, the beer gardens in Germany devoted to family enjoyment – all reflect the eternal rhythms of community enjoying life. Some are sordid, some are sad; some riotous, some just filled with the joy of life. All bring to light a part of the spectrum of pleasure and enjoyment that arises out of a community celebrating life in its myriad forms.

Other passions in our communities have evolved out of unexpected twists of history. Rome's extravagant fountains, pouring forth music, beauty, and coolness at every corner, have their root in the ancient Roman celebration of its engineering genius. The Romans constructed aqueduct after aqueduct to bring water to the city and to feed its ever more extravagant public baths during the Empire. Over time, those same sources were tapped to feed celebrations of civic beauty, with sponsor, sculptor, and architect competing against each other during the Renaissance.

Another important part of the power of great places, particularly urban ones, is the shape of a community livelihood which grew out of unique environmental, historical, cultural and technological conditions. Venice and Amsterdam both were centers of international ocean trade at a time when boats were the most effective way to move goods. Consequently, canal systems developed in both cities.

New England mill towns, in contrast, developed around the conversion of water into mechanical power to run manufacturing operations. In both cases, once other means developed

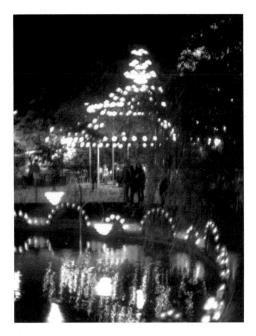

Part of the magical world of Tivoli at night

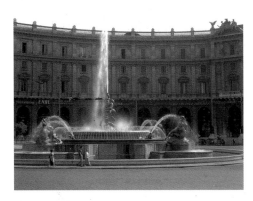

One of the innumerable public fountains gracing the city of Rome, fed by aquaducts since Roman times.

Water, rather than highway transportation, gives cities like Venice, Amsterdam and Bangkok a different pace and energy.

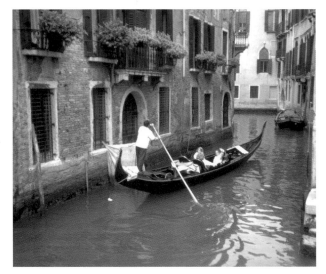

to fuel the commercial passions which brought them into being, the dams, millponds, canals, mills, and workshops have been discovered to have qualities of their own which can contribute to the specialness of life in that place. They have become a free gift of the past to the life of the community today.

History lives in us. Even on the smallest scale, time and history have the power to affect our lives. A house on an island in Maine that has been in the same family for seven generations shows the mark of all those lives and years. In it, we can feel the happiness, pain, care, or neglect of each generation whispered to us from every worn step and handrail, every coat of paint or wallpaper, every piece added, taken away, or changed.

Boston, Philadelphia, or Charleston – like many of the great cities of all enduring cultures – are enriched, and enrich our lives in turn, though layering of the patterns and passions, dreams and failures of era upon era.

Our links with our past or future can either be deepened or weakened, depending on the respect our communities pay (or the breach they make) with tradition, the honor they give to our ancestors, the kind of legacy they create for our descendants, and the trees they plant to give shade to their grandchildren. Those links fuse us to the rest of human and other life, which together form the stream that fills the banks of our river of community.

Harmony with our cosmology needs to be reflected in all our actions. The Palace of Versailles in France and the military-inspired boulevards of Paris alike reflect the cosmology of the supreme power of an absolute monarch. The incredible water and temple systems of the Khmer capital of Angkor illustrate a different cosmology and sense of the role of Kingship. Similarly, the great cities of China and Mesoamerica have been built on images of the cosmos, the nation, nature, and our place as part of it. This gives unique and potent meaning to the lives of their inhabitants.

At worst, what is expressed through the complex interaction of public and private, individual and group actions can weaken our communities if it is at odds with our cosmology and beliefs. At best, it can powerfully strengthen the energy focused on our actions and dreams, and give them coherence and meaning.

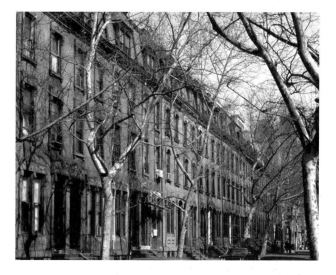

Philadelphia brownstones. The building and living patterns of different cultures and climates evolve into distinctive settings for living. Human communities adapted to those settings become distinctive in themselves, and part of the ecological community specific to that place.

A plan of the gardens and palace of Versailles – geometry imposed on nature. A vision of power-over, not power-from.

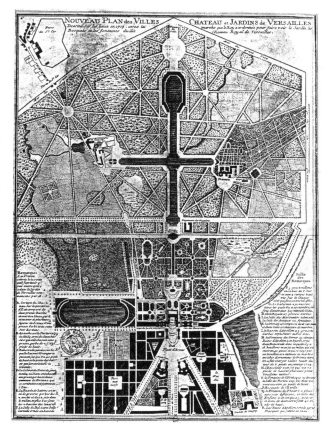

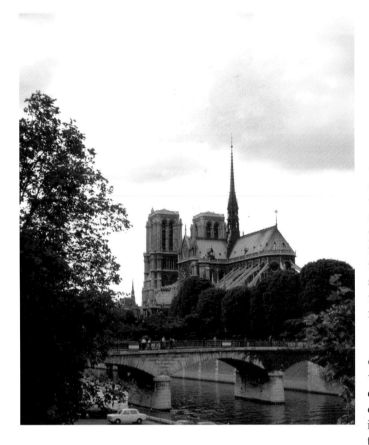

Any well-loved city has evolved immense richness in the interconnections between individual, family, and community; body, mind, and soul; the sacred and the mundane; the everyday world and the community's vision of the Universe.

Perhaps the most important function that our communities fulfill is that of sustaining our will and marshaling our inner forces to worthy goals. Giving place instead to simplistic objectives such as bigger freeways, better police protection, or greater corporate freedom from taxation, forfeits the endurance of our communities. Restoring that role requires opening ourselves to our deeper instincts, giving primacy to things of the heart, and giving our hearts to greatness rather than greed.

In knowing deeply any of the dimensions of community and its passions and connections, we come to love it, its location, and its crazy-quilt expression of our dreams and the possibilities of our time and place. Loving it, we come to hold it inviolate, which is the thread of sacred connection that embraces and underlies the unity of all creation.

There is more to life than TV and packaged breakfast cereal. Our communities can play a vital role in connecting us with that deeper power of life. The sound of a city of temples like Kyoto, Luxor, Uxmal, or Mecca, with bells resounding and prayers and songs of celebration filling the air, can never be confused with the sound of a city solely of commerce.

FINDING A PASSION

We can see how the beliefs and passions of others have given special form and qualities to their communities. But how do we find passions for our own communities?

The Makah Indian Museum is located at Neah Bay in the extreme northwest corner of Washington's Olympic Peninsula. The museum contains remarkable objects made by the tribal ancestors, preserved by a mudslide for over a hundred years.

Like most tribal lands, this is a poor one. The museum has restored a vital sense of their history, achievements, and self-esteem. As well, it has brought in tourist dollars and seeded an empowering cycle of development. Most striking about the museum is the tone of young and old alike proudly sharing the achievements of their families and ancestors, in contrast to the academic and institutional feeling of most museums.

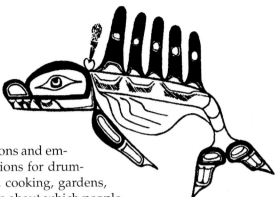

If even a small village with few resources, like Neah Bay, can empower itself, how can the same community passions and empowerment be brought to other villages? What about passions for drumming, singing, dancing, storytelling, woodcarving, boating, cooking, gardens, furniture-making, or quilting? There are thousands of things about which people become passionate, which give them a shared interest, and which can attract the respect and interest of others.

Any community, large or small, can develop such passions. It takes only a few people excited about something, getting together to invite someone to teach a workshop, then developing their own skills, inviting other communities to festivals and competitions, and bringing together outstanding people with the same passion. Soon the community becomes known for that passion and it shapes their lives, their spirits, and the physical and emotional structure of their community. Port Townsend, Washington, is known now for its wooden boat building, and Pendleton, Washington, for its Roundup. In the process a whole community becomes something unique and wonderful for others to visit, share, and experience.

The unique art and passons of every culture and community evolve from an interweaving of individual passions and visions and the overarching community response and melding of those energies.

The town of La Patrie, in Quebec, Canada, when faced with the collapse of its timber industry through overcutting of its ancient forests, decided to use the remaining high-quality, vertical-grain timber to higher use. The community retrained itself to make guitars and other musical instruments that depended on that wood, finding a new passion, new skills, and a new sense of self through a deeper connection to its resources. Towns such as K'san and Hazelton in northern British Columbia, Canada, have become known as the Cities of Totem Poles, through salvaging and re-erecting abandoned poles, and sponsoring and training new carvers in the skills and values of celebrating their culture and traditions in wood.

Delving deeply into any interest gives us a sense for things done well and thoroughly. It makes us aware of how much more we can achieve and what we gain personally from *everything* we do. It becomes a touchstone in our own experience by which we can weigh the depth of understanding and rightness in talk or action on *any* subject.

Anything deeply delved into brings forth wisdom, weirdness, and wonders. All are worth aspiring to.

A community that has no passions, which does not enjoy itself, does not enjoy life. It has no great enthusiasms, and dreams only small dreams. Such a community has not learned the incredible drama of life of which we are part, and is not capable of creating sustaining bonds within itself, with its neighbors, and with the natural world in which it is embedded.

So make our communities places to love. That is the sustaining force of life. When we have communities we are passionate about, we will want them to endure and will assure the changes in infrastructure, land use, building practices and patterns of living essential to that survival.

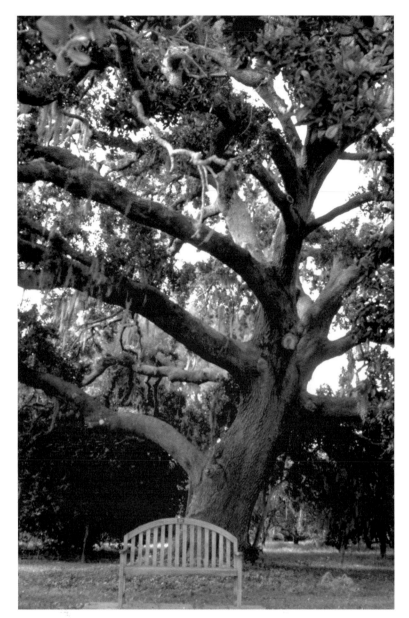

The beginnings of a sacred place at a Hospice House in Florida. Rescued from construction debris at a forgotten corner of the property by families of Hospice residents, the towering oak gives solace and energy to residents, families, and staff alike.

CHANGING COMMUNITY CHI

There is another kind of chi, community chi, which is often ignored when we focus solely on the energetics of our personal living and working places. Community chi is the glue of culture – the result of values, beliefs, and energy reflected back to us from our human surroundings. It is the joy or fear we feel walking down a street at night or being approached by a lover or a stranger in the dark. It is the dread or excitement we feel as we enter a school, hospital, or government building. It is the emptiness or fullness we feel as we leave a church, shrine, or temple. It is the shared meaningfulness or emptiness of our lives which we gain from our surroundings, communities, and culture. That, in turn, comes from how profoundly they embody a relationship with the rest of Creation and a role of value in our universe.

It is not only what our surroundings reflect but what they *don't* reflect which conveys to us our community chi, creates resonance in our hearts, and nurtures our personal and community health. Those gaps and silences, those darknesses where nothing is reflected when something should be reflected, are possibly the most essential aspects of community chi to be dealt with if we are to create wholeness in our lives and society. Let's look at a few of the silences where changes can transform our lives:

CELEBRATE DEATH

Death is an essential part of the cycles of life. It is the gateway between the material and energetic planes of existence. It is the place where we often feel most deeply our bonds with people and things that suddenly are no longer part of our material world. And in a culture of growth and materialism, where newness and youth are worshipped, death is feared, fought, denied in all possible ways, and dealt with in frightening superficiality when it inevitably occurs.

Only when we acknowledge the wonder and value of death can we begin to see how we have shunned it in every aspect of our surroundings. We begin to see, then, how to honor and celebrate it and bring greater richness to our lives and communities. We begin to design buildings which become richer and more mellow under the patina of time and aging. We begin to design gardens and landscapes that honor the full cycles of life, blossoming and fruiting, ripening, aging, death, and rebirth.

We begin to give proper prominence and design to hospices, memorial chapels, and other facilities that deal with death. We learn to create them as gateway structures – places where we can reflect, summate, say our farewells, grieve, and honor the losses, the gains, and the lives of both the living and the dead. We give proper place and settings to the rituals of departure.

We can also begin to create places which assist connection between our world and the spirit world – where we can connect with the wisdom of our ancestors and other life. We begin to acknowledge and honor the lives of the materials given up in the making of our places and our lives. In acknowledging the constant feeding upon and giving of life to other life through death, we begin to offer our own lives and deaths in that spirit. Ending this one silence alone begins to transform our connection with all life and to bring our own lives into harmony with reality.

Clear signs of cultural values and institutions out of harmony with life. When such sign persist, they give even deeper messages of cultural ill-health.

HEAL PLACE-RAPE

We have ignored the essential role of energy in the health of place as much as we have in that of people. We know now the indelible marks that rape, abuse, or destruction of self-esteem have on an individual. We are only beginning to acknowledge, however, that those same imprints are left on the physical and psychic bodies of both human and ecological communities that have suffered pillage, rape, murder, or abandonment.

There is a similarity in the feeling of an abandoned New England mill town, a logged-out California lumber town, a fished-out Oregon coastal village, a corporatized Midwestern farm community, or a mined-out Appalachian town. The human population is left without a source of livelihood; left with the debt and costs of infrastructure and mortgage payments on now-valueless homes; left with injury, sickness, and hopelessness. The soils, forests, waters, and earth are ravaged, and no longer able to support the needs of their community of life There is a sense of defeat, abandonment, grief, bewilderment. There is, as with individuals, massive damage to the psychic bodies of the community and the land.

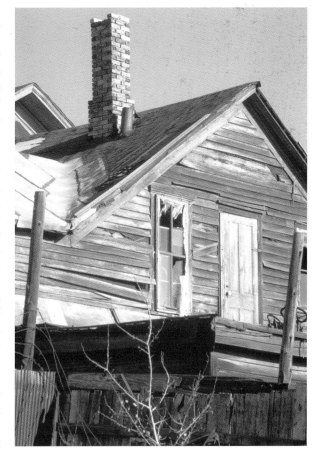

The power to cleanse and restore wholeness to places comes in part through time. It comes in part through the renewal of faith of an individual, then a group, and then the community. It comes from tapping the infinite power of the earth to heal, which makes even its own grievous pains insignificant. It comes through actions of individuals to forgive, release, and set free the memory of those who caused the damage. It comes from a community's intention to heal its energetic and physical body.[5]

Like those of individuals, damaged energy bodies of communities cause physical manifestations of illness. They show the same kind of rupture, clogging, displacement, and disconnection from their sources of energy that individual auras do from traumatic events. They can attract and contain the same negative spirits that an individual can have. Intentional healing can be performed on the chi of a place or community to begin restoration of the energy source of the community well-being.

Paying attention to the energy of relationships is vital for health. Here, neighbors distraught by clearing of trees on an adjacent property were given trees for a visual screen by the owner. Their caring about their impacts on the neighbors was more important than the gift itself.

Individuals, a group, or preferably the community itself, can raise healing energy and feed it into the energy body of the community or the place. Rituals offering acknowledgment, release, and healing to unwanted spirits that have come to reside there can be performed. We can restore the ongoing cycles of ritual and celebration that generate and sustain the energy of a community and empower individual acts of healing. When their energetic roles are more deeply understood and acknowledged, existing rituals such as births, graduations, weddings, funerals, and Independence Day parades can be transformed to contribute to community energetics.

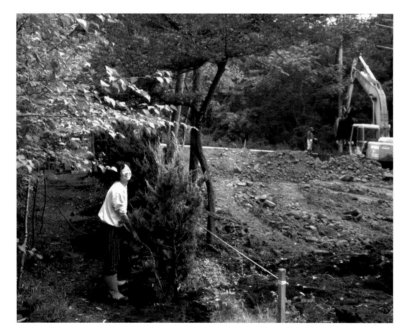

At the same time, we need to perform physical acts of healing – planting trees, restoring streams and wetlands, creating fish and wildlife habitat, removing sources of toxins, and creating meaningful work and self-respecting lives for the members of the community. Any acts of caring and taking responsibility – from sweeping sidewalks to picking up trash and removing junked autos and equipment to painting, fixing up, planting flowers or just a song and a smile – can begin the process of healing. Avoiding institutional patterns and practices which exploit people, place, and things is essential.

---

[5] Malidoma Somé's OF WATER AND THE SPIRIT, Tarcher/Putnam, 1994, gives an outstanding account, from the heart, of the role and value of community ritual. His RITUAL: Power, Healing and Community, Swan, Raven & Co, 1993, and THE HEALING WISDOM OF AFRICA, Tarcher/Putnam, 1998, go more extensively into the intellectual framework and specific examples of community ritual and how energy sustains a community. Starhawk's THE SPIRAL DANCE, Harper SF, 1979, is an excellent resource on raising energy through group ritual. Barbara Brennan's LIGHT EMERGING, Bantam Books, 1993, Chapter 17, gives more energy-specific detail on group hara energy and techniques to enhance and build it. Denise Linn's SACRED SPACE, Ballantine Books, 1995, though focused on energy in a home, contains many things that work as well on a community level; Chapter 15 is on ghostbusting. Various feng shui books give rituals for release of ghosts or spirits, or, to counteract negative energies in a place. Machaelle Small Wright's PERELANDRA GARDEN WORKBOOKS contain sections dealing with war and battlefield energy.

MAKE THE SACRED VISIBLE

The act of publicly acknowledging what we deeply value is vital to our social health and to the sustainability of culture and place. When we hold something sacred – in community – *and make that sacredness visible* in our public places, our whole culture is able to embody and reflect the sacred dimension of life. Places dedicated solely to the sacred provide a locus for individual and communal nurturing, grounding, and harmonizing. They focus and accumulate chi in place so we can more easily bring our energy into resonance with it. They reinforce the sense of the sacred within us essential for it to imbue all of our public and shared institutions and places.

Create shrines. Honor the sacredness of place, of other life, of all Creation, and of our dreams. Fill that absence in our communities with the presence of joy and celebration.

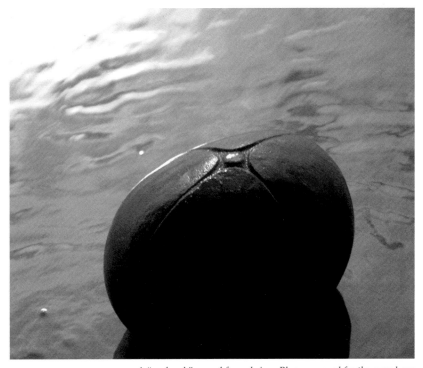

A "seed rock" carved for a shrine. Places reserved for the sacred can be visually identified and marked in many different ways.

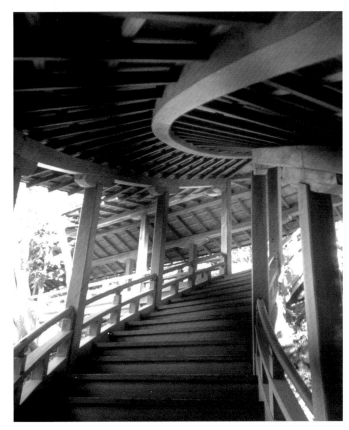

MAKE WORK SACRED

Work – or any action that employs our skills and joins them together with those of others to bring forth the gifts of joint action – is vital for the fellowship of community to develop and be sustained. When held sacred, work honors, joins, expands, and enriches our own nature and that of the community of life.

In sacred work, all serve and are served. None are servants. Its outward product in our community becomes a celebration of the heights our individual and joined capabilities can attain. Its inward product provides the individual health and capacity to open and give to others in community. Sacred work becomes encouragement to others and an acknowledgment of a coming together and uplifting in concord.

Deep skill is rarely visible until we grasp the profundity of the task attempted. To most people, this is just a beautiful stairs. To a carpenter, the curved wood beams, unsupported ridge beam, and flawless joinery stand as testimony to the immense skill of the builders.

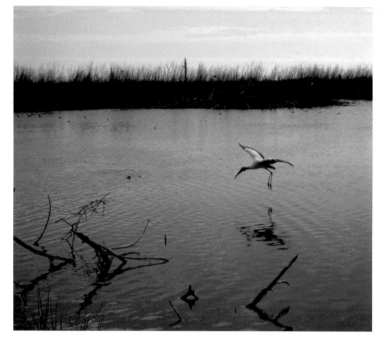

A wildlife refuge is a small space left for the rest of Creation to live with less pressure from our actions.

TRANSFORM ROOT INTENTIONS

Love and giving are the fundamental principles upon which any viable society or community is formed. Their absence, and the lack of even acknowledging their existence and importance, are gnawing silences in our communities which clash with our inner root impulses. An intention to have *community* rather than an *economy* produces a different world.

HONOR OTHER LIFE

Our communities and their energy speak almost exclusively of ourselves. The rest of Creation, their needs, their dreams, and the greater community we form together have been yet another void of silence in the places where we live. We can make room for other life in our communities – for its own sake, not for our enjoyment or recreation. We can honor other life when we build. We can, like other cultures, live intimately with other life, open our souls to their special gifts and wisdom, and live intimately with those gifts through spirit totems, shrines, and other ways to manifest and connect with that energy.

Open corridors for wildlife migration. Create room for the song of birds and insects, and the beauty of moonlight and shadows. Make places where other life is held sacred and our presence proscribed. Ask into our lives the wisdom and gifts of other forms of life. Limit our numbers and appetites. Celebrate and honor other life in the making and use of our places.

MAKE SPACE FOR NEW CREATION

These silences in our community energy are silences of purposeful omission. They are the silences of *shunning* and intentional ignoring of fundamental elements of a society which nurtures life and shares in the evolution and creation of an ever more wonderful community of life.

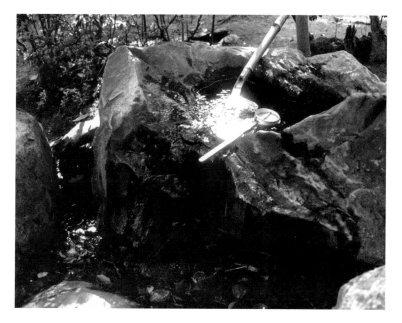

A place made for us to open our hearts and allow ourselves to be filled with the energy of life and creation.

There is also a silence – that silence from which new creation emerges – awaiting behind the desperate staccato of our media-filled lives. Allow that silence. Breathe! Create stillness, emptiness, and openness. Make room out of which new creation can arise in our lives. Generate a soul in our places and our communities which provides the energy to feed new creation. There is a music to silence and a dance within stillness which is lacking in our lives and communities. And there is a depth and wonder in the act of true creation that it allows, which brings incredible joy and meaning to our lives.

Community is born and its energy nurtured through many, often subtle, things. A coffee shop next to the post office where news passes, friendships are nurtured, and new things spark into being; the percentage of people on the street whom we know and care about; song; hardship and joy shared; passage of life together.

The examples above help us see the role which the community chi we generate plays in our lives, as well as some of the voids and gaps in the energetics of our communities. Our actions, no matter how small, can have a transformative impact on restoring wholeness and resonance to our communities.

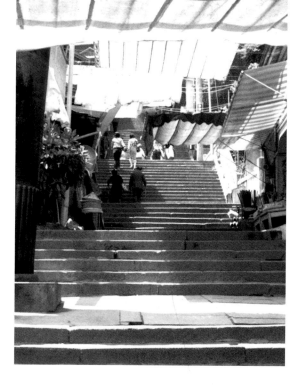

A gift of shade from neighboring shopkeepers to pilgrims climbing the eight hundred steps to the Konpira Shrine.

12 *SACRED PLACES*

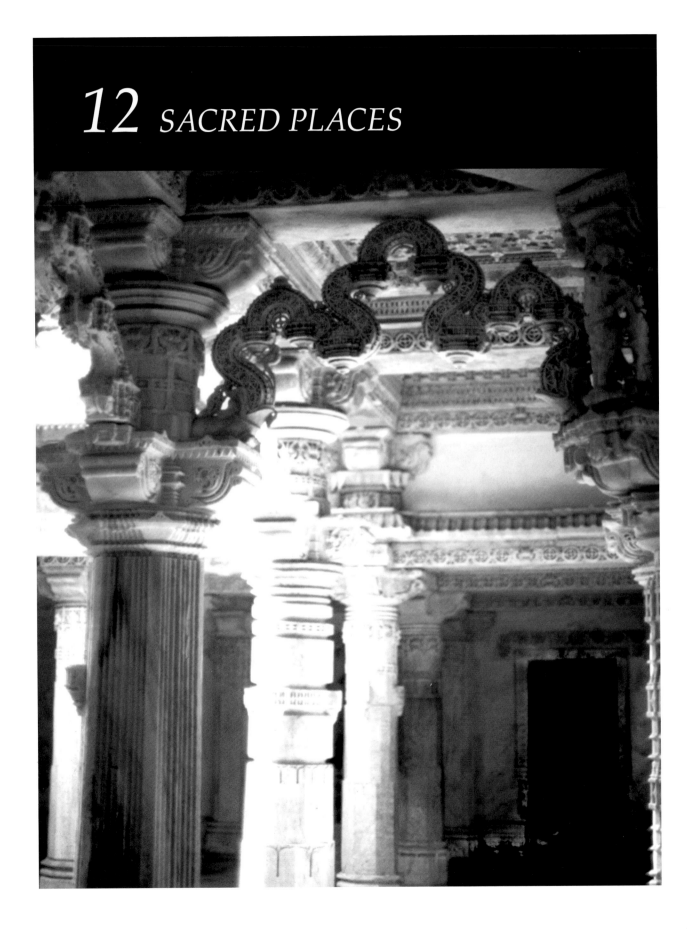

HOLDING PLACES SACRED

Sacred places are vital to our lives. While the idea of sacred places may seem alien to our culture, now more than ever we need to hold *all* our places sacred. Places draw sustenance from how they are held in our hearts. How we feel toward them nurtures them, and they in turn nurture us.

We need to hold places sacred, because we need to hold ourselves and all else sacred in order to be whole. Holding places sacred opens our hearts to hear and to speak what is "whole-ly." We need *special* sacred places because we need to be able to touch the immensity of power in nature, and the energetic roots of events and beliefs which we value.

Opposite: The Dilwarra Temples at Mt. Abu transform stone into magical traceries, held deep in the hearts of visitors and pilgrims.

A friend once commented that tourism was destroying the cathedrals of Europe. "Each person comes," he said, "and takes away a little of the cathedral – in their camera, in their mind, or in their conversation – and now nothing remains."

All places live through the reverence with which we hold them. Without that reverence, they crumble apart unloved, unmaintained, abandoned and destroyed. That reverence is the glue that binds the stones, the blood that sustains the life of a place, and the power that raises the funds for its upkeep. And it is that reverence first which is taken away, piece by piece, flashbulb by flashbulb, tour bus by tour bus. Without it, a place has nothing to give to those whose lives it must sustain, and they in turn fall into the same dereliction.

Some spiritual traditions have devices to enchance connection with sacred places from a distance and through time.

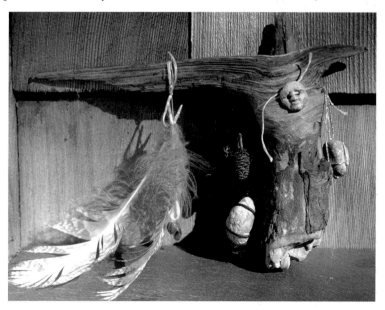

Far different is the visit of a pilgrim. Pilgrims bring love and respect, and their visits leave behind a gift of their reverence for others to share.

We lessen the soul of all places, and ourselves as well, when we take without giving. We all lose when we come to a place without reverence for life and land, for people and place, for ourselves and the Creation of which we are part. This is the destructiveness of tourism, but by the same token it is the arena where we can find a healing power for our land and our lives.

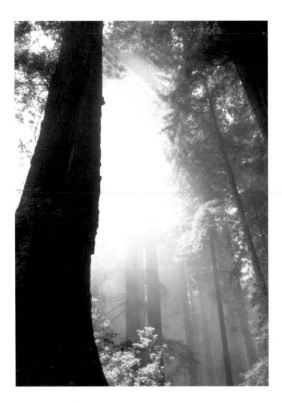

There is a wisdom in trees that have stood in one place for a thousand years, that is important for us to hear.

The power of intention alone, in the Pyramids of Giza, is enough to create a powerful sacred place.

VARIETIES OF SACRED PLACES

There are many kinds of sacred places, and many reasons for holding places sacred:

Some are physically special places, with unusually powerful patterns of nature, which draw us apart from our everyday lives and into awareness of primal forces. Mountains, rivers, oceans and lakes rarely fail to make a powerful impact on us. Many are "edges" – places of meeting and joining of water and earth, earth and sky.

Some places are sacred purely because our actions don't dominate them, such as the Redwoods, Glacier, or Yosemite National Parks, or wilderness areas. These places allow us to shed the self-centeredness and self-importance of our actions and dreams and become aware of the greater context within which we are embedded.

Special places enhanced by enlightened building can embody particularly powerful visions of our universe and our place in it. The Chess Pavilion perched among the clouds on the granite shoulder of Hua Shan in China conveys an unsurpassed sense of "life among the Gods." Zen gardens in Japan convey a depth of action and knowing. The Itsukushima Shrine in Japan, built on posts out into a bay on its island, or the Pyramids of Giza reflecting the pattern of the stars in Orion's Belt alongside the Milky Way River-in-the-Sky, generate wonderful senses of connectedness.

The feng-shui of Chinese pagodas or Alpine village churches communicates balance and peace with nature. The Kailasa Temple at Ellura, carved out of living rock, conveys an unmatched intimacy with our planet, an economy of means, and the confident power of sacred imagery. Together, these suggest the special power which can, on occasion, be evoked through our buildings, gardens, and shaping of the landscape.

Other places, by merely placing a limit on our actions, remind us in unequivocal terms of the necessity to limit our dreams and use of power. The sacred cows of India and the Ise Shrine in Japan both represent this powerful kind of statement. By saying "no" to actions or by denying access, they convey by very different means the significance of limits – of not letting us or anything else become all-powerful.

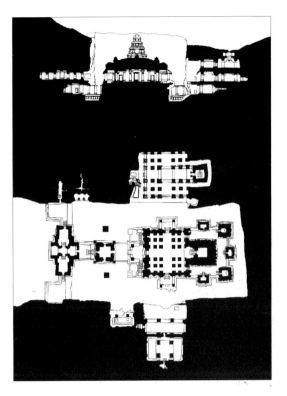

Quite differently, *places of important history or context hold before us events, actions, lives, and places that have stood witness to values we hold high.* Think of the Dome of the Rock, the Lincoln Memorial, the Agora in Athens, or the birth or death places of saints. Oracular sites, such as Delphi, and any places long held sacred are particular examples of how our act of holding sacred creates sacredness itself.

Places with special electromagnetic or chi energy have also long been held sacred. Hawaiian birth centers, favorable Chinese feng-shui locations, English cathedrals, "vision-quest" sites, and Ohio's famous Serpent Mound all give documentary evidence of the proven ability of places with unusual energetic conditions to favorably influence human activities materially and through our belief systems.[1]

❖

The Kailasa Temple at Ellura, carved out of native rock, maintains a powerful unity with the energy of the site.

This variedness of sacred places suggest how powerful sacred places can be, but also that their real significance may not lie in the places themselves. *Our act of "holding sacred" has the most enduring impact on a place's energy, not what caused us to choose that particular place.*

The true power of sacred places lies in their role of marshaling our inner resources and binding us to our beliefs. In holding a place sacred, we grant power *to* that place and acknowledge the power *of* the place. As an icon, or through its own inherent patterns, we acknowledge its ability to impact our awareness of certain relationships and their value to us.

The act of excluding people from the inner precincts of the Ise Shrine in Japan is a potent reminder of the importance of saying "No" to our limitless desires, and of reserving a place for the spirits alone.

The human uses to which sacred places are put are many. Jim Swan lists traditional cultural uses of sacred places as including graves, cemeteries and burial grounds, purification places, healing sites, sacred plant and animal sites, quarries for ritual objects, astronomical observatories, shrines, temples and effigies, oracular sites, historical sites, places of spiritual renewal, mythic and legendary sites, vision questing and dream places, rock art

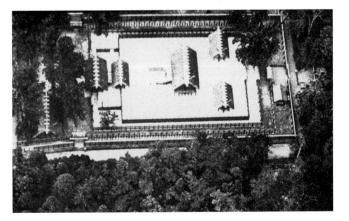

---
[1] Martin Gray's PLACES OF PEACE AND POWER, 1997, provides a related categorization, as does Swan, below.

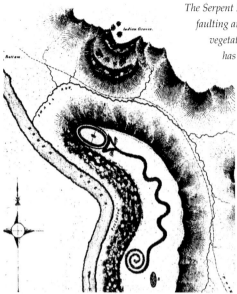

The Serpent Mound, in Ohio, is located on a site of massive geological faulting and vertical shifting. Exposed rocks, resultant soil chemistry, vegetation, and energy differ radically from surrounding terrain. It has been held as a sacred place for millennia.

places, fertility sites, and sunrise ceremonial sites.[2] Our interaction with such places and events augments both our own energies and those of the place.

Sacred places thus forge and strengthen bonds between us and the universe. They empower us by affirming the wholeness of the universe we see revealed about us, and by reflecting our chosen place and role in that universe. The inviolability of sacred places is essential. Through the act of holding things sacred, we affirm the primacy in our beliefs of the values they embody.

Great achievements in creating sacred places, such as Borabudur in Java or Chartres Cathedral in France, give us a sense of the possible. Equally important, however, is to know that the same basic possibilities lie within the scope of our own actions. Few of us have the power of an absolute monarch, the real estate of Yosemite, or the honed skills of a Zen master. Yet what each of us has is more than enough. There is opportunity in every action to show what we love and hold sacred.

Making sacred places requires only that we look for ways to make our surroundings connect us more powerfully to each other and to the life that surrounds us. That first step unfolds the next, and that, in turn, what follows.

We can make our places sacred by making them at home in the universe. As we perceive a certain harmony in the world, we can reinforce that harmony in our building. We thereby strengthen our confidence in an overarching harmony and rightness in the universe – and in our ability to positively influence the mysterious forces affecting our lives and marshal them to our needs. The way we organize our places expresses our own sense of order and creation in the universe. Immutable Euclidean geometry, topological organization, or fractal growth rhythms speak of different awareness of growth and relationships.

In learning to honor others as we make our surroundings, we touch the sacredness of both people and place. The English build a parlor to honor guests. The Japanese place an honored guest in front of their tokonoma so that others will associate the

The Royal Mosque in Isfahan is largely an empty outdoor space. But the power of intention, geometry, and ornament in the surrounding enclosure give it powerful impact on our souls.

2   James Swan, SACRED PLACES, Bear & Co., 1990.

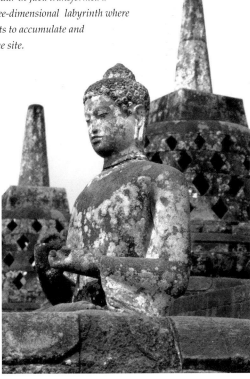

The Stupa of Borobudur in Java transformed a mountain into a three-dimensional labyrinth where pilgrims' passage acts to accumulate and enhance energy of the site.

guest with the specialness of the flowers and art. By using the traditional design wisdom of a region, we honor the work, insights, and hard lessons of the past. By planting trees, we honor a will to have a future. Providing opportunity for birds to nest, wildflowers to grow, and squirrels to play, we honor the other lives with which we share our world. Whatever we honor – a TV, children, or a good cook – is made manifest in the way we design and use our buildings and their surroundings. It speaks forth clearly of where we place our values.

By putting sacredness into all of our relationships, and making all places sacred, we align ourselves with the incredible power that generates the wonder we see revealed around us.

EXPRESSING SACREDNESS

The luminosity of the stained glass at S. Chapelle in Paris transforms a stone structure into an expression of the sacred light experienced in ecstacy.

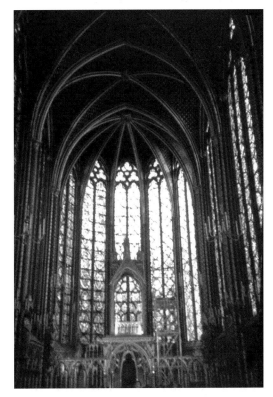

In the Middle Ages in Europe, the church spire towering over a community was a measure of the role of the sacred in that society. Today, the economic world of greed competing for dominance of the sky cannot be matched by any sacred place. Each age has to find appropriate vehicles for demonstrating the sacred in our lives in ways which cannot be matched by other beliefs.

Today, that expression must come out of dimensions of design that are able to move our hearts with little cost in resources or dollars; ones that are able to connect us to sources of energy unavailable from other beliefs; and ones that can bring us back into connection with the rest of Creation. Is that a garden rather than a cathedral? Is it a hidden place of prayer opening between the worlds, rather than a large church sanctuary? Is it the song of love and happiness in a community, or the glimmer of spider webs sharing space with our lives? Finding those answers is part of finding true expression of our time, our place, and ourselves.

THE SHRINE OF THE MOUNTAIN
AND THE WATERS

It might be useful here to shift gears a bit and try to give a sense of what it is like to *do something* outrageous, unprecedented, and totally outside of anything we've ever been taught to do . . . like create sacred space for our community.

Words and theories help little when we are faced with marshaling our own courage, coming up with a *real* idea of what to do in *our own* very real community, getting a group of people committed to an idea, and actually showing up and *doing* it. So here's a story of what happened a few years ago when we made the Shrine of the Mountain and the Waters:

✧

It's a long way from the beach to the top of the mountain with a rounded two-hundred-pound boulder continually slipping out of your hands. I asked myself again and again why on earth we would be doing such a crazy thing. But inside, I knew; we all knew: we were making a shrine.

A shrine-maker? I certainly never saw that before in my career plan. So it surprised me as much as everyone else when suddenly the urge overcame me and my family.

I couldn't even have told you very clearly what a shrine was. I had no idea how one makes a shrine, or what it should look like. I have always flinched a bit inside every time I heard the term *"shrine"*; it somehow seemed to carry with it a connotation of some primitive religious thing with "the meager offerings of the natives to their gods," of spaced-out hippie rituals, or of people pretending something. This feeling didn't totally leave me until we had actually founded shrines and experienced what the act of doing so with a pure heart could do.

✧

To me, like most people in our culture, shrines seemed to be an anachronism from an age of superstition. Yet here I was, preparing to make shrines. Where did such a curious urge begin? And *is* it so curious once we have learned the power that lies within such an act?

Most deeply, for me, the shrines grew out of a realization that to help cure the diseases of the spirit of our society, it was necessary to affirm a *giving* and healing presence in our own surroundings. To have that presence, our surroundings must reflect and be shaped out of the creative force in our lives that gives them meaning and power.

Another root of our shrine-making was the physical impacts of greed and growth encroaching on our mountain. Until recently, our community was a back-

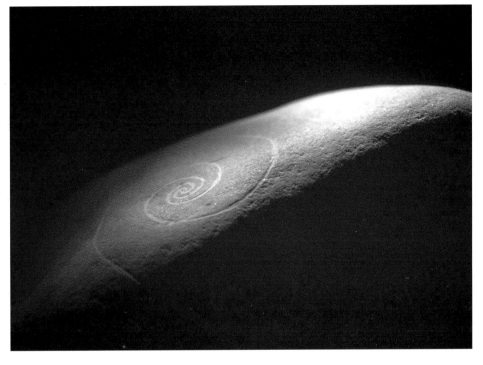

water unreached by the excesses of modern culture. It survived on care for each other and love of place. A few years ago that changed, as development pressures bent on the exploitation of people and place impinged on our community. The cutting of forests, blasting of roads, development of subdivisions, and franchising of consumerism brought with it the twisted anger, greed, and selfishness of modern civilization.

Seed rock of the Shrine of the Mountain – a two hundred pound basalt beach boulder carved with a double spiral and hand-carried to the top of the mountain.

I realized that if our surroundings showed only the scars and ravages of greed, then greed would unquestionably become the heart value of our community. But if we ensured that, in some way, our surroundings showed and kept alive the reverence for all Creation in the midst of the onslaught of greed, our community would at least have an alternative basis on which to chart its future.

A final root was my growing knowledge of the role that chi plays in generating and sustaining the power of people and places. Important to that power of chi is the role of focal places, such as shrines, to concentrate that energy and increase our ability to connect with it.

✦

In beginning to imagine the shrine, the past seemed to have little to offer us. We can't wear the clothes of another era; they don't fit our changed bodies and souls. Making a Gothic shrine or a Buddhist temple felt about as apt as wearing a suit of armor or a monk's robes to the office. To fit, and to have power, a shrine must come out of what *we* are and the changes we are making in ourselves – today. But how were we to find that?

Shrines have existed in every culture, in every possible configuration, in every age. We can find them anywhere, once we start to look: atop mountain passes, in the forest, on a city street, tucked between the piers of a church; over a doorway, within a home, in small and great buildings of their own.

In a stone village in the Spanish Pyrenees, the Christian Virgin appears everywhere – a reflection of the people's prayers, hopes, beliefs, and values. In a town in the Austrian Alps, a statue of the Black Madonna stands in the town center, and small wooden shrines dot the surrounding mountain forests. On an island in Japan, straw ropes with shide paper prayers distinguish a particular rock, tree, or pool in the forest; they bind together huge rocks at the ocean's edge, and adorn a black boulder at the curb of a busy urban intersection.

In India, in Mexico, in Africa, simple yet honored shrines line the sides of roads and paths. In traditional cultures the world around, shrines have festooned busses, trucks, and cars, homes and public places. In Cambodia and Indonesia, the sluice-gates of the Khmer irrigation canals became shrines because of the role of the sacred in regulating the flow of the chi-filled water throughout the kingdom. In Washington, D.C., the Vietnam Memorial is a place of poignant emotion for visitors to the capital, serving an important need; other memorials stand forgotten.

What shrines show us is what we hold sacred, what we value so greatly as to hold inviolate. They have made visible the depth of feeling and meaning that a place or person has. They show us the empowerment of our connection with the rest of nature and the breath of life that infuses it.

✧

Expressions of the sacred in other cultures may be magnificent and very moving, yet they will not fit our space and time wholesale. Ours is a time of gathering in, testing, and using what fits together well to express our time and world.

When the spiritual core of a culture is clear and strong, conventions exist for the making of a shrine. At times when we are reforging the spiritual dimensions of our lives, we have to fashion anew the expression of that spiritual nature. This is particularly true when we want a place to be accessible to all people, without blockage by religious symbolism which is uncomfortable for them.

Where does one begin to do something like this, which has no precedent? In our case, we began by talking with our friends about what in our community could become an affirmation of sacredness. What could express our holding inviolate the health and well-being of people, place, and things? Two things came repeatedly to our minds: the mountain and the waters by which we live.

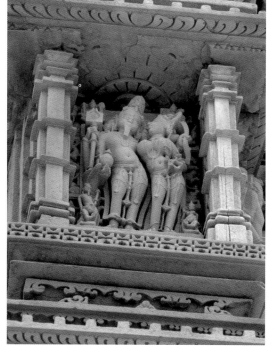

Neahkahnie Mountain, upon which we live, has been sacred from time immemorial. Its name means "'place of the gods." It has been honored and held sacred by hundreds of generations who have lived within its compass. It rises directly from the Pacific Ocean, and at its foot lies the bay of the Nehalem River, channeling back to the ocean the hundred-plus inches of rain we receive every year. The Mountain and the Waters. The relationship we have lived with them led eventually to a plan for a double shrine, to honor both the mountain and the waters and the complementary forces of nature which they represent.

What we decided to do was to take a rock from the beach, worn and rounded by the waves, and place it on top of the mountain. We then would take a rock from the mountain and place it by the waters of the bay. Like the yin/yang symbol, each rock connected to and was a seed of its opposite. These rocks would form the nucleus of the shrines, and link them together.

Why a rock? We wanted something lasting, something without monetary cost, and something natural. But more than that, rocks had come to have special meaning. Our bodies are made of rock – fragmented into soil, organized into plants, and become mobile as animals. The rock that is our planet is made of the ashes of long-dead stars. The stars of today are in fact our cousins, and rocks under our feet are our geological grandparents. They are our genealogical link with the canopy of stars overhead. What better could we use in making a shrine than the rocks that stand as our historical connection with the rest of life?

The form a shrine takes comes in part from its chosen location. In this case, the knife-edge summit of the mountain was out as a location; it was intensively used by hikers, and recently desecrated by the state park's installation of commercial, for-profit cellular phone apparatus. There was a grove of trees, though, on the saddle of the mountain, which did have a special feel and power to it – on top, yet closed in by ancient sitka spruce, survivors of winds sometimes reaching 120 mph. The grove focused inward on the mountain, not out at the view.

The site for the shrine of the waters came more slowly, out of more options. We finally found a place on the bay side of the sand spit between the river and the ocean that was accessible, yet rarely visited, and which held a special beauty and peacefulness. Between the high, tree-covered dune and the bay itself was a wonderful area of giant driftwood logs, sculpted tree roots, birds, elk, water and sky. Nearby were the almost-vanished remains of an old Indian village, whose spirit seemed to still protect the area. At the edge where the dune met the beach and the marsh grasses, there it was: a remarkable enclosure of driftwood, living branches, and wild roses. They said, "Here is the place!"

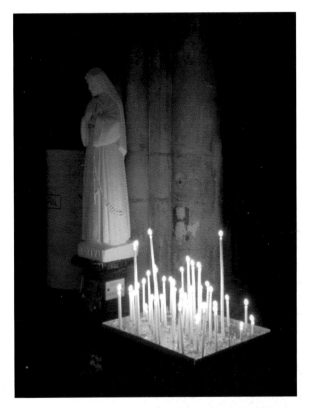

Both the grove of trees on the mountain and the enclosure by the bay had power and beauty of their own. Both could accommodate individuals or small groups. Neither needed to be "gussied up." The shrine-making required only the seed rocks and some fine-tuning to create memorable and potent places.

We found the rocks: a boulder from the beach and a rock from a rockfall high on the mountain. And now we had homes for them. I felt the need to mark the rocks in some way – to have them clearly express our intention. It seemed they needed to be the product of human as well as other natural process, and to convey a measure of the meaning we felt and acknowledged in our world. What we decided to carve in the rocks was a spiral. Not just any spiral, but the specific *fibonacci* spiral of growth found in the development patterns of pine cones, cabbage, sunflowers, and tree branches. It is a geometry of the linkage through which life ties into and uses the energy fields in our surroundings.

But a spiral alone wasn't right; it didn't have the right balance. Suddenly a pair of spirals leapt to mind, coiling or uncoiling around each other in balance. Here again the dual nature of the shrine manifested itself: double spirals uncoiling to the left on one rock and, mirrored, uncoiling to the right on the other one. Here

What we take home from other places may be as little or as great as learning that some legacy we leave behind us – be it candles, paper prayers, piled rocks, or steps worn and polished by thousands of feet – tells the next visitor that others have come and found wonder in the place.

was duality again, the spirals sometimes appearing to coil inward – in the inner-focusing of meditation and centering – and sometimes to uncoil outward – in the ancient pattern of growth and becoming. Breathe in, breathe out. Duality and balance. It felt right in the head, in the heart, and in the stone.

And so they were carved.

Then another question arose. The carved rock felt somehow too intrusive, too visible, on the mountain. So I said, half joking, "Well, let's bury it!" And suddenly that felt terribly right. It dealt well with the issue of intrusiveness. But it felt even more right for a totally different reason: visualizing the rock with its spiral in contact with the chi of the earth had much more rightness and power than as just a visible "sculpture" to be looked at. Knowing of its unseen presence rather than seeing its face, we could feel the difference between inner and outer qualities and the importance of those often hidden inner ones.

We decided that we would open the rock to the air every year in a ceremony of renewal. Thus we could acknowledge its presence, honor it, bring it into touch with the world above the ground, and then return it to its placement connected inward to the earth for another year. At the same time, we could renew our connection with it and the meaning it held in our hearts. It is amazing the tortuous paths by which right-feeling decisions wend their way into existence!

The rightness of this revealed itself in the reaction of people who saw the rock before we placed it, or who were at the placing ceremony and didn't know our plans to face it into the earth. Everyone seemed to agree that the rock was beautiful and powerful. But their faces transformed as they learned that we were placing it *into* the ground. Somehow it stopped being a crazy prank, and became something which was true, right, and powerful. It truly affirmed our belief in chi, our belief that this shrine was important enough to put a lot of effort into making, and that it would influence our lives.

✦

Would anyone help? You could see it on some faces: "It's a wonderful idea, but I don't think I could get *myself* to the top of the mountain, to say nothing of dragging a two-hundred-pound rock with me." Or, "Yeah, it would be fun to get together and do something, but no way am I going to do such a crazy thing in public."

Yes, that is what it was about: going public about loving and holding sacred our selves, our neighbors, our world. About doing, not talking about. About making it okay for others to do both. About making visible an alternative to letting fear and deceit rule our entire lives.

Even though an access road up the mountain was temporarily open, we had decided to carry the rock to the top of the mountain. This project wasn't about the world of machines. It was about the changes in us and in our surroundings that come about through the process of doing it with our bodies. It wasn't a question of macho, it was a question of community, of accomplishing something together that we were unable to do alone. So we improvised a sling to carry the rock, and invited our friends to join us. On the evenings of the full moon and the new moon, we planned to move the rocks into place.

A few did come – enough to get the rock two-thirds of the way to the top of the mountain the first evening. (Even with four people carrying at a time, it *was* heavy.) We got to the top the next weekend, and carried the second rock to the water shrine on the third. So it did happen, with drums and Oreos and kids and barking dogs, with the sacred and the mundane tripping over each other's feet as they always do. And our individual doubts as to our ability to accomplish the job were replaced by a real *knowing* in every sinew of our bodies that together we could accomplish handily and with joy what we hardly dared dream of alone.

Once at the sites, there was a final step to the process of founding the shrines. That was installing the rocks in their new homes, and with that the installation in our hearts of new meaning. This ritual was something we both looked forward to and dreaded. Was it going to work, physically and ritually? How do you do it? The library, strangely, didn't have any books on founding shrines to mountains and rivers.

Was it going to feel like playing at something, or would it have the depth and power of meaning we sensed lay in wait? Founding something new is always awkward, like a new colt struggling to its feet for the first time. Later, in our memories, it may become smooth and powerful. The things that didn't quite work are easily forgotten in the potency of the memories of those that did. But it's rarely that way at the time.

Morning sunlight filters through the fog at the Shrine of the Mountain.

The dogs underfoot made sure we kept a balance of humor and seriousness, of laughing at ourselves at the same time we were doing something profound. One tiny dog not only made it to the top of the mountain, but appointed herself to dig the hole for us to set the rock in! If we thought we were running the show, she straightened us out right away.

I started the ceremony by explaining why we had wanted to make the shrines. I said we had no idea of the right way to do it. "Lacking experience," I said, "we are doing the only thing we can do: following our hearts." We welcomed anyone to contribute, and to participate as they wished. If they felt uncomfortable actively taking part, we were thankful for their presence and witnessing. That seemed to make us all feel more at ease.

Then we spread out in a circle around the shrine, and stood gently absorbing the silence, aligning our own energy with its abundance. We smudged ourselves and the site with sage, and placed Japanese folded paper prayers (*shide*) around the perimeter, creating a circle of small temporary markers.

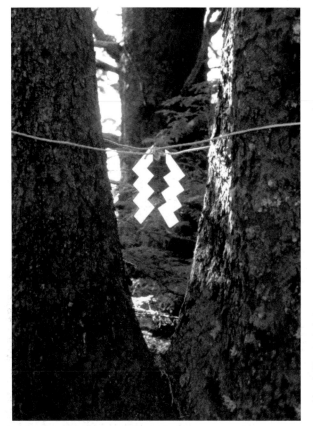

We were surprised and pleased that many people had brought something personal to leave as part of the shrine. That let us know that the idea of the shrine had already found deep-rooted meaning and value – enough that other people wanted to put a piece of their heart into it. They were there in the same spirit as we were, which brought a new level of power to the ceremony. Somehow, we had created a safe and sacred space where unprecedented intimacy could happen with a group of people. We shared – sometimes with tears all around – the meaning of our gifts. As we did so, the significance of the shrine to all of us expanded and deepened.

We each talked about our dreams, our fears, our love, our thankfulness for what each had been given by the others. In silence we meditated on the trees, the water, the power of the places. We sang. Individually and together, we blessed the place and the rocks. We avowed our intention to have a place which showed the love we held for our community and our surroundings. We cleansed our minds and the energy of the rocks with fresh spring water from the mountain. Again the duality came together: the rock and the water, the resistant and the yielding.

Paper prayers hung at the Mountain Shrine for its annual celebration.

We focused and connected our personal chi together, and to the rock, and the place, and through it to the other shrine. At the end, I passed out small carved rocks and prayers, as a memento of the occasion. As we walked away, we looked back and saw something that had never existed before, something we had created. We carried it with us in our memory.

✦

It was done: two shrines. One in a vigorous mountain top grove of towering trees, the other in a serene enclosure nested in the wetlands at the edge of the bay. Both with their seed rocks establishing, affirming, and linking their purposes. We stood in the silence, awestruck at the power of the places and the changes we had created within us.

It did work. It worked because we knew in our hearts that it was right and that it would succeed. It worked because our spirits were clear and focused on creating something that was true, not on our own aggrandizement. It worked because we spoke from our deepest feelings, and felt our way humbly toward what would work. It worked because we were there, open and vulnerable in our desire to take a vital step to heal the wrongness that was destroying the world on both sides of our skin.

Looking back at the sources of the shrines and their ceremonies, *everything* was borrowed: Native American customs, Shinto prayers, Chinese feng-shui, Christian song, Earth Goddesses, Buddhist meditation, "fake petroglyphs," Hindu kundalini, and a friend's dog; there was a little of everything. Yet, together, those pieces had come together into two shrines, unprecedented and potent.

The only thing that really mattered in all that hodge-podge was, "Is it whole, does it fit, is what it creates *right*?" If it fit, we used it. If something else worked better, we used that. This *is* a time of cross-fertilization, of growing, borrowing, adapting, and intuiting powerful new things that fit specific and unprecedented contexts. It is the final rightness that matters, not the source of the pieces.

✧

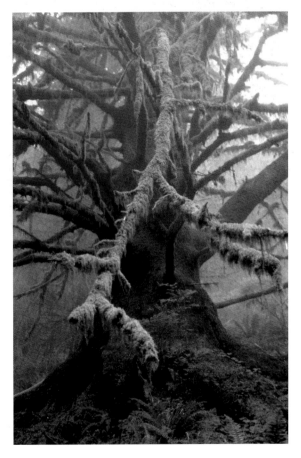

The Mothertree, now surrounded by the mature forest which it seeded.

The shrines were made, but had yet to unfold and reveal themselves in their fullness. That has happened and continues, as always, in unexpected and wonderful ways. The Shrine of the Mountain immediately expanded in our minds from the rock itself to the tree, to the whole grove which surrounded it. A double "guardian" tree to the north became a part. Other trees ringing the rock's tree offered sitting places among their roots which people have begun to use. The wildflower understory within this ring became a part of the setting, as well as the wonderful silence of the place. It has become a place for people to scatter the ashes of their loved ones. The wind and fog streaming through seem to carry the energy of the place outward to the other shrine and to our community below.

Attuned to the sacredness of place, our eyes began to see the entire mountain differently. We rediscovered a tree we had found on the mountain long ago, part way up the trail to the top. Ancient and massive, this tree stood with limbs spread wide and covered with moss, within a forest of lesser trees standing shoulder-to-shoulder straining skyward in competition for the sun. It was a survivor from the past, from days when the first local tribes burned the south face of the mountain to provide pasturage for the elk. It must have stood solitary then in a great and wind-blown mountain meadow, with limbs spread unencumbered reaching for sunlight. Now it was the mother tree; having spawned the entire surrounding forest, it deserved to be honored in its own right.

At the Shrine of the Waters, it took several adjustments of the rock before things felt right – we ended up finally totally burying the seed-rock. There, the entire shrine site is itself constantly changing. The waters in the bay and marsh rise and fall silently twice each day, tied to the rhythm of the sun and the moon, covering even the rock itself at high flood stage. Then they recede again, allowing us, for short periods, to be present in this special place. Sometimes, going to the shrine, we find that the giant driftwood logs surrounding it on the water side have been silently raised by the tides and rearranged in our absence.

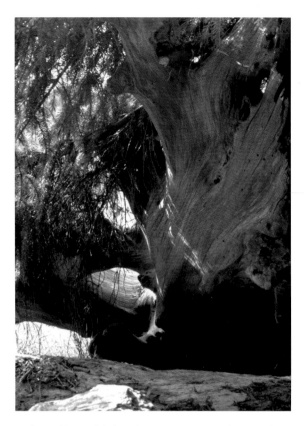

Sculptured forms of driftwood spruce roots give enclosure to the Shrine of the Waters, and place for birds to nest and new plants to grow.

Seed rock for the Shrine of the Waters – a mountain rock carried down to the Bay, carved with the double spiral of growth.

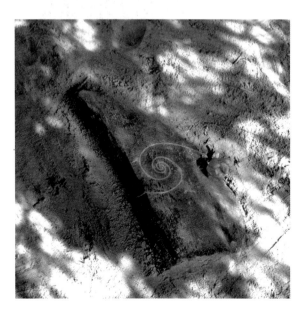

The chi of the mountain shrine seems to be a vertical chi – a power plunging down through the heart of the mountain to the center of the earth, and up the trees to the stars above. It is the energy of becoming, of creating new material manifestations of the energy of life. The Shrine of the Mountain feels connected with the emergence of the unforeseen and totally new. It seems to bond us again with the dynamism of the primal energy of life.

The *chi* of the water shrine feels, in appropriate contrast, to be a horizontal one. It spreads outward on the waters, encompassing and embracing all things on the interface between the earth, the waters, and the air. The mountain rock invites our touch and direct connection to its chi. The water rock draws us to the bay and the water-filled sand upon which the rock rests, rather than to itself.

The Shrine of the Waters feels connected with life, fecundity, death, and rebirth. The dead trees hold nests, new tree sprouts, shelter for the birds and animals. Deer sleep in the shrine. Grouse – the birds of the spiral dance of rebirth, according to local Indian legends – send their haunting, thrumming hoot from the woods around. The mud flats teem with growth and dying; and out of that death, a richer life emerging.

People in our community have gone to the shrines at sunrise, during the full moon, in fog, rain and snow. From them, we've watched the moon rise over the bay in full eclipse, and seen a comet in the night sky. We've gone there alone and together; for comfort and inspiration and thanksgiving; in grief and joy. With each visit, the gift the shrines have given us increases and deepens, and what they represent to us becomes more encompassing.

One day, almost a year after creating the shrines, I was channeling chi through the rock on the mountain. With a jolt, I suddenly felt a laser-like beam of golden energy shooting out from the rock directly to the rock at the other shrine on the bay below. They had broken through an area of bad chi that had existed for years in between, and were linked!

The shrines have become more than physical places. People go to them for silence, to rest, to meditate or pray, or to be in the presence of an affirmation of the sacred. People say that images of the shrine's, and the knowledge of their existence, surface in their minds with a deep and warm feeling even when they are far away. New people keep discovering the shrines. We're stopped on the street with tears and thanks by strangers who have been deeply touched by the shrines' existence. The shrines are becoming touchstones – in our hearts and our community – of the sacred and of the power of the breath of life.

What does the future hold for these shrines? I don't know. They may be forgotten, they may be seeds for all sorts of change. It really doesn't matter; they have changed us. Anything more is a bonus.

The shrines have let us become conscious of ourselves as part of a wonderful process of creation. They have confirmed to us that loving and holding inviolate all of Creation is essential for healing us and our world. They have shown us that the act of holding something sacred is a vehicle for restoring our connectedness with all of that Creation. We now carry this within us into the rest of our lives and our future.

If they were created again, or in a different place, the shrines would emerge in a different form. This was a small community in a rural area, with its own unique conditions. Yet in the most crowded urban area there are niches and places accessible to everyone that can become shrines with equal power. I saw one in Venice once – there wasn't room on the street, so the shrine had been built into the wall of a building, ten feet off the ground, visible only from a bridge that crossed the canal there.

The act of frankly affirming sacredness, and opening ourselves to the connectedness that sacredness engenders, is what becomes enshrined. It is that which empowers and transforms us and our communities.

The prayer said at the founding of the shrines said it another way:

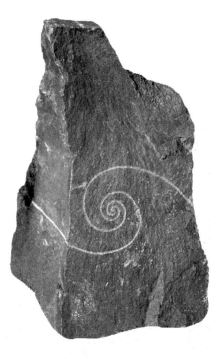

From stillness
comes intention
then manifestation.

Our stars, our sun,
our rocks, our dreams
are all stardust –
the ashes of stars before.

The chi of life permeates, joins,
and sustains all.

Open our hearts.
Purify us, heal us, sustain us.

Honor and celebrate all creation.
We are one.

We are One!

Some people have asked how to tell what places are sacred or which ones have strong energy. At this point I can only answer, "Trust your tummy." If a place feels good to you, it is good for you. If you don't feel anything at a place, it doesn't have anything for you right then. I used to ask myself the same thing in Japan, seeing a straw rope marking a totally unexceptional place in the forest. When asked, a local priest said it was the abode of an earth spirit. How can we tell if such a spirit is present? Someone once asked Denise Linn how she could tell if fairies or other spirits are present in the woods or a garden. "Well, I *see* them!" was her reply.[3] For those of us yet unblessed with such vision, we have to trust our tummies and deal with what we *can* feel.

So, where did the making of these shrines leave me, my community, and my friends? Looked at a few years later, interesting things have happened. Carving the rocks got me into carving other rocks. One of those inspired a potter friend to do a whole series of "egg" sculptures; and other friends were inspired to use rock carving to mark sacred places. I've learned a lot about ritual, celebration, and the energy flows that are created in making and using sacred space.

And the community? The stories of the shrines has wended its way through the local grapevine. One friend gave a talk about it at a local ecology workshop. The local historian put a story about it into a time capsule being buried on the

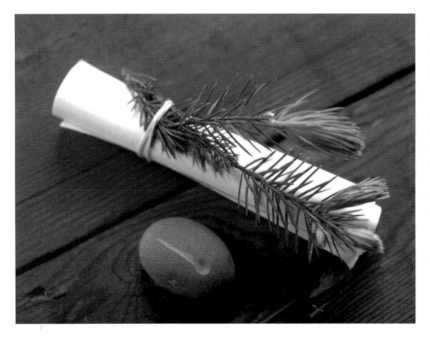

Mementos given each participant at the founding ceremonies for the Shrines of the Mountain and the Waters – a copy of the prayer, a hand-carved rock to maintain connection with the shrines, and a symbol of new growth.

town's 50th anniversary. The paths to the shrines have become more visible as more people find and use them. People have started asking for help in making shrines at their homes and businesses. A group wants to build a temple to the Earth Goddess. There's even some talk about other community celebrations.

Places like this within our communities act as touchstones to hold the patterns and relationships of our ecological communities in a clear and powerful way that helps us deepen our connection. In the rain country, a "Rain Garden" in the center of the city can honor and show water in its myriad powerful patterns – or there can be fountains and waterways throughout the community celebrating water. In the desert, a place of emptiness and silence can be created in the middle of community. In the forest lands, a place can allow us to commune with the Standing People.

3 Denise Linn, SACRED SPACE, Ballantine Books, 1995.

We can create places of incredible power honoring, celebrating, and bringing our hearts in touch with earth, rock, and the primal process of planetary tectonics – the life-dance of our Earth Mother. We can create a Shrine to the Waters of the World, to Fire, to Air, to Spirit. In touching our hearts and learning to love these things more deeply, we bring ourselves piece by piece back into oneness with all of Creation.

We need sacred places in our lives and communities. We need them in our homes, to honor our beliefs and give us places to trigger the grounding and nurturing of our own energy. We need them in our neighborhoods, or within walking distance, as places to meditate, or to find a moment of peace, or to restore our energy in deeper and more powerful ways than we can do in our homes. We need special sacred places available to our entire communities. And we need to make our communities into places that honor the sacredness of all Creation.

13 TAKING ACTION

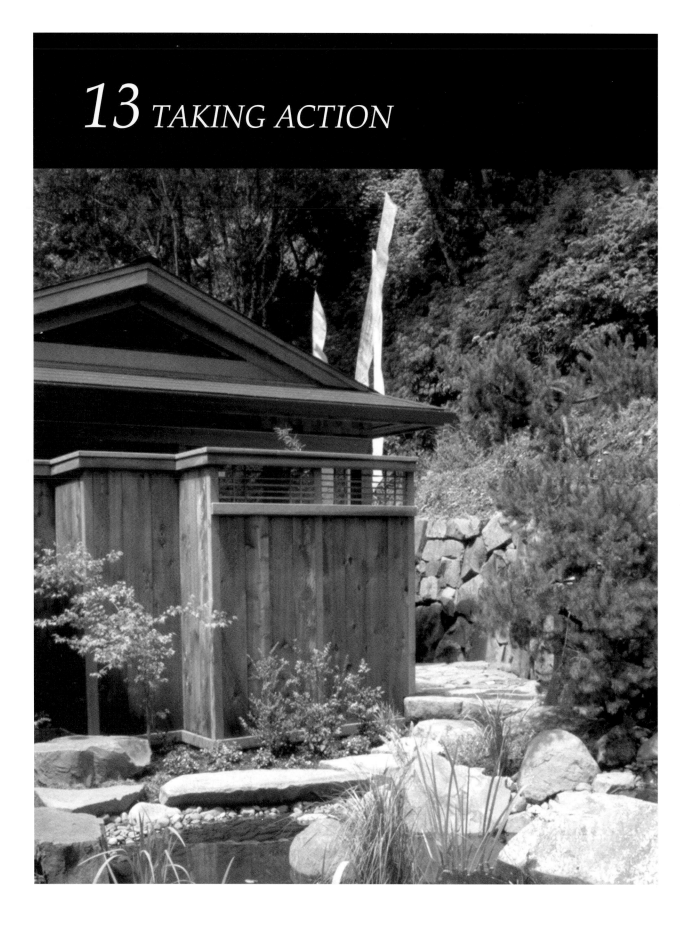

Some Personal Notes on Implementing Energetics of Place

Successful achievement of a new way of relating to and shaping our surroundings is, of course, where the proof of these concepts lie. In this culture, that accomplishment is yet in its infancy. Throughout this book, and in *Silence, Song & Shadows*, are examples that provide a tangible sense of the possibilities.

Taking action means changing what we do, as well as changing how we are. It involves chi, and intention. It involves how our feet touch the earth, and how we shape the earth to better touch our feet. In the real world there is no separation – only interweavings of chi, intention, love, honoring, respect, celebration, ancestors, the past and future, what we have been and what we are becoming.

SEWAGE IS ART!
Healing of Place with Chi and Li

This study was done as an entry in a design competition for a new Museum of Korean Art and Culture (KOMA) to be built in Los Angeles, California. In this case, site choice was not an option. The site was already determined: a commercial ghetto in a smog-ridden, automobile-dominated urban area of Los Angeles, filled with racial and class tensions and a history of rioting and arson. The site was rubble-strewn and barren, with virtually no trace of the natural ecological community remaining. The site starkly reflected the results of a society based on greed, on self-centeredness and materialism, on taking rather than giving. This provided an appropriate challenge to find what could be given to a place and its community to nurture and improve its life, and to tackle head-on the issue of healing the places most damaged by our actions.

Rather than the conventional owner's demands of "I want . . . , I want . . . ," this study really began with the question, "What is the *most* we can *give* to users of the place, to its surroundings and community, to the future, and to all of life?" It suggests that a *giving-centered* design process can generate the greatest power of a place to affect us, to heal and enhance our lives and community.

Some traditional practices of place energetics constituted a highly competitive search to obtain and flaunt the most geomantically favorable site or de-

Opposite: The quality of chi energy in our homes, gardens, and communities has little direct connection with the physical design, and cannot be enhanced by focus on that dimension. Our energetic intention is primary – out of that will flow both the energy of the place and the placement of elements that lead us to connect with that energy.

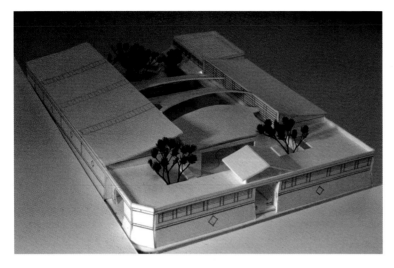

A model of the KOMA design, showing gardens, courtyards, daylighted galleries and meeting spaces.

sign, to give comparative advantage to one's life or success. Such sites had the most dominant views and positions, favorable breezes, exposures, terrain, and neighbors. In contrast, good energetics practice seeks improvement of the qualities of physical surroundings which can benefit an entire community.

Our energy connections with a place occur through our bodies, our minds, and our hearts. No matter how beautiful we make it, nobody will visit a museum if its neighborhood is too scary to enter. If our surroundings reflect only the values of greed, lack of caring, and failure, we are unlikely to become caring, giving, successful people. But if we initiate caring for a place and its people, honoring a belief in a good future, it will come to reflect those values, too, and become a support for the people who live within it.

✦

One basic strategy chosen was to take what we consider waste, honor it, and turn it into wealth which can enrich the community. This was probably the most unexpected action possible: taking the community sewer and rerouting it onto the site. The sewage of the neighborhood would be pumped onto the roof of the museum, and given advanced biological treatment. Its nutrients would then be used to support rooftop produce gardens to provide fresh produce to the neighborhood. The produce would be sold at a greengrocer incorporated in the public area of the site, which would provide incentive and opportunity for everyone in the neighborhood to drop in, linger, relax, and obtain fresh, healthy produce.

The wastewater from the produce gardens would then be used to irrigate street-tree plantings of native California live oaks. This would help restore greenery, shade, and some of the native ecology back to the area, while decreasing temperature swings. It would also provide groundwater aquifer recharge, demonstrating that a community can take action to improve itself.

This may at first seem to be far removed from the mission of an art museum and culture center. It is a potential gift, however, which is inherent in any facility in a neighborhood that has community consciousness and a large roof area. It also has a particular appropriateness in KOMA's case. KOMA does not have a traditional museum's goal of just storing old objects. Its goal is to honor its cultural heritage, transmit its skills and values, heal tensions in the community, and stimulate a positive new synthesis of culture.

In order to succeed in that primary role, however, the center has to show leadership, become a valued part of the community, and draw people into its activities. Vitality is a goal of art, and any tool which helps achieve that vitality is appropriate. The resultant roof gardens, street landscaping, and facility gardens are a true form of art as well as wealth. In this context, sewage truly is art, and the neighborhood an appropriate canvas!

A community that enriches and empowers itself by discovering its least likely source of wealth can be a leader in synthesizing a new and vibrant culture. It also provides several concrete benefits: recapture and savings of sewage treatment and disposal costs, avoiding use of chemical fertilizers, keeping nutrients and food production in the neighborhood, and providing an attraction to bring more than just Korean neighborhood residents into the project.

The proposal turns unused roof areas – that typically contribute only to climate extremes – into green, productive areas. It provides areas of economic value on the property beyond those limited by city zoning codes. Perhaps most importantly, it demonstrates a commitment to improving the quality of the community, and concern for the health and well-being of all members of the community – human and otherwise.

This first level of energetic design was to change the energy and intention of the neighborhood, replacing destructive values, then setting in motion ones that support and restore life, diversity, caring, and giving.

The KOMA forecourt – open to the community – was ringed by shops, meeting hall, studios, and the performance hall. That hall sloped up to the upper level traditional garden, surrounded by display galleries, library, and breakout space.

✦

A second level of energetic design for KOMA was to change the ecology of the site itself. In addition to the rooftop produce garden, four other garden or green elements were designed into the project: a traditional Korean garden in the heart of the site; a community-use "forecourt" garden area; an outside neighborhood "pocket garden" along the sidewalk adjacent to the west entrance to the project; and the native street tree plantings surrounding the site. These were planned to quiet the site, to freshen and improve the oxygen/carbon-dioxide balance in the air, to provide food and home for birds, butterflies, bats, and other forms of life.

Other water features were part of the design: a gurgling, splashing "moat" surrounding the building; a waterfall and pond in the traditional garden; fountains at the building corners and at the "spirit wall" at the south entrance; and fountains and water features at the entrances. They were used to cool and refresh the air, provide a counterpoint to street noise, and to increase the levels of negatively-charged ions in the air to counter the "Santa Ana" winds.

The forecourt area, while people-intensive and necessarily hard-

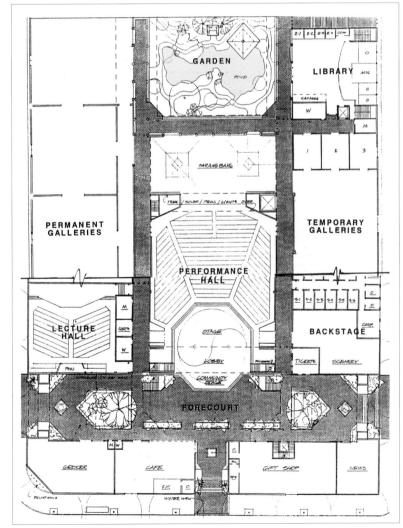

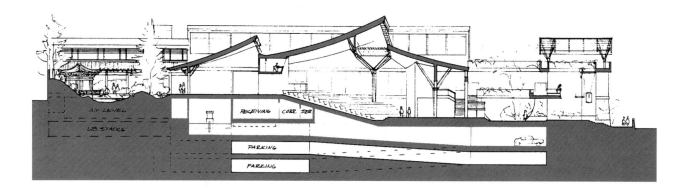

A section through the building shows the garden, performance stage opening to both the performance hall and the forecourt, natural lighting, and biological sewage treatment on the roof.

paved, was designed to be shaded by trees. Moss would cover the undersides of overhead structure, and ivy-covered walls and planters in guardrails and court areas would soften the impact of the buildings. These green areas were all designed to be watered and fed by the wastewater system.

The traditional Korean garden was located in the core of the building, which was devoted to understanding and conveying the roots, values, and achievements of traditional Korean culture. The garden was ringed by a research library, museum galleries devoted to the traditional arts of Korea, and a performance hall for traditional art forms. While providing a serene "breakout" space, the garden gave an intensive experience of traditional Korean garden and architectural arts. This garden also held a central role of symbolically affecting the chi of the place, partly by being nurtured by the community wastewater, and partly due to its special location in the arrangement of the facilities.

Together, these gardens would help visitors share the place with other life, delighting in the beauty, richness, and diversity of the natural community. Equally important, the gardens could help people rediscover a sense of fit and rightness of the natural community that evolved in that place over the ages.

✦

The third and perhaps most powerful level of energetic design involved the minds and hearts of the visitors. This level dealt with the internal arrangement, design, and symbolic meaning of elements of the facility. In traditional Korean city and home planning, the position of energetic power is the north end of the central north-south axis. Here, the ruler or owner faced and received power and warmth from the sun in the south, and became the local source of energy in the complex. In this project, that pattern of arrangement was honored; that prime location was given to tradition, to nature, and to ancestors, in the form of a traditional garden.

Within the garden, in the position of greatest importance directly on this axis, was placed a physically non-imposing, but symbolically vital element: a shrine to the ancestors. This was to contain earth and icons brought from sacred places in Korea. Its role was to honor the tradition, the land, and the ancestors who created the Korean culture and brought it to this place. It formed a touchstone for members of the community who had come from Korea or whose family still live there, and a place to scatter the ashes of those with deep ties to the "old country."

This is not of small importance. If a museum and cultural center can demonstrate, through its own design and function, the *continuing* validity of the principles underlying a culture, it becomes an order of magnitude more successful than one which can only preserve fragments of a tradition it is unwilling to embrace.

Around this shrine, representing the active and passive, yang and yin powers of nature, were a mountain, a waterfall, a central pool of water, and a traditionally-designed garden pavilion – representing the participation of people in the balance of life. From the roof, the sun-purified waters were conducted to the mountain and waterfall, to the still waters of the pond, and then flowed outward, carrying the energy to the rest of the project and out into the surrounding community. At the core of the facility, the garden provides a place of silence and emptiness and a reflection of the primal source out of which all Creation arises.

On the same north-south axis are the main activity spaces of the center: the performance hall; a breakout space for its audience, opening into the garden; a unique stage arrangement with operable walls allowing a variety of combinations of public and private use; and the community forecourt which permits a more public, community, people-oriented gathering space connected with the various parts of the facility.

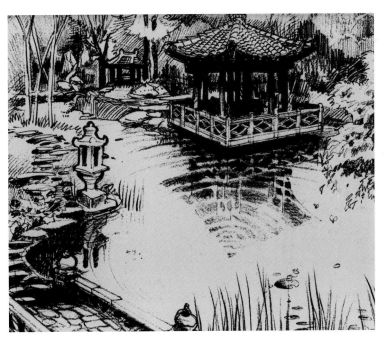

The arrangement of the stage area and the performance hall was planned to give opportunity for flexible and public community use. It restores events to the simple effectiveness of natural lighting, open air performance, and audience participation. The foyer walls slide aside, merging the performance hall thrust stage and the public performance area in the forecourt into a single circular stage for large community events, which can play to the hall, the forecourt, and the balconies around it.

✦

Sustainability requires that something be held close to our hearts so that we value it enough to devote the resources needed to its continuance. It also requires that such maintenance be affordable, and not press heavily on other life. Energetics recognizes the importance of wisely channeling the renewable energies of nature to heat, cool and light a building. All of the elements of this KOMA design were to be naturally lighted, heated, and cooled. Except for the permanent exhibit areas for fragile artifacts, they were designed for open-air use tied to the garden areas during the majority of the year. This reduces conventional energy needs by an order of magnitude. The buildings would also be constructed of natural and traditional building materials of the area.

The traditional garden, based on principles of feng shui, placed the Shrine to the Ancestors on the main axis, balanced by a pavilion and a hill, and with quiet water to the south.

The design for the facility was also based on the energetic principle of *durability*. The savings from durability permit a generosity of design that gives comfort, repose, and fullness to its elements and its users. The expression of that goal of durability also conveys a firm belief in the future and creates a gift of the facility to that future, acknowledging that our own lives are built upon the gifts of the heritage we have inherited.

This core – of permanent and temporary museum galleries, performance hall, gardens, library, greengrocer, bookstore, and newsstand – was all contained within the traditional form of a walled enclosure. This building form is found not only in the Korean tradition, but in many of the Latin, African, and early Southwest traditions – the roots of other community residents. It was a particularly appropriate form for safekeeping of cultural treasures; for protection from the noise, confusion, and wrongness of American urban streets; and for a sense of security in a tension-filled community. This "enclosure" was combined with curved roof forms that embody the sense of effortless, floating support provided by traditional Korean roof construction.

The "moat" and "wall" distinguish the facility from surrounding areas, defining it as an honored or "sacred" area. They particularly acknowledge this difference at points of public entry. At these points, the four elements of life – earth, air, fire, and water – are honored. A gong is located in the central entry, acknowledging the power of air, vibration, and sound in the organization of life from energy. Fire, in the form of sunlight, is honored in the form of the plant life it makes possible. Earth is honored in the placement of special rocks, which remind us of our kinship with the earth, the rocks themselves, and the stars. Water is honored everywhere at entrances for its central role in the creation and unfolding of life.

Incorporation of traditional principles of design acknowledges their value, and therefore the value of the culture of which they were part. Demonstrating their effective power in new materials, technologies, climate, culture, and context not only gives greater meaning and effectiveness to the design itself, but further enhances the credibility and contemporary value of those traditions.

✦

By asking the prime question, "What can we *give*?" we see what can be gained and created in the course of meeting the specific needs of a facility. Here, careful arrangement of facilities and creation of ancillary services would allow the community to use facilities outside of museum hours. The performance hall, meeting rooms, studios, bookstore, newsstand, greengrocer, cafe, and courtyard could all have double uses. The gardens, trees, and fresh vegetables became gifts to the community and a new *intention* of caring, expressed via something as unthinkable as turning sewage into gardens, trees, and the song of birds.

Rediscovering the effective design principles of a tradition and finding successful contemporary expression of them became a give-back and honoring to that tradition and those born in it. The respect and honor we give that tradition affects, in turn, our own self-esteem and mutual respect. By asking what we can give, we create an opportunity for the community to grow, learn, give, share, and enjoy. A community without joy is without life.

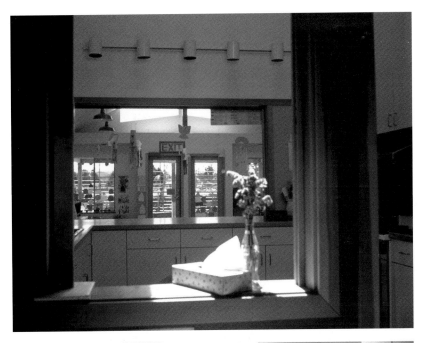

INSTITUTIONS HAVE HEARTS

Our intention toward a place can totally change the lives of others. Out of an intention of making a Head Start Center good for kids, I asked the staff what would make us feel best if we were kids coming in the door. "The smell of good food!" was the unanimous response. This led us to put the kitchen right in the middle of the building, open to all the class-rooms and the entry.

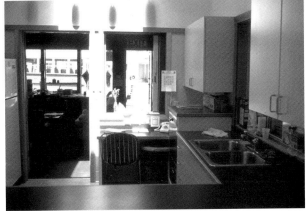

It works wonderfully, giving immediate plea-sure and a sense of rightness to everyone who comes in the door. It also gives parents a place to stop for a cup of coffee and a chat, and to peek around the corner to see how their kids are doing. It allows the cook to be an extra friend and a source of snacks and hugs for the kids, and a backup pair of eyes for the teachers.

What we didn't realize until later was how much our intention totally changed the job of being a cook in this place! Cooking is usually a "back-room" job, tucked out of sight in service areas near the loading dock. In contrast, putting the cook in the *middle* of everything, and in contact with everyone, makes the cook a whole person, and part of everything that goes on!

At this Head Start Center, we unmarginalized people, honored them, and changing their working context. The right-design of place intermingles, enhances, and enriches the lives of *everyone* concerned. The design tradi-tion of putting kitchens in the back corner, behind closed doors, and next to the loading dock relegates cooks' lives to the background. It deprives both the cooks and the rest of the people of contributions those people could make to the whole.

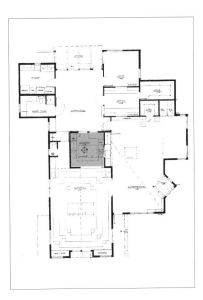

An architect later asked me what I would do if the Center was larger and needed a bigger kitchen and loading dock. The answer was simple: "You've just defined too big!" A change in intention – from wholeness and people-centeredness to optimizing mechanical function – is usually what underlies our gut feeling of wrongness when something becomes too big.

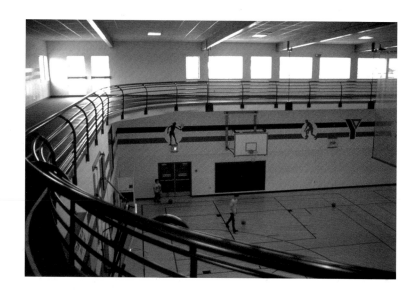

THE RICHNESS OF EDGES

I did a very low budget expansion for a YMCA on the Oregon Coast several years ago. Their national office did all the programming and preliminary design, giving local architects an already designed layout that only had to be "gussied up" and engineered. But it felt as if something important was missing.

It was. All of the *programs* were planned for – swimming classes, basketball games, and exercise rooms – but there was no planning for *people!* What about the shy new kid, who was more than a little apprehensive about some program and wanted to scope it out a bit before committing to join it? What about people who wanted to sit around and rest after a hard game and watch other people play? What about the kids who came to spend the day, and needed a place to sit with friends and eat their sack lunch? What about a place to sit around during the bigger kids' play time and learn some good moves? What about a place to sit and replay an exciting game, or to just jaw and make friends? None of those places were in the program!

With some hard stretching, it was possible to enrich the edges to give space for such "people stuff." Wide spaces in the corridors were provided with chairs and full-length windows into the gym. The entrance lobby was widened to provide room for lunch tables and vending machines. A balcony corridor at the handball courts was added so that non-players could watch the games. Wherever a usable corner could be found, lights, windows, seating, carpet, or whatever was needed were added to turn it into a people place.

The success of these places acknowledged the psychological, emotional, and interpersonal dimensions of human lives that rarely show up on a planning program. The edges where one thing ends and something else begins are special places with important values of their own.

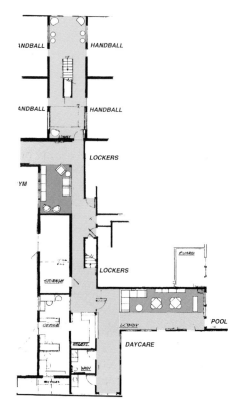

Circulation space was stretched out, wherever possible, to create people-spaces connected with the various program spaces such as the pool, gymnasium, handball courts and daycare; and around the edges of the gym and running track.

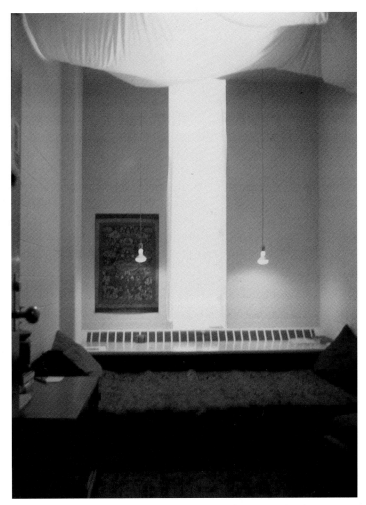

TRANSFORMING A WORKPLACE

Imagine being held captive in a 20th century architecture-school faculty office: concrete block walls, metal desks and windows, asphalt tile floors, fluorescent lights. Stark, functional, depressing to the soul. Sounds an awful lot like a prison cell, doesn't it?

Then imagine that you are teaching some courses in non-Western architectural history, with different concepts of space use, an eye for rich and subtle color combinations, lighting, mood, spirit of a space. Something would have to give way.

We're usually blocked from making institutional space feel good more by our own perceptions of what is "allowed" than by what is actually possible.

It did. The department secretaries were startled when the desk was pushed out into the hall. Their eyes *really* rolled when a mattress was dragged in from a second-hand store. A trip to the dusty storerooms in the basement of the building turned up a wall sculpture and an old samovar. A lucky find of a worn Oriental carpet in a rag store, a coat of warm-white paint, a tricot ceiling, and a couple of $2 spotlights – and the architecture prison was gone!

In its place was something closer to a nomad's tent. There was room for *people* – to sit and talk as equals on a comfortable carpeted platform with pillows. Soft lighting; shoes off; tea and quiet music; a low shelf for a desk. Hierarchical office and interpersonal patterns wouldn't work.

This is about *experiencing* a different way of living and being, not *talking* about one. Our acceptance of conventions of space use is often more limiting than the institutional restrictions put on us as users.

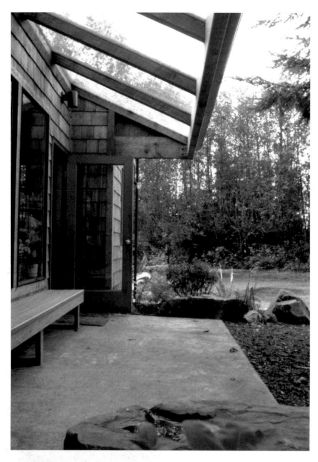

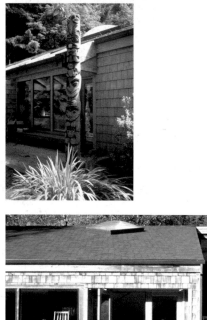

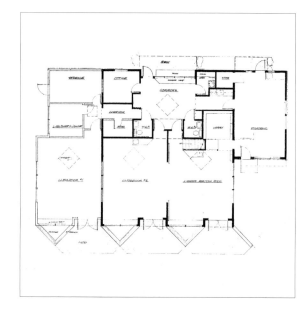

THEIR OWN PLACE TO LEARN

It is rare that we actually consider and honor *children* in the design of schools. It is usually classrooms, teachers, support staff, program activities, and code requirements that get attention. We designed this elementary school as a place *for children* – to give them access to resources, guidance, enthusiasm, and love of others.

As a result, windows are placed where kids can see through them, open them, and make window seats in them. Library and supply shelves are open and accessible so that everyone can find what they need. Outdoor places are made to be used by groups and individuals in good weather. Classrooms have lofts, where kids can go off by themselves (yes, out of sight of teachers) to read, nap, or work on projects. Doors have glass window panes so that kids can see what is happening inside or outside. A small kitchen lets

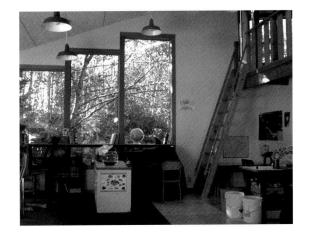

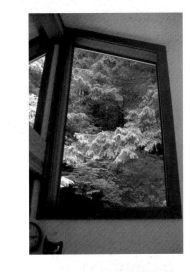

them make their own lunches. The surrounding forest provides real-time nature labs. Windows allow us to keep an eye out for interesting things happening in those woods – hummingbird nests, hailstorms, or visiting elk.

A Commons provides space for small-group meetings or projects outside of the classrooms. The classrooms have different sizes and configurations. In real life, student/teacher ratios are never exact, classes are different sizes, class groups are combined in different patterns, and different projects have different space needs. Two classrooms have sliding doors between them so they can be used together, or as a stage for plays.

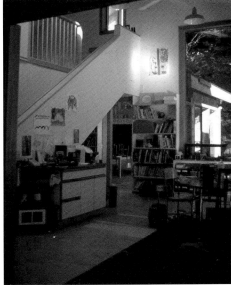

The school was built by the families, with the kids helping to nail framing and raise walls in what turned out to be a very wet "barn-raising." Daylighting and sunshine is provided to all interior spaces.

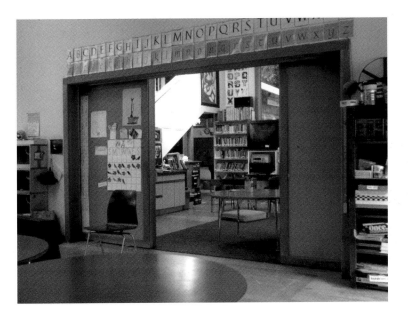

FINDING THE FREEDOM TO GIVE

This is a simple exercise to remind us how big the gap is between our wants and our real needs. It is best done in a group, or a least with one other person.

Sit down, the first thing in the morning, with a piece of paper and pencil. Make a list of what you need to get done before noon, and why.

Then look at the list and cross off the things that really aren't essential. You could skip work. You could sluff off on getting the kids to school. Getting dressed? Breakfast? Do you really need to earn that much money? Trade lists with someone else, and see what else could be whittled down on their and your lists.

When we did this at a conference in Australia, the only thing that ended on the For-Sure list was: *Breathing;* On the Fairly-Sure list: *Taking a pee.*

Try some other lists — a weekly or monthly one, a list of what would bring true fullness and joy into your life, a list of what you could give to others.

Giving becomes possible when we find freedom in our lives, and see what is truly important. It is one of the seeds of fullness in our hearts out of which a rewarding life grows.

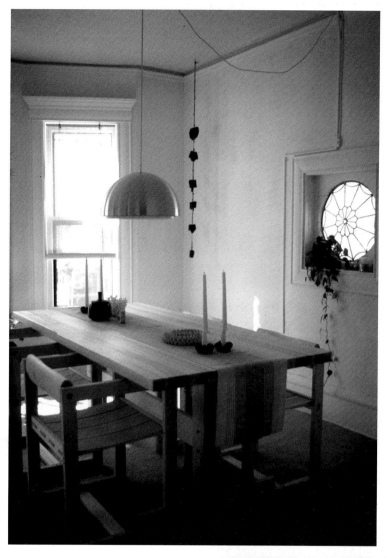

THE COLOR OF LIGHT

As renters or visitors, we are more restricted than owners in what we can do to improve the energy of a place. With stark white walls being typical to most rental spaces, other means need to be used to provide warmth, color, and richness in a space.

One of the simplest and most effective means is to use light reflecting off colored fabrics. Spotlights on an orange bedspread casts an instant golden glow within a room. Sunlight on a rich-colored rug reflects a warm ambiance into the room. Inexpensive fabric bedspreads can be used as wall hangings. Wide and inexpensive colored fabrics such as tricot can be used to create a soft, billowing ceiling that diffuses harsh built-in lighting and hides an ugly ceiling. The same fabric, or shoji paper, can be used as window coverings to let in diffuse light while hiding an ugly view. Folding screens or bookcases can create privacy at an entrance.

Crystals in a sunlit window can refract rainbows deep into a room. Plants, of course, can bring the richness of life into otherwise stark spaces, and the sound of wind chimes or a small fountain can give pleasant sound.

Above: A gold ceiling and an orange carpet rolled out over the existing grey wall-to-wall carpet brought a warm glow to this room on snowy days.

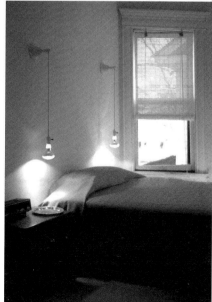

Right: Here, light reflecting off of a rich-colored bedspread changed the energy of a bedroom.

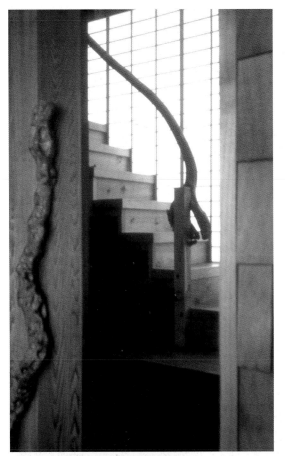

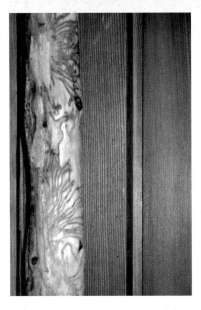

The lives of materials put into our buildings can contribute richness and meaning to those spaces.

HONORING THE SPIRITS OF ALL LIFE

It is wonderful to discover how much our hearts are moved when we find ways to honor other life in our buildings. It started for me, I think, with a spruce root found on the beach years ago that we made into the handles on our front door. The root had squeezed its way among the pebbles on the beach, which had left their imprint on its contours. Some pebbles were still enfolded into the root!

With another twisted piece of driftwood as a handrail on the stairs, coming into the entry in the evening had a particularly moving quality, hard to decipher. What we realized finally is that through the contortions of their shapes, the root and the driftwood were still telling the story of their lives. Like the wrinkles and stoops of an old person, each told of a battle won or lost, a lesson learned, an impasse surmounted. We were feeling the history of their lives, and the stories were worth experiencing. When we do something because it feels good, eventually it teaches us why it felt good.

As time went on, I started trying to have at least one place in buildings I designed where the past lives of the materials were not sawn, ground, split or otherwise taken away. In one house, it was a single driftwood arch – not much work, but something that *everyone* entering the house fell in love with! In another place, it was a pair of natural boulders forming the end of a quarried stone retaining walls – honoring their past lives, untouched, as part of a new place.

Now I often make door handles of driftwood or bug-chewed wood, where the traces of the insects' paths add a singular beauty to the wood. Recently, I've been finding ways to honor other spirits in making a house. It's hard to define the difference between doing this and adding "art" or "sculpture" to a building, but it is very different. It all comes back, again, to *intention*.

On one house, situated on the edge of a slough of the Columbia River, we had the projecting ridge beams of the roof carved into bird heads. The eagle head happens to be visible from inside through a clerestory window. Unexpectedly, the lightness and shape of the roof, combined with the carved head, gives a subtle feeling to the room underneath of being sheltered under the wings of this powerful spirit! This is how, perhaps, we should feel connection with the spirits of all life around us.

TAKE CARE WHAT MIRRORS REFLECT

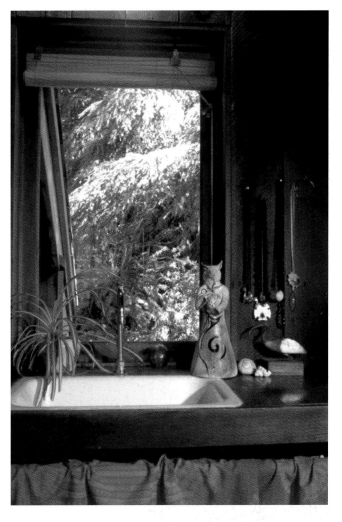

Mirrors are often used in modern buildings to give an *illusion* of greater space. Using anything to *delude* people into believing something untrue damages the energetics of a place. It's better to design a *good* small room than to use mirrors to give the illusion of a space twice as large.

Mirrors are often used geomantically as a cure for negative qualities of spaces. They may have some effect in reflecting light into dark spaces, or on movement of subtle energies, but their symbolic value can be achieved better through other means, and their actual use often worsens the qualities of the place.

Our family once stayed in a rental apartment in Florida that had mirrored walls everywhere. Waking up in the middle of the night to use the bathroom, we got disoriented in the reflections and non-existent hallways, frightened by the intruders we bumped into around every corner (our own reflections, it turned out). Mirrors reflect *confusion*, not comfort.

We also use mirrors compulsively to check on how we *look*. In the process, they focus our attention on surface appearances, rather than inner qualities, of ourselves and others. We tend to use them at times of day when we are our bleary-eyed worst, with subsequent damage to our self-esteem. Without their reminders of externalities, we stop thinking about ourselves, stop being so concerned with outside packaging, and become more attuned and responsive to important inner qualities.

There is value in avoiding bathroom mirrors – putting them on the inside of medicine cabinet doors or on the back of bathroom doors, where they can be available when needed, but out of the way otherwise. If we're stuck with non-removable mirrors, we can hang fabric over them when not in use, stick pictures on them, or otherwise diminish their effect. How much better to have the view of a garden from a bathroom sink, rather than a mirror! How delightful to start our day seeing beauty and nature – rather than a mirror image of our packaging.

Mirrors can be used beneficially in certain cases: to reflect light or sunshine into an otherwise dark space; to give us a glimpse of something hidden around corners or out of sight; for playful accents of sparkle, lightness, or incongruity; or to give us a glimpse of someone approaching from a blind direction who could unexpectedly interrupt our privacy. More commonly, however, they disturb the congruence of a place and probably should be avoided.

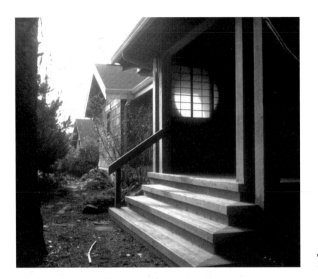

THE PEACE OF SANCTUARY

What a building becomes or doesn't become emerges from the nature of the owner, designer, builder, site, budget, and the times. As I understand intention more clearly, I've been able to look back at past projects and see the subtle yet vital impact that the intention of the owner has on a project. In one project there was lack of trust, and the results turned out competent but uninspiring. In another, the client exuded trust, respect, caring and clarity. What resulted had real soul. With a third client, their lack of caring held me back from doing things that would have resulted in a more moving building. In another case, the client's expectation that I could do more than I thought I could resulted in spectacular improvement in the building's sensitivity.

This one house, in ways I don't fully grasp, powerfully and instantly affects everyone who enters it. The patterns are good: porch and entry as welcome, kitchen as a place to gather around food, living space as connection between people and between people and place, bedrooms as sanctuaries. But there is something else – the generosity and love of the owner? – that is reflected in it and which causes people to feel it a haven immediately upon entering.

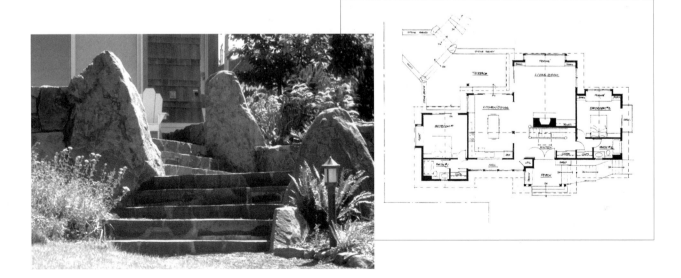

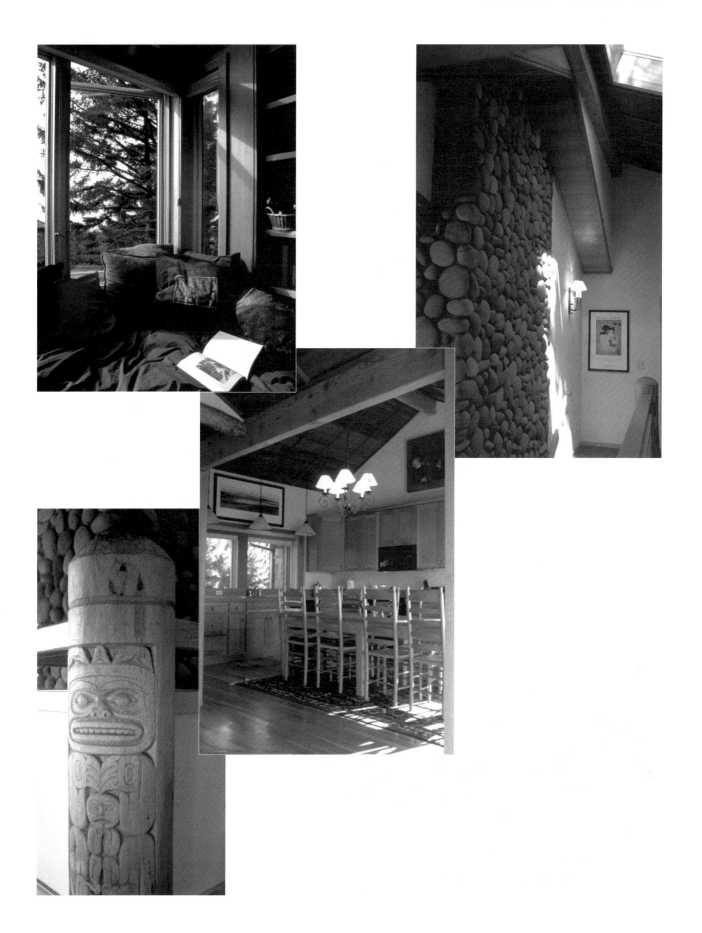

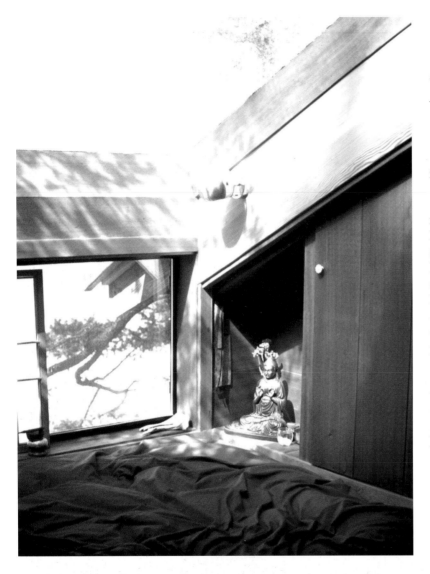

SILENCE AND INTENTION

One of my richest memories is of silence.

It is a memory of a full-moon night inside the dome of the Taj Mahal, filled with the reverberation of singing. Near midnight, most people left, and silence filled the majestic space.[1] The dome magnified the silence as it had magnified the sound, and our breathing and our hearts fell deeper and deeper into the rich and powerful silence. . .

Ever since, I have listened for that silence – and the harsh mechanical noises of TV, toilets, refrigerators, dishwashers, clothes washers, and heating systems have jarred me to the core.

In our house, more than twenty years ago, I set out to regain that silence. Flush toilets were replaced by a compost toilet. Heating was provided by the sun and by

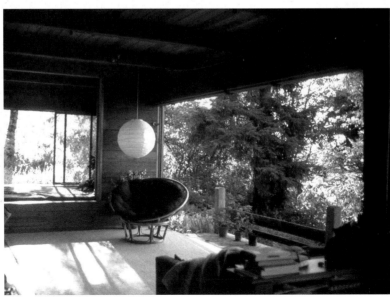

wood. An insulated cupboard, or cool box, in the kitchen captured the cool night air, eliminating need for a refrigerator. Earphones supplement audio speakers. There is no TV. And we have only one house rule: quiet has priority over noise.

The silence of the Taj returned, and grew deeper. It was enriched by the wind and waves, by birdsong, by the dainty footsteps of deer in the night. It filled with the sound of snowfall, and of moonlight on the water.

That silence made a space for clear attention and intention, for working from the heart and touching the heart of what was being worked with. It opened a closeness with the world outside, between people, and with our inner selves. It began the journey that has become this book.

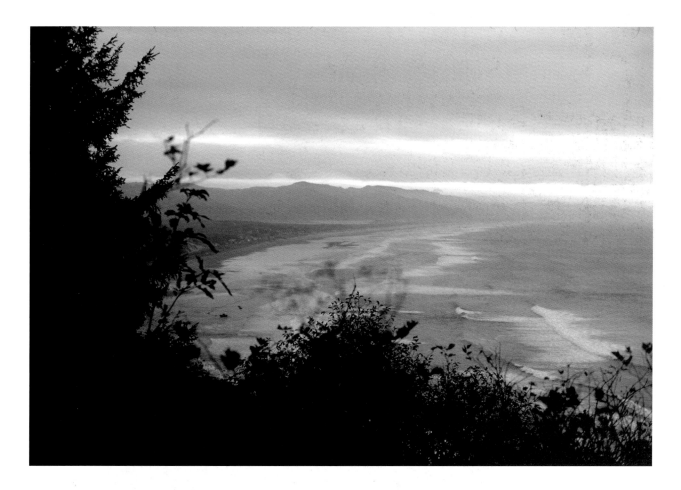

---

[1] Paul Horn's recording, INSIDE THE TAJ MAHAL, gives a feeling for the wonderful acoustic power of this space.

*B*IBLIOGRAPHY

Alexander, Christopher - A PATTERN LANGUAGE, Oxford Univ. Press, 1977.
ANTIQUITY, 1964, 1968 and 1969 - Newgrange excavations.
Ater, Bob - AMERICAN SOCIETY OF DOWSERS QUARTERLY, Spring and Fall, 1997, Spring 1998.
Azby Brown, S. - THE GENIUS OF JAPANESE CARPENTRY, Kodansha International, 1989.

B

Batra, Ravi - THE GREAT DEPRESSION OF 1990, Simon & Schuster, 1987.
Bear, Greg - BLOOD MUSIC, Ace Books, 1986.
Beardsley, Richard, Hall, J. & Ward, R. - VILLAGE JAPAN, Univ. of Chicago Press, 1959.
Beasley, Victor - YOUR ELECTRO-VIBRATORY BODY, University of the Trees, 1978.
Becker, Robert O. - CROSS CURRENTS: The Perils of Electropollution, The Promise of Electromedicine, Tarcher, 1990.
_____, and Gary Selden, BODY ELECTRIC: Electromagnetism and the Foundation of Life, Morrow & Co, 1985.
Beckinsale, R. P. and Houston, J.M. - URBANIZATION AND ITS PROBLEMS, Barnes & Noble, 1968.
Beier, Ulli - THE RETURN OF THE GODS, Cambridge University Press, 1975.
Bender, Tom - *"Amazon Married Student Housing,"* 1994.
_____, - *"Bamberton,"* 1993.
_____, - *"Borrowing Trouble,"* 1990, IN CONTEXT, Issue 44, July, 1996 (www.context.org).
_____, - *"Building Real Wealth,"* 1993, IN CONTEXT, Issue 44, July, 1996 (www.context.org).
_____, - BUILDING VALUE, Office of the California State Architect, 1976.
_____, - *"Building with a Soul,"* in DIALOGS WITH THE LIVING EARTH, James & Roberta Swan, 1996.
_____, - *"Building with the Breath of Life,"* FENG-SHUI JOURNAL, Summer 1997.
_____, - *"Economic Value of Coastal Forest Lands,"* 1994. IN CONTEXT, Issue 44, July, 1996 (www.context.org).
_____, - *"Eco-Building II,"* May 1996, reprinted in ENVIRONMENTAL BUILDING NEWS, July 1996 and IN CONTEXT, Issue 44, July, 1996 (www.context.org).
_____, - *"Endgames,"* IN CONTEXT, Issue 44, July, 1996 (www.context.org).
_____, - ENVIRONMENTAL DESIGN PRIMER, Schocken Books, 1973.
_____, - *"Feng-Shui,"* THE URBAN ECOLOGIST, 1994 #3.
_____, - *"Feng-Shui: A Place for Your Home,"* EAST WEST JOURNAL, July 1984.
_____, - *"Feng-Shui: Energy and Place,"* 1972. Reprinted as *"Feng-Shui: Earth Acupuncture,"* EAST-WEST JOURNAL, July 1973.
_____, - GARDENS OF THE SPIRIT, 1991.
_____, - *"Hidden Costs of Housing,"* 1984. RAIN, Mar. 1984; UTNE READER, Summer 1984; SUN TIMES, Nov. 1984; ALTERNATIVE PRESS ANNUAL, 1984.
_____, - *"It's Oil Right, Folks! There's Good Times Ahead,"* Solar '96 Solar Energy Association of Oregon Conference, October, 1996, reprinted in IN CONTEXT #44, July '96.
_____, - *"Living Lightly,"* 1973.
_____ - *"Making Places Sacred,"* in THE POWER OF PLACE, James Swan, ed. Quest Books, 1991.
_____, - Sacred Roots of Sustainable Design," Sept. 1995.
_____, - *"Sharing Smaller Pies,"* NEW AGE JOURNAL, Nov. 1975; THE FUTURIST, 1976; RESETTLING AMERICA, Gary Coates, ed. 1981; and UTNE READER Fall 1987.
_____, - *"Shedding A Skin That No Longer Fits,"* Mar. 1996. Reprinted in IN CONTEXT #44, July '96.
_____, - *"Some Questions We Haven't Asked,"* 1996. IN CONTEXT, Issue 44, July, 1996.
_____, - THE HEART OF PLACE, 1993.
_____, - *"The Pantheon Revisited,"* Oct. 1990.
_____, - *"The Sacred Art of Building,"* IN CONTEXT, Autumn 1986. Reprinted in UTNE READER, Feb/Mar 1986; WHOLISTIC LIVING NEWS, Oct/Nov 1985, (www.context.org).
_____, - *"Their Population, Our Problem,"* Nov. 1996.
_____, - *"Transforming Tourism,"* 1993. EARTH ETHICS, Summer, 1993. IN CONTEXT, Issue 44, July, 1996 (www.context.org).

____, - *"Unexpected Gifts - The Real Rewards of Sustainable Communities,"* Solar '96 Solar Energy Association of Oregon Conference, October, 1996. Reprinted in IN CONTEXT #44, July, 1996.

____, - *"Vitality and Affordability of Higher Education,"* 1993. IN CONTEXT, Issue 44, July. 1996 (www.context.org).

Benton, Itzhak - *"Micromotion of the Body as a Factor in the Development of the Nervous System,"* in Snanella, Lee, KUNDALINI EXPERIENCE, Integral Publishing, 1992.

Berliner, Helen - ENLIGHTENED BY DESIGN, Shambhala, 1999.

Binder, Tim & Russell, Walter - IN THE WAVE LIES THE SECRET OF CREATION, Univ. of Sci. & Philos., 1995.

Boner, Alice - PRINCIPLES OF COMPOSITION IN HINDU SCULPTURE, E.J. Brill, 1962.

____, and Sharma, S. Rath - RAMACANDRA KAULACARA - Silpa Prakasa, E.J. Brill, 1966.

Boyd, Andrew - CHINESE ARCHITECTURE AND TOWN PLANNING, Univ. of Chicago Press, 1962.

Bradsher, Keith - *"Gulf widens between wealthy and poor,"* NEW YORK TIMES NEWS SERVICE, April 20, 1995.

Brennan, Barbara - HANDS OF LIGHT, Bantam Books, 1987.

____, - LIGHT EMERGING, Bantam Books, 1993.

Broday, Warren - *"Biotopology 1972,"* in RADICAL SOFTWARE 4, Raindance, 1972.

Bruyere, Rosalyn - WHEELS OF LIGHT, Fireside Books, 1989.

C

Cauville, Sylvie - LE TEMPLE DE DENDERA, Bibliotheque Général, 1990.

Chang, Dr. Ching-Yu - *"Japanese Spatial Conception,"* THE JAPAN ARCHITECT, 1984.

Chang, Sen Dou - *"Some Observations on the Morphology of Chinese Walled Cities,"* ANNALS, ASSOC. OF AMERICAN GEOGRAPHERS, Mar. 1970.

Chia, Mantak and Maneewan - AWAKEN HEALING LIGHT OF THE TAO, Healing Tao Books, 1993.

Ch'ien, Ssu-ma - "Basic Annals of Qin," in RECORDS OF THE GRAND HISTORIAN OF CHINA (Shiji-Qinbenji), Vols. 1 & 2, Burton Watson, trans., Columbia University Press, 1961.

Chuen, Lam Kam - FENG SHUI HANDBOOK, Henry Holt, 1996.

Clow, Barbara Hand - THE PLEIADIAN AGENDA, Bear & Co., 1995.

Coates, Callum - LIVING ENERGIES, Gateway Books, 1996.

Coates, Gary - ERIK ASMUSSEN, ARCHITECT, Byggfolaget, 1997.

Coedes, George - ANGKOR, AN INTRODUCTION, Oxford Univ. Press, 1963.

____, - *"La destination funeraire des grands monuments khmers,"* BULLETIN DE L'ECOLE FRANCAISE D'EXTREME-ORIENT, 1940.

Cohen, Kenneth S. - *"Chinese Geomancy,"* YOGA JOURNAL, 1980.

Collinge, William - SUBTLE ENERGY, Warner Books, 1998.

Creasy, Rosalind - THE COMPLETE BOOK OF EDIBLE LANDSCAPING, Sierra Club Books, 1982.

Critchlow, Keith - ISLAMIC PATTERNS: An Analytical and Cosmological Approach, Schocken Books, 1976.

Crowley, Brian & Esther - WORDS OF POWER: Sacred Sounds of East and West, Llewellyn Publications, 1991.

D

Davis and Rawls - MAGNETISM AND ITS EFFECTS ON THE LIVING SYSTEM, Exposition Press, 1974.

Davis, Wade - SHADOWS IN THE SUN, Island Press, 1998.

Day, Christopher - PLACES OF THE SOUL, Aquarian, 1993.

Devereux, Paul - EARTH MEMORY, Llewellyn Books, 1992.

____, - PLACES OF POWER, Blanford Books, London, 1990.

Diamond, John, M.D. - YOUR BODY DOESN'T LIE, Warner Books, 1979.

DuBoulay, Shirley - TUTU, Archbishop without Frontiers, Hodder & Stoughton, 1996.

Dumitrescu, I. and Kenyon, J. - ELECTROGRAPHIC IMAGING IN MEDICINE AND BIOLOGY, Neville Spearman, 1983.

Duncan, Richard - *"The Energy Depletion Arch...,"* 1995.

E

Eden, Donna - ENERGY MEDICINE, Tarcher/Putnam, 1998.
Elkin, A.P. - ABORIGINAL MEN OF HIGH DEGREE, 1946, Inner Traditions International, 1994.
Ellis, Normandie - AWAKENING OSIRIS, Phanes Press, 1988.
____, - DREAMING ISIS, Quest Books, 1995.
ENVIRONMENTAL BUILDING NEWS, Sept./Oct. 1995.
Eitel, Ernest J. - FENG-SHUI: The Rudiments of Natural Science in China, Lane, Crawford & Co, 1873.
        Reprinted Synergetic Press, 1993.

F

Farallones Institute - THE INTEGRAL URBAN HOUSE, Sierra Club Books, 1979.
Feuchtwang, Stephan D.R. - AN ANTHROPOLOGICAL ANALYSIS OF CHINESE GEOMANCY,
        Editions Vithagna, Laos, 1974.
Fidler, J. Havelock - LEY LINES: Their Nature and Properties, Turnstone Books, 1983.
Fisher, Jeffrey - THE PLAGUE MAKERS, Simon & Schuster, 1994.
Freedman, Maurice - "Geomancy," PROCEEDINGS OF THE ROYAL ANTHROPOLOGICAL
        INSTITUTE, 1968.
____, - "Geomancy and Ancestor Worship," CHINESE LINEAGE AND SOCIETY, Athlone Press, UK, 1971.
Freidel, David; Schele, Linda; and Parker, Joy - MAYA COSMOS: Three Thousand Years on the
        Shaman's Path, Wm. Morrow & Co., 1993.

G

Gendlin, Eugene - FOCUSING, Bantam, 1988.
Gerber, Richard - VIBRATIONAL MEDICINE, Bear & Co., 1996.
Gilman, Robert - Plenary Talk, HOPES '97 Conference, University of Oregon School of Architecture and
        Allied Arts.
Goloubew, Viktor - "L'Hydraulique Urbaine et Agricole a l'Epoque des Rois d'Angkor," in BULLETIN
        ECONOMIQUE DE L'INDOCHINE, 1941 fascicule 1, or abbreviated in CAHIERS DE
        L'ECOLE FRANCAISE D'EXTREME ORIENT, vol. 24 (1940).
Govinda, Lama Anagarika - THE WAY OF THE WHITE CLOUDS, Shambhala,1966.
Gray, Martin - PLACES OF PEACE AND POWER, 1997, from PO Box 4111, Sedona AZ 86340.

H

Hale, Gill - THE FENG SHUI GARDEN, Story Books, 1998.
Hancock, Graham - FINGERPRINTS OF THE GODS, Three Rivers Press, 1995.
____, & Robert Bauval - MESSAGE OF THE SPHINX, Three Rivers Press, 1996.
Hawkins, Gerald - STONEHENGE DECODED, Doubleday, 1965.
Heckler, Richard Strozzi - IN SEARCH OF THE WARRIOR SPIRIT, North Atlantic Books, 1992.
Horn, Paul - INSIDE THE TAJ MAHAL, CD, CBS Records, 1979.
Houston, Jean, - THE PASSION OF ISIS AND OSIRIS, Ballantine, 1995.

I

Itoh, Teiji - JAPANESE ENVIRONMENTAL DESIGN, Vol. 2 - Architecture, draft, School of Architecture,
        University of Washington, 1965.
Ivanhoe, L. F. - "Future world oil supplies: there is a finite limit," WORLD OIL, Oct. 1995.
____, - "Oil Reserves and Semantics," Newsletter of the M. KING HUBBERT CENTER FOR PETROLEUM
        SUPPLY STUDIES, Colorado School of Mines, Aug. 1996.

J

Jenny, Hans - CYMATICS, 1967; and CYMATICS, Vol 2., 1974, Basilius Presse.
____, - "Cymatic Soundscapes," and "Cymatics" videos available from MACROmedia, P.O. Box 279,
        Epping NH 03042 USA.

K

Katz, Richard. - "Education for Transcendence: Lessons from the !Kung Zhu Twasi," JOURNAL OF
        TRANSPERSONAL PSYCHOLOGY, #2, 1973.

_____,BOILING ENERGY: Community Healing among the Kalahari Kung, Harvard University Press, 1982.

Kelley, Kevin - THE HOME PLANET, Addison-Wesley, 1988.

Knaster, Mirka - DISCOVERING THE BODY'S WISDOM, Bantam, 1996.

Korn, Joey - DOWSING: A PATH TO ENLIGHTENMENT, Kornucopia Press, 1998.

Kramrisch, Stella - THE HINDU TEMPLE, University of Calcutta, 1946.

Kubiak, W. David - *"Ki and the Arts of Sex, Healing and Corporate Body Building,"* KYOTO JOURNAL, Winter 1988.

L

Lambert, Johanna - WISEWOMEN OF THE DREAMTIME, Inner Traditions International, 1993.

Lansing, John Stephen - PRIESTS & PROGRAMMERS: Technologies of Power in the Engineered Landscape of Bali, Princeton University Press, 1991.

LaViolette, Paul - BEYOND THE BIG BANG, Park St. Press, 1995.

Lawlor, Robert - VOICES OF THE FIRST DAY: Awakening in the Aboriginal Dreamtime, Inner Traditions International, 1991.

Lee, Thomas - *"Kan Yu - the Book of Change Concept in Environmental and Architectural Planning,"* GREENING TO THE BLUE CONFERENCE, Yale University, 1996.

Linn, Denise - SACRED SPACE, Ballantine Books, 1995.

Lip, Evelyn - FENG SHUI - A Layman's Guide to Chinese Geomancy, Heian International, 1979.

____ , - FENG SHUI FOR THE HOME, Heian International, 1986.

Lonegren, Sig - SPIRITUAL DOWSING, Gothic Image, 1986.

Lovins, Amory - *"The Super-Efficient Passive Building Frontier,"* ASHRAE JOURNAL, June 1995.

____ , Lovings, L. Hunter, and Hawken, P. - NATURAL CAPITALISM, Little, Brown & Co., 1999.

____ , Lovings, L. Hunter, and von Weizsäcker, Ernst - FACTOR FOUR: Doubling Productivity, Halving Resource Use, Earthscan, 1997.

Lusseyran, Jacques - AND THERE WAS LIGHT, Parabola, 1987.

M

MacKenzie, James - *"Oil as a Finite Resource,"* WORLD RESOURCES INSTITUTE, March, 1996.

March, Andrew L. - *"An Appreciation of Chinese Geomancy,"* JOURNAL OF ASIAN STUDIES, 1968.

McDermott and Biayak - MASTERING FEAR, Frog & Latte, 1996.

Merz, Blanche - POINTS OF COSMIC ENERGY, C.W. Daniel Co. Ltd., 1983, 1995.

Meyer, Jeffrey F. - PEKING AS A SACRED CITY, Orient Culture Service, 1976.

Moodey, Raymond A. - LIFE AFTER LIFE, Bantam, 1988.

Morgan, Marlo - MUTANT MESSAGE, HarperSF, 1995.

Morehouse, David A. - PSYCHIC WARRIOR, St. Martin's Press, 1998.

Motoyama, Hiroshi - MEASUREMENTS OF KI ENERGY, DIAGNOSIS AND TREATMENTS, Human Science Press, 1998.

____ , and R. Brown - SCIENCE AND THE EVOLUTION OF CONSCIOUSNESS: CHAKRAS, KI, AND PSI, Autumn Press, 1978.

Mus, Paul - BARABUDUR, Bole, Kees W., 1978.

Myers, Fred - PINTUIP COUNTRY, PINTUPI SELF, Smithsonian Press, 1986.

Myss, Caroline - ANATOMY OF THE SPIRIT, Harmony Books, 1996.

N

Nasr, Seyyed H. - SCIENCE AND CIVILIZATION IN ISLAM, Kazi Pubns., 1996.

Naydler, Jeremy - TEMPLE OF THE COSMOS, Inner Traditions International, 1996.

Needham, Joseph - SCIENCE AND CIVILIZATION IN CHINA, Vol. 2, Cambridge University Press, 1956.

____ , - THE SHORTER SCIENCE AND CIVILIZATION IN CHINA, Vol 1, Colin Ronan, ed., pp 239-40, Cambridge University Press, 1978.

Nelson, R., G. Bradish, Y. Dobyns, B. Dunne and R. Jahn - *"Field REG Anomalies in Group Situations,"* JOURNAL OF SCIENTIFIC EXPLORATION, 1996.

Norbeck, Edward - TAKASHIMA, University of Utah Press, 1954.

Northrop, Suzane - THE SEANCE, Dell Publications, 1994.

O

Orloff, Judith - SECOND SIGHT, Warner Books, 1996.

P

Parent, Mary Neighbour - THE ROOF IN JAPANESE BUDDHIST ARCHITECTURE, Weatherhill/
    Kajima, 1983.
Pennick, Nigel - THE ANCIENT SCIENCE OF GEOMANCY, Thames and Hudson and CRCS
    Publications, 1979.

R

Radin, Dean - THE CONSCIOUS UNIVERSE, HarperSF, 1997.
Rael, Joseph - BEING AND VIBRATION, Council Oak Books, 1993.
Raymond, E.A.E - THE MYTHICAL ORIGIN OF THE EGYPTIAN TEMPLE, Manchester Univ. Press,
    1969.
RECLAIMING QUARTERLY, Fall 1998.
Rees, Bill - *"Ecological Footprints and Appropriated Carrying Capacity . . .,"* in INVESTING IN NATURAL
    CAPITAL, Island Press 1994.
____, - *"Revising Carrying Capacity. . . .,"* in POPULATION AND ENVIRONMENT: A Journal of
    Interdisciplinary Studies, Jan 1996.
Rich, Peter - Presentation, DESIGN HAS NO BOUNDARIES CONFERENCE, Brisbane, AU, 1995.
Rocky Mountain Institute - GREENING THE BUILDING AND THE BOTTOM LINE, 1994.
Rose-Neil, S. - *"The Work of Professor Kim Bong Ham,"* The ACUPUNCTURIST, 1967.
Rossbach, Sarah - FENG SHUI - The Chinese Art of Placement, Arkana Books, 1983.
Rousseau, David - HEALTHY BY DESIGN, Hartley & Marks, 1997.

S

Schele, Linda and Freidel, David - A FOREST OF KINGS, Wm. Morrow & Company, 1990.
____, and Mathews, Peter - THE CODE OF KINGS, Scribner, 1998.
____, and Pérez de Lara, Jorge, HIDDEN FACES OF THE MAYA, A.L.T.I., 1997.
Schumacher, E.F. - A GUIDE FOR THE PERPLEXED, Harper & Row, 1977.
____, - SMALL IS BEAUTIFUL, reprinted Hartley & Marks, 1999.
Schwaller de Lubicz, R.A. - THE TEMPLE IN MAN, Inner Traditions International, 1949, 1977.
Schwartz, Gary and Russek, Linda - THE LIVING ENERGY UNIVERSE, Hampton Roads Pub. Co.,
    1999.
Sheldrake, Rupert - SEVEN EXPERIMENTS THAT COULD CHANGE THE WORLD, Riverhead
    Books, 1996.
Shukla, D. N. - VASTU-SHASTRA, vol 1, Bharatiya Vastu-Shastras Series, Punjab University, 1960.
Sitchen, Zacheria - THE TWELFTH PLANET, Bear & Co, 1991.
Somé, Malidoma - OF WATER AND THE SPIRIT, Tarcher/Putnam, 1994.
____, - RITUAL: POWER, HEALING, AND COMMUNITY, Swan, Raven & Co, 1993.
____, - THE HEALING WISDOM OF AFRICA, Tarcher/Putnam, 1998.
Somé, Sobonfu - THE SPIRIT OF INTIMACY, Berkeley Hill Books, 1997.
Spear, William - FENG SHUI MADE EASY, HarperSF, 1995,
____, - THE FENG SHUI HOUSE BOOK, with Gina Lazenby, Watson-Guptill Publications, 1998.
Spencer Brown, G. - LAWS OF FORM, George Allen and Unwin, Ltd., 1969.
Srinivasan, T.M., ed. - ENERGY MEDICINE AROUND THE WORLD, Gabriel Press, 1988.
Starhawk - THE FIFTH SACRED THING, Bantam, 1993.
____, - THE SPIRAL DANCE, Harper SF, 1979.
____, & NightMare, M. Macha - PAGAN BOOK OF LIVING AND DYING, HarperSF, 1997.
Steiner, Rudolf - EURYTHMY AS VISIBLE SPEECH, Rudolf Steiner Press, 1984.
Stillman, Ed - *"Dowser's Brainwave Characteristics,"* AMERICAN DOWSER QUARTERLY, Winter '97,
    Spring '98.
Suda, Fumio and Carpenter, Colin - *"House Reading: A Spiritual Approach to Residential Design in
    Traditional Japan,"* in Swan, DIALOGUES WITH THE LIVING EARTH, Quest Books, 1996.
Swan, James - SACRED PLACES, Bear & Co., 1990.
____, - ed, - THE POWER OF PLACE, Quest Books, 1991.

____, and Swan, Roberta, ed. - DIALOGUES WITH THE LIVING EARTH, Quest Books, 1996.

T

Tange, Kenzo - ISE: Prototype of Japanese Architecture, MIT Press, 1965.
Taut, Bruno - HOUSES AND PEOPLE OF JAPAN, Sanseido Co, Ltd., 1937.
Tice, Chris - *"A Ritual for Empowering Statues,"* SHAMANIC JOURNEYS NEWSLETTER, 1998.
Tiller, William - *"Some Energy Observations in Man and Nature,"* in Krippner, S. and Rubin, D. eds., THE
        KIRLIAN AURA, Doubleday, 1974.
____, - *"A Gas Discharge Device for Investigating Focused Human Intention,"* JOURNAL OF SCIENTIFIC
        EXPLORATION, 1990.
____, - SCIENCE AND HUMAN TRANSFORMATION: Subtle Energies, Intentionality And
        Consciousness, Pavior, 1997.
Tompkins, Peter - SECRETS OF THE GREAT PYRAMIDS, Harper & Row, 1971.
Tuan, Yi Fu - *"A Preface to Chinese Cities,"* in Beckinsale and Houston, URBANIZATION AND ITS
        PROBLEMS, Blackwell, 1968.
Tyng, Anne Griswold - *"Geometric Extensions of Consciousness,"* ZODIAC 19.
____, - *"Urban Space Systems as Living Form,"* in ARCHITECTURE CANADA, Nov, Dec. 1968 and Jan.
        1969.

U

Underwood, Guy - THE PATTERN OF THE PAST, Pitman Publishing, 1969.

V

van Eyck, Aldo - in Smsithson, Alison, ed., TEAM 10 PRIMER, 1964.
Venolia, Carol - HEALING ENVIRONMENTS, Celestial Arts, 1988.
Video of research results available from World Research Foundation, 15300 Ventura Blvd., Suite 405,
        Sherman Oaks, CA 91403.
Vilenskaya, Larissa - FIREWALKING, Bramble Co., 1992.
Vitousek, Erlichs, and Matson, *"Human Appropriation of the Products of Photosynthesis,"* BIOSCIENCE 36:
        368-74. 1986.
Volwahsen, Andreas - LIVING ARCHITECTURE: INDIAN, Grosset & Dunlap, 1969.

W

Wackernagel, Hans, and Rees, William - OUR ECOLOGICAL FOOTPRINT, New Society Books, 1995.
Walters, Derek - THE FENG SHUI HANDBOOK, Harper Collins, 1991.
Wampler, Jan - *"People and the Places They Build,"* ARCHITECTURE PLUS, July/Aug '74.
Wang, P., X. Hu, and B. Wu - *"Displaying of the Infrared Radiant Track Long Meridians on the Back of the
        Human Body,"* CHEN TZU YEN CHIU ACUPUNCTURE RESEARCH, 1993.
Watterson, Barbara - THE HOUSE OF HORUS AT EDFU, Tempus, 1998.
West, John Anthony - SERPENT IN THE SKY, Harper & Row, 1979.
Wheatley, Paul - THE PIVOT OF THE FOUR QUARTERS, Aldine, 1971.
Wiener, Jonathan - PLANET EARTH, Bantam, 1986.
Wolff, Edward - TOP HEAVY, Twentieth Century Fund Report, 1995.
Wong, Eva - FENG-SHUI, Shambhala, 1996.
Woods, Walter - LETTER TO ROBIN: A Mini-Course in Pendulum Dowsing, 1990-96.
Wright, Machaelle Small - CO-CREATIVE SCIENCE, Perelandra Ltd., 1997.
Wright, Machaelle Small - PERELANDRA GARDEN WOORKBOOK I & II, Perelandra Ltd., 1993, 1990.
Wu, Nelson - CHINESE AND INDIAN ARCHITECTURE, George Braziller, 1963.

Y

Yoon, Hong-Key - GEOMANTIC RELATIONSHIPS BETWEEN CULTURE AND NATURE IN KOREA,
        Orient Culture Service, 1976.

Z

Zangshu, THE BURIAL BOOK OF QUO-PU (AD 276-324), quoted in PARABOLA 3, Issue 1, 1978.

INDEX

A

Aboriginal, 136, 168
Acupuncture, 18
    Meridians, verification, 18-19
Ancestors, 39-40, 66-67, 69-75, 77-79
Angkor, 69-75
Asmussen, Erik, 76
Astrology, 37, 137-138

B

Bali, water temples, 75
Bear, Greg, 145
Birth stones, 84
Brennan, Barbara, 112-113
Broday, Warren, 125-126
Brown, G. Spencer, 125, 130-131
Building with the breath of life, 32-41
Buildings with souls, 186-199
    building from inside, 197-199
    characteristics, 187-189
    entries, 192—196
Bushmen, 46

C

Calling and Moving Place Energy, 162
Chang'An, 68
Change, qualities of, 121-128, 134-135
Chi
    acknowledgment of, 18-19
    actions, relative significance, 117-121
    and acupuncture, 18
    and cities, 214-233
    and cosmology, 40-41, 69-75, 137, 225
    and education, 76, 262-263
    and electromagnetic fields, 36, 108-109
    and environmental health, 37-38
    and geometry, 65, 122-133
    and health, 35-42, 110, 144
    and history, 44-85
    and interconnection, 13, 20-22, 28, 53, 80-83
    and landforms, 134-136
    and Pacific Northwest Indians, 80-81
    and past and future, 39-40, 66-67, 71, 77-79
    and place, 27-28, 45-85, 103, 126, 215-226
    and sacred, 25, 41, 96-98, 123-133, 128, 231
    and sound, 50-51
    and sustainability, 86-103
    and sustainable design, 34-35
    and the Australian Aboriginals, 136, 168
    and the Kalahari Bushmen, 46
    and the Khmers, 69-75
    and the Maya, 59-63
    and warfare, 22, 60-61
    and water, 69-75
    and words, 50-51
    and work, 16, 231, 259, 261
    as element of energy of place, 116-118
    changing community chi, 228-233
    characteristics, 23
    clearing and moving place energy, 162
    clearing energy in a space, 164
    design tools, 141-169
    design with, 29
    experiencing personal, 21
    factors influencing in place, 170-184
    filling a place with soul, 191
    healing place with chi and li, 253-258
    healing place-rape, 229-230
    implications for society, 17-18
    in China, 66-68, 105-106, 108-110, 119, 121-138
    in education, 262-263
    in Egypt, 48-57, 82, 137
    in India, 64-65, 124-125, 128-129
    in Japan, 58, 84-85, 126, 159-160, 182
    in material world, 121-138
    in our bodies, 18-24
    in world cultures, 14-15
    names for, 14-15
    other cultures, 14-15
    principles of energy design, 35-42
    researchers, 18-20th centuries, 15
    sensing chi in a place, 176-177
    significance of actions, 115-119
    working with, 30-31, 161-163
Chih Chung, 137-138
China, 66-67, 121-138
    Chang'An, 68
    Chih Chung, 137-138
    Chu Hsi, 109, 119
    feng shui, 13, 66-68, 77
    Five Elements, 134-135
    Hexagrams, 127-128

Hsing, 134-136
Kuo-p'u, 106
Li, 109-110
Lo Shu, 128-129
Ming Tang, 67
Qin Shihuang, 66
So, 123-133
Chu Hsi, 109, 119
Clearing Energy in a Space, 164
Cities, 214-233
    celebrating death, 228-229
    changing community chi, 228-233
    chi of place, 215-226
    community intentions, 218-220
    finding a passion, 226-227
    healing place-rape, 229-230
    honoring other life, 232
    layout, 68, 69, 75, 130
    making space for new creation, 232-233
    making the sacred visible, 231
    making work sacred, 231
    of passion, 214-233
    resources and community, 141-142
    roots of community passions, 220-226
    transforming root intentions, 232
    what makes a city lovable, 215
    wildness in, 220
Co-creation Conference Calls, 146
Critchlow, Keith, 65

D

Dagara, 16,46-47, 77-79
Day, Christopher, 76
Death, 206-208
    celebrating death, 228-229
Diseases, of the spirit, 94
Divination, see Dowsing
Dowsing, 169
    Brainwaves in, 24
    earth energy, 167-168
    locating religious structures, 84-85
    working with, 167-169
DuBoulay, Shirley, 102-103
Duration, 114-119

E

Eden, Donna, 26
Egypt, 48-57, 137
    and chi, 48-57
    energized images, 82-83
    genealogy, 56
    historic linkages, 56
    intention and mass, 53-55
Eitel, Ernest, 13, 77
Empowering Images, 82-83
Energetic design tools, 141-169
    affirming the world we believe in, 143-144
    becoming native, 141
    clear goals, 141
    free nature, 142-143
    resources and communities, 141-142
    what does Gaia want. 144-145
Energetic design, 29, 253-257, see also Chi
Energetic tools, 153-169
    earth energy, 167-168
    intention and chi, 167
    ritual, 156-159
    rituals in building, 159-160
    rituals of relationship with place, 160-161
    spiritual centering, 153
    trance design, 154-156
    working with chi, 161-165
Energetics of place
    elements, 116-118
    implementing, 253-271
Energized images
    Hathor, 53,
    Pacific NW Indians, 80-81
    working with, 82-83
Energy medicine, 18-20
Entries, 192—196
Environmental Building News, 141-142
Exercises, 11
Experiencing Personal Chi, 21

F

Factor-Ten efficiencies, 90-101
Feng shui, 13, 66-68, 77,
Feuchtwang, Stephan, 110
Filling a Place with Soul, 191

Finding the Freedom to Give, 264
Five Elements, 134-135
Forms, outward, of nature, 134-136
Fuller, R. Buckminster, 147

G

Gaia, 144-145
Gardens
    cloud gardens, 209-211
    homes for our spirits, 201-202
    computer zen gardens, 205-206
    of celebration, 209-212
    of death, 206-208
    of the spirit, 200-213
    of time, 208-209
    spirit of place gardens, 202-205
    wind, water, and star gardens, 205
    wind gardens, 211-212
    winter gardens, 203-204
Geometry, 64-65, 124-133
Getting to know a place, see Site analysis
Giving
    economy of, 95
    -based design, 253-258
Goals, 141-141
Greed, letting go of, 98-99
Group Energy in Ritual, 158
Growth
    changing dimensions of, 88-93
    costs of, 92-94
    limits to, 88-90

H

Hathor, Temple of, Dendera
    enclosure, 53
    energy fields, 53
    Healing Temple, 51
    hidden crypts, 54
    sculpture, 53
Head Start Center, Seaside, 259
Healing place with chi and li, 253-258
Hexagrams, 127-128
Hindu Temples, 64-65
    and geometry, 64-65, 124-125, 129-130
    and sculpture, 65
    Kailasa Temple, 65
Honoring
    honoring the spirits of all life, 266
    other life, 80-81, 232
Hsing, 134-136

I

I-Ching, 34
In-between spaces, 95
Injunction, 130-131
Institutions
    edges, 260
    KOMA, 253-258
    structure, 143-144
    workplace, 261
Intention, 108-112, see also *Li*
    changes lives, 259
    community intentions, 218-220
    intention and chi, 167
    setting intention of a space, 165
    silence and intention, 270-271
    transforming root intentions, 232
    working with, 166
Intuition, 115-116
Itoh, Teiji, 159-160
Izumo Shrine, 58

J

Japanese temple roof construction, 182
Jenny, Hans, *12*, 121

K

Kailasa Temple, 65
Kami, 58
Katz, Richard, 46
Kawakiutl, 80-81
Khmers, 69-75
Kinesiology, **26**
Kiyomizu Temple, 84-85
Kleinforms, 125-126
KOMA, 253-258
Korn, Joey
    and Izumo, 58
    clearing and moving place energy, 162
Kuo-p'u, 106
Kurashiki Inn, 126

L

Lambert, Johanna, 136, 168
Landforms, 134-135, 175, 217
Lansing, John Stephen, 75
Lawlor, Robert, 136
Lee, Thomas, 122
Letting Go of a Greedy World, 98-99
Li, 108-112, see also Intention
    healing place with chi and li, 253-258

in Chinese philosophy, 109-110
in our personal energy field, 110
of place, 111-112
Linn, Denise, 156-157,165, 250
Lo Shu, 128-129
Love
what makes a city lovable, 215
living from the heart, 97-98

M

Magic squares, 128-129
Maya
community portals to spirit world, 59-63
plazas, 59, 61, 63
spirit guides, 59-63
Merz, Blanche, 53, 84-85
Mesa Verde, 45
Mind tools, 147-151
following the threads, 150-151
looking at the world whole, 147
Ming Tang, 67
Mirrors, 267
Myss, Caroline, 90

N

Names, 150
Nasr, Seyyed H., 124
Numbers, 123-133
and design, 124-129
qualitative aspects, 123-128

P

Pennick, Nigel, 127
Place tools, 151-153
maintenance and caring, 153
x-ray vision and empty minds, 151-152
Planetary energy fields, 36
Plugging in to the Energetic Universe, 30-31
Possessions, 183-184
Privacy and intimacy, 215

Q

Quantum teleportation, 20

R

Rael, Joseph, 216
Remote viewing, 20
Rented space, 261, 265
Resonance, 123-133, 128
Resources, inner, 100

Right duration, 114-115
Ritual, 156-159, 230
and community, 46-47
and Maya, 59-63
and Khmer, 69-75
and Egypt, 48-57
and work, 16
group energy in, 158
in building, 159-160
of relationship with place, 160-161

S

Sacred
and chi, 25, 41
expressing sacredness, 239
holding places sacred, 235
making the sacred visible, 231
making work sacred, 231
society, 97
surroundings, 96-98
Sacred places, 234-251
expressing sacredness, 239
holding places sacred, 235
the Shrine of the Mountain and the Waters, 240-251
varieties of sacred places, 236-239
Sanctuary,
peace of, 268-269
Sensing Chi in a Palace, 176-177
Setting Intention of a Space, 165
Schele, Linda and Matthews, Peter, 63
Schumacher, E.F., 149-150
Sewage, 253-258
Shrine of the Mountain and the Waters, 240-251
Silence, and intention, 270-271
Site analysis, 170-185
connections and barriers, 178-180
human elements, 173
inside buildings, 180-182
invisible forces, 173-174
natural features, 171-173
neighborhood, 174-175
people - past and present, 178
possessions, 183-184
site and building, 175-184
surroundings, 171-174
topology and topography, 175-178
So, 123-133
Somé, Malidoma, 16, 46-47, 77-79, 157-158
Somé, Sobunfu, 47
Songlines, 136, 168
Spirit of place gardens, 202-205
Steiner, Rudolf, 76
Surroundings as mirrors, 33-34

Sustainability, 86-103
    and design, 34-35
    characteristics of, 101-102
    material basis, 90-93
    non-economic benefits, 93-101
Suzanne Wenger, 78
Swan, Jim, 13

T

Taking action, 252-271
    intention changes lives, 259
    honoring the spirits of all life, 266
    sewage is art, 253-258
    silence and intention, 270-271
    take care what mirrors reflect, 267
    the color of light, 265
    the peace of sanctuary, 268-269
    the richness of edges, 260
    their own place to learn, 262-263
    transforming a workplace, 261
Tiller, William, 23
Totems, 80-81
Trance design, 154-156
Tummi, 113-114
Tutu, Desmund, 102-103
TV, 144
Tyng, Anne Griswold, 131-132

V

Values
    in our surroundings, 33
Vibration, 50-51, 123-133, 128
Volwahsen, Andreas, 65, 124-125, 130

W

Water temples, 69-75
Wealth,
    true, 93
    non-economic dimensions, 93-102
    sustainable, 86-102
Wenger, Suzanne, 78-79
Wildness, 220
Wind, water, and star gardens, 205
Winter cities, 219
Work
    as spiritual path, 41
    making work sacred, 231
    intention changes lives, 259
    transforming a workplace, 143-144, 261
Working with Intention, 166
Wright, Machaelle Small, 26, 145-146

Y

Yin and *yang*, 122-123
    transcending dualities, 149
Yoruba, 78-79

*I*LLUSTRATIONS

Illustrations, other than noted below, are by the author:

p6 (and other miscellaneous graphics) - Dover Pictorial Archives; p12 - *Cymatics,* from p 104, CYMATICS, Vol. 1, Hans Jenny, Basilius Presse, 1967. MACROmedia, PO Box 279, Epping NH 03042. www.cymaticsource.com; p18 - *Acupuncture Meridians,* see ACUPUNCTURE, Felix Mann, 1978; p19 - *Chakras,* see YOGA: THE METHOD OF REINTEGRATION, Alain Danielou, 1949; p24 - *Dowsing EEGs* - Dowser's Brainwave Research Project, Ed Stillman and Dr. Matthew J. Kelly, courtesy of The American Society of Dowsers, PO Box 24, Danville VT 05828; p27 - *Kinesiology Hand Test,* drawing by Brian Torian; p52 - *Egyptian Dowsing Drawings,* courtesy of American Society of Dowsers, PO Box 24, Danville VT 05828; *Stele and Block Statue of Sihathur,* Items #569 & 570, © copyright The British Museum; p53 - *Dowsing Map of Temple of Hathor, Dendera,* POINTS OF COSMIC ENERGY, Blanche Merz; *Ceiling fresco of Nut, Temple of Hathor, Dendera,* courtesy of Deutsches Archaeologisches Institut, Cairo; p56 - *Section Drawing of Foundations, Temple of Montu, Karnak,* THE TEMPLE IN MAN: Sacred Architecture and the Perfect Man by R. A. Schwaller de Lubicz, courtesy of Inner Traditions International, Rochester, VT 05767. Translation copyright © 1977 by Autumn Press, Inc.; p58 - *Dowsing Maps of Izumo Shrine,* courtesy of Joey Korn; p59 - *Diviner Figurine,* courtesy of National Museum of the American Indian, Smithsonian Institution (22.5598); p59-63 - *Maya Line Drawings,* A FOREST OF KINGS and MAYA COSMOS, Linda Schele and David Freidel, courtesy of the Foundation for Advancement of Mesoamerican Studies, Inc.

p64 - *Plan, Temple of Konarak,* after Archeological Survey of India; p 65 - *Space and Time Geometries,* PRINCIPLES OF COMPOSITION IN HINDU SCULPTURE, Alice Boner; p67 - *"The Great Wall of China,"* CHINA, Vol. 1, Thomas Allom; *Ming Tang Diagram,* see LIVING ARCHITECTURE: CHINESE, Michèle Pirazzoli-T'Serstevens; p68 - *Chang-An Plan,* see LIVING ARCHITECTURE: CHINESE, Michèle Pirazzoli-T'Serstevens; *"The Western Gate of Peking,"* CHINA, Vol. 3, Thomas Allom; p69 - *Angkor Plan and Map,* "L'Hydraulique Urbaine et Agricole a l'Epoque des Rois d'Angkor," BULLETIN ECONOMIQUE DE L'INDOCHINE, Viktor Goloubew; p71- *Bayon Plan,* after L'Ecole Francaise D'Extreme Orient; p76 - *Nant-y-Cwm Steiner Kindergarden,* PLACES OF THE SOUL, Chris Day; *Culture House, Järna, Sweden,* by Eric Asmussen, drawing by Susanne Siepl-Coates, from ERIK ASMUSSEN ARCHITECT, Gary J. Coates, Byggförlaget, Stockholm, 1997; p78 - Aiyedakun, *Original and New Yoruba Shrine by Suzanne Wenger,* see RETURN OF THE GODS, Ulli Beier; p80 - *"Raven House, Gwayasdums Village,"* courtesy of the Royal British Columbia Museum, Victoria, British Columbia; *"Beam Ends of the Eagle House in Tanu Village",* courtesy of Field Museum of Natural History; p81 -*"Bear House Post from Kitamaat,"* A1790, courtesty UBC Museum of Anthropology, Vancouver, Canada; p84 - *Hawaiian Birth Stones,* photo by Kathleen Bender; p85 - *Kiyomizu Plan,* after JAPANESE URBAN SPACE, Dec. 1963; p106 - *Magnetosphere Diagram,* EARTH'S ELECTRIC ENVIRONMENT, 1986; *"Dying Storm north of Hawaii,"* courtesy NASA; p107 - *Lizard Mounds State Park Plan,* courtesy of James P. Scherz.

p114 - *Beam Bridge, Fukien Prov., China, 1053 A.D.,* HISTOIRE DES ARTS ANCIENS DE LA CHINE, Vol. 4, Osvald Siren, or SCIENCE AND CIVILIZATION IN CHINA, Vol. 4, JOSEPH NEEDHAM; p123, CYMATICS, see p12 above; p122 - *Ground Plan Development,* LIVING ARCHITECTURE: Indian, Andreas Volwahsen; *Somnathpur Plan,* after ARCHEOLOGICAL SURVEY OF INDIA; p127 - *Parthenon,* THE POWER OF LIMITS: Proportional Harmonies in Nature, Art and Architecture, by György Doczi, © 1981. Reprinted by arrangement with Shambhala Publications, Inc., Boston, www.shambhala.com; p129 - *Temple Plan,* p130 - *City Plans,* see LIVING ARCHITECTURE: Indian, Andreas Volwahsen; *Jaipur Plan,* after Archeological Survey of India; p134 - *Feng Shui Site Diagrams,* see FENG SHUI, Eva Wong; *Feng Shui Landscape Types,* see THE FENG SHUI HANDBOOK, Derek Walters; p 135 - *"Imperial Palace at Tseaou-shan",* CHINA, Vol. 1, Thomas Allom; p137 - *Orion/Pyramids Diagram,* from MESSAGE OF THE SPHINX, Graham Hancock and Robert Bauval, copyright © 1996 by Graham Hancock and Robert Bauval. Reprinted by permission of Crown Publishers, a division of Random House, Inc.; p163 - *Newgrange,* see ANTIQUITY, 1964; p167 - *Westminster Abbey Dowsing Diagram,* THE PATTERN OF THE PAST, Guy Underwood; p168 - *Dowsing Diagram* by Brian Torian; p170 - photo by Kathleen Bender; p173 - *"The Foochun Hill, Che Keang,"* CHINA, Vol. 2, Thomas Allom; p182 - *Temple Roof Section,* after THE ROOF IN JAPANESE BUDDHIST ARCHITECTURE, Mary Parent; p184 - *House Plan,* after THE JAPANESE HOUSE, Heinrich Engel; p210 - *Cliff/Clouds Photo* by Kathleen Bender; p216 - *"A Feast Day at Acoma Pueblo,"* Edward S. Curtis, see PORTRAITS FROM NORTH AMERICAN INDIAN LIFE, Promentory Press; p217 - *"Lake See-Hoo and Temple of the Thundering Winds, from Vale of Tombs,"* CHINA, Vol. 1, Thomas Allom; p219 - *Isfahan Plan,* see PERSIAN GARDENS AND GARDEN PAVILIONS, Donald Wilber; p222 - *Adalej Step-well Section,* Archeological Survey of India, via FORMAL STRUCTURE IN INDIAN ARCHITECTURE exhibition, Klaus Herdeg; p225 - *Versailles Plan,* Biblioteque Nationale; p237 - *Kailasanath Plan,* after Archeological Survey of India; p238 - *Serpent Mound,* E.G. Squier & E.H. Davis; p257 - *KOMA Garden Sketch* by Don Osborne.

FIRE RIVER PRESS

Quick Order Form

Telephone Inquiries: (503) 368-6294
Email Inquiries: fireriverpress@nehalemtel.net
Postal Orders: *FIRE RIVER PRESS,* PO Box 397, Manzanita OR 97130
Please send payment with orders.

PLEASE SEND THE FOLLOWING BOOKS:

( ) copies of *Silence, Song & Shadows* @ $27
( ) copies of *Building with the Breath of Life* @ $28

SHIPPING: US – $4 FOR THE FIRST BOOK, $2 FOR EACH ADDITIONAL BOOK.
INTERNATIONAL – $9 FOR FIRST BOOK, $5 FOR EACH ADDITIONAL BOOK. (ESTIMATE)
NAME: _____

ADDRESS: _____

CITY: _____ STATE: _____ ZIP: _____ COUNTRY: _____

TELEPHONE: _____ E-MAIL ADDRESS: _____

FIRE RIVER PRESS

Quick Order Form

Telephone Inquiries: (503) 368-6294
Email Inquiries: fireriverpress@nehalemtel.net
Postal Orders: *FIRE RIVER PRESS,* PO Box 397, Manzanita OR 97130
Please send payment with orders.

PLEASE SEND THE FOLLOWING BOOKS:

( ) copies of *Silence, Song & Shadows* @ $27
( ) copies of *Building with the Breath of Life* @ $28

SHIPPING: US – $4 FOR THE FIRST BOOK, $2 FOR EACH ADDITIONAL BOOK.
INTERNATIONAL – $9 FOR FIRST BOOK, $5 FOR EACH ADDITIONAL BOOK. (ESTIMATE)
NAME: _____

ADDRESS: _____

CITY: _____ STATE: _____ ZIP: _____ COUNTRY: _____

TELEPHONE: _____ E-MAIL ADDRESS: _____

FIRE RIVER PRESS

Quick Order Form

Telephone Inquiries: (503) 368-6294
Email Inquiries: fireriverpress@nehalemtel.net
Postal Orders: *FIRE RIVER PRESS,* PO Box 397, Manzanita OR 97130
Please send payment with orders.

PLEASE SEND THE FOLLOWING BOOKS:

( ) copies of *Silence, Song & Shadows* @ $27
( ) copies of *Building with the Breath of Life* @ $28

SHIPPING: US – $4 FOR THE FIRST BOOK, $2 FOR EACH ADDITIONAL BOOK.
INTERNATIONAL – $9 FOR FIRST BOOK, $5 FOR EACH ADDITIONAL BOOK. (ESTIMATE)
NAME: _____

ADDRESS: _____

CITY: _____ STATE: _____ ZIP: _____ COUNTRY: _____

TELEPHONE: _____ E-MAIL ADDRESS: _____